D1759290

STAFF EDUCATION CENTRE
LIBRARY, RAMPTON HOSPITAL

LIBRARY RAMPTON HOSPITAL

R71853L0532

Clinical Methods
in Transcultural Psychiatry

Clinical Methods in Transcultural Psychiatry

Edited by

Samuel O. Okpaku, M.D., Ph.D.

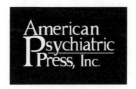

WASHINGTON, DC
LONDON, ENGLAND

Note: The authors have worked to ensure that all information in this book concerning drug dosages, schedules, and routes of administration is accurate as of the time of publication and consistent with standards set by the U.S. Food and Drug Administration and the general medical community. As medical research and practice advance, however, therapeutic standards may change. For this reason and because human and mechanical errors sometimes occur, we recommend that readers follow the advice of a physician who is directly involved in their care or the care of a member of their family.

Books published by the American Psychiatric Press, Inc., represent the views and opinions of the individual authors and do not necessarily represent the policies and opinions of the Press or the American Psychiatric Association.

Copyright © 1998 American Psychiatric Press, Inc.
ALL RIGHTS RESERVED
Manufactured in the United States of America on acid-free paper
01   00   99   98   4   3   2   1
First Edition

American Psychiatric Press, Inc.
1400 K Street, N.W., Washington, DC   20005
www.appi.org

Library of Congress Cataloging-in-Publication Data
Clinical methods in transcultural psychiatry / edited by Samuel O.
  Okpaku.—1st ed.
      p.   cm.
    ISBN 0-88048-710-0 (alk. paper)
    1. Psychiatry, Transcultural—Methodology.   2. Psychotherapy—
  Social aspects.   I. Okpaku, Samuel O.
    [DNLM: 1. Psychiatry—methods.   2. Mental Disorders—ethnology.
    3. Cross-Cultural Comparison.   WM 100 C6394 1998]
    RC455.4.E8C58   1998
  616.89—dc21
  DNLM/DLC
  for Library of Congress   97-47207
                                                                              CIP

British Library Cataloguing in Publication Data
A CIP record is available from the British Library.

*To my mother
and the memory of my father*

Contents

Section III: Treatment Approaches, 211

Section IV: Recent Research and Special Topics, 299

Section V: Education and Training, 337

Section VI: Women and Children, 363

Contributors

Sayed Ahmed, M.D., M.P.H., Dr.P.H.
Assistant Professor, Department of Family Medicine, East
Dayton Health Center, Wright State University, Dayton, Ohio

Goffredo Bartocci, M.D.
President, Italian Institute of Transcultural Mental Health,
Rome, Italy

Irma J. Bland, M.D.
Clinical Professor and Associate Chair for Clinical Affairs,
Department of Psychiatry, Louisiana State University Medical
Center, New Orleans, Louisiana

Claude Charles, M.A.
Assistant Professor, Department of Psychiatry, University of
Miami School of Medicine; Director of Haitian Services, New
Horizons Community Health Center, Miami, Florida

Thi Hong Trang Dao, M.D., F.R.C.P.C.
Staff Psychiatrist, Reddy Memorial Hospital, Montreal,
Quebec, Canada

Simon Dein, M.R.C.Psych.
Consultant Psychiatrist, Essex and Herts Community NHS
Trust, Princess Alexandria Hospital, Harlow, Essex, England

**Vincenzo F. DiNicola, M.Phil., M.D., Dip.Psych.,
F.R.C.P.C.**
Chairman, Division of Child and Adolescent Psychiatry, and
Professor of Psychiatry, Pediatrics, Psychology, and
Community Health and Epidemiology, Queen's University,
Kingston, Ontario, Canada

Timi Edeki, M.D., Ph.D.
Resident, Department of Medicine, University of Louisville,
Louisville, Kentucky

Solvig Ekblad, Ph.D.
Associate Professor of Transcultural Psychology, Karolinska
Institute; Director of Unit for Immigrant Environment and
Health, National Institute for Psychosocial Factors and
Health, Stockholm, Sweden

M. Fakhr El-Islam, F.R.C.P., F.R.C.Psych.
Professor Emeritus, Department of Psychiatry, Cairo
University, Cairo, Egypt

Teresa di Fonzo, M.D.
Consultant, Inpatient Department ASL RM/6 Monterotondo,
Rome, Italy

Edward Foulks, M.D., Ph.D.
Sellars-Polchow Professor, Department of Psychiatry and
Neurology, and Associate Dean for Clinical Affairs and
Graduate Medical Education, Tulane University School of
Medicine, New Orleans, Louisiana

Luigi Frighi, M.D.
President, Society of Medicine and Migration, Rome, Italy

Charles C. Hughes, Ph.D.[†]
Department of Family and Preventive Medicine, University of
Utah, Salt Lake City, Utah

Bengt Jansson, M.D.
Emeritus Professor of Psychiatry, Department of Clinical
Neuroscience and Family Medicine, Huddinge University
Hospital, Karolinska Institute, Stockholm, Sweden

J. David Kinzie, M.D.
Vice Chairman and Director of Clinical Services, Oregon
Health Sciences University, School of Medicine, Department
of Psychiatry, Portland, Oregon

Laurence J. Kirmayer, M.D., F.R.C.P.C.
Associate Professor and Director, Division of Social and
Transcultural Psychiatry, McGill University, Sir Mortimer B.
Davis–Jewish General Hospital, Montreal, Quebec, Canada

[†]Deceased.

Robert Kohn, M.D.
Assistant Professor, Department of Psychiatry and Human
Behavior, and Director of Psychiatric Epidemiology Research
Program, Brown University, Butler Hospital, Providence,
Rhode Island

Irvin Kraft, M.D., P.A.
Emeritus Professor of Mental Health, University of Texas
School of Public Health; Clinical Professor of Psychiatry,
Baylor College of Medicine, Houston, Texas

Nicola Lalli, M.D.
Director of Department of Psychiatry and Psychotherapy,
University "la Sapienza," Rome, Italy

David Larson, M.D., M.S.P.H.
President, National Institute for Healthcare Research,
Rockville, Maryland

Harriet P. Lefley, Ph.D.
Professor of Psychiatry and Behavioral Sciences, Department of
Psychiatry and Behavioral Sciences, University of Miami School
of Medicine, Jackson Memorial Hospital, Miami, Florida

Alexander H. Leighton, M.D.
Professor of Social Psychiatry Emeritus, Harvard School of Public
Health, Cambridge, Massachusetts; Professor of Psychiatry and
Professor of Community Health and Epidemiology, Dalhousie
University, Halifax, Nova Scotia, Canada

Maurice Lipsedge, F.R.C.Psych.
Consultant Psychiatrist, Department of Psychological
Medicine, Guys Hospital, London, England

Francis Lu, M.D.
Clinical Professor, Department of Psychiatry, School of Medicine,
San Francisco General Hospital, San Francisco, California

M. Sharda Menon, M.D.
Director, Schizophrenia Research Foundation, Madras, India

Larry Merkel, M.D., Ph.D.
University of Virginia, Student Health Services,
Charlottesville, Virginia

Mary Greenwold Milano, B.A., MGM
Research Coordinator, National Institute for Healthcare
Research, Rockville, Maryland

Usha S. Naik, M.D.
Professor of Psychiatry, Niloufer Hospital, Osmania Medical
College, Hyderabad, India

**Samuel O. Okpaku, M.D., Ph.D., M.B., Ch.B.,
M.R.C.P.I., F.R.C.P.C.**
Associate Clinical Professor of Psychiatry, Vanderbilt
University School of Medicine, Nashville, Tennessee

Danilo E. Ponce, M.D.
Professor of Psychiatry, John A. Burns School of Medicine,
University of Hawaii, Honolulu, Hawaii

Raymond H. Prince, M.D., M.Sc.
Emeritus Professor, McGill University, Division of Social and
Transcultural Psychiatry, Montreal, Canada

Giangiacomo G. Rovera, M.D.
Full Professor, University of Turin, Turin, Italy

Perminder Sachdev, M.D., Ph.D., F.R.A.N.Z.C.P.
Clinical Director, Neuropsychiatric Institute, School of
Psychiatry, University of New South Wales, Prince Henry
Hospital, Sydney, Australia

Mercedes Cros Sandoval, Ph.D.
Professor of Anthropology, Miami Dade Community College;
Adjunct Professor (Associate) of Psychiatry, University of
Miami School of Medicine; Former Director of Hispanic
Services, New Horizons Community Mental Health Center,
Miami, Florida

Jurg Siegfried, Ph.D.
Private Practice

André Smith, M.S.W.
Ph.D. candidate, Department of Sociology, McGill University,
Montreal, Quebec, Canada

Karen Ta, M.D.
Assistant Professor, Department of Psychiatry, Ramsey
Medical Center, University of Minnesota, St. Paul, Minnesota

Myriam M. M. P. Van Moffaert, M.D., Ph.D.
Professor, Department of Psychiatry and Psychosomatics,
University Hospital, Gent, Belgium

Joseph Westermeyer, M.D., Ph.D.
Chief, Psychiatry Service, and Professor of Psychiatry and
Adjunct Professor of Anthropology, University of Minnesota,
V.A. Medical Center, Minneapolis, Minnesota

Marta Young, Ph.D., C.Psych.
Assistant Professor, Center for Psychological Services,
University of Ottawa, Ottawa, Ontario, Canada

Acknowledgments

It is impossible to be exact about the circumstances that have led to the conceptualization of this volume. Less difficult is the recognition of those individuals who have contributed their time and effort in listening to my views on transcultural psychiatry and who were willing to consider and support each perspective. In that regard I would like to express my gratitude to all of the contributors and reviewers of the earlier drafts, including Virginia Abernathy, Janie Adams, Sayed Ahmed, Ariel Arieli, Goffredo Bartocci, Irma Bland, Jean Carlin, Michelle Clark, Lee Combrinck-Graham, Joop DeJong, Bincenzo DiNicola, M. Fakhr El-Islam, Giuliana Fedeli, Ed Foulks, Thomas Gregor, Charles Hughes, Wolfgang G. Jilek, David Kinzie, Arthur Kleinman, Robert Kohn, Joan Koss-Chioino, Irvin Kraft, Robert Kraus, William Lawson, Barbara Lex, Keh-Ming Lin, David McGill, M. Sharda Menon, Larry Merkel, Laurie Moore, Usha Naik, Anire Okpaku, Aubrey Okpaku, Temisan Okpaku, Danilo Ponce, Homero R. Sanchez, Jurg Siegfried, Veida Skultans, Helen Ullrich, Myriam Van Moffaert, Vijoy Varma, Don Williams, and Harry Wright. In addition, I would like to offer exceptional gratitude to Anita Proctor, Marilyn Daniels, and Jeanine Miller, M.A., who in their multiple roles as secretarial staff, editorial assistants, and friends, made numerous telephone calls at home and abroad tracking down the various contributors and making sure the deadlines were met.

I also would like to thank Patrice Mayo-Ligon, Ph.D. candidate, for her editorial contribution in proofreading and revising the entire manuscript. Additionally, I would like to mention my sons, Anire, Aubrey, and Temisan, whose critical comments enhanced the quality of the work. Finally, I would like to express my appreciation to Carol Nadelson, M.D., and the American Psychiatric Press in supporting the publication of this volume.

If I have inadvertently omitted anyone from this list, it is not by design but by chance, and I offer my most heartfelt apologies.

Introduction and Background

SAMUEL O. OKPAKU, M.D., PH.D.

Although earlier psychiatrists, notably Jung and Kraepelin, alluded to possible cultural factors in the etiology of mental disorders, the field of transcultural psychiatry began to gain strong momentum only about 40 years ago, as evidenced by the proceedings of a Ciba Foundation symposium held in London, England, in 1965. The symposium participants were eminent social scientists and psychiatrists, including Margaret Mead, E. D. Wittkower, A. Hollowell, T. A. Lambo, G. M. Carstairs, H. Murphy, G. A. De Vos, and M. Fortes. The symposium focused on the definition of transcultural psychiatry—the boundaries of the field, its subject areas, issues of research methodology, and treatment modalities. The panel discussed the then-current gaps and shortcomings in the field and suggested further directions.

Since that conference, major developments in clinical practice and research have filled in some of the gaps. These efforts include the international studies of schizophrenia, depression, and disability; the construction of manuals such as the DSM-IV (American Psychiatric Association 1994); and the development of research instruments for depression, schizophrenia, and other psychiatric disorders. From the clinical perspective, awareness of the need for more cultural sensitivity in treatment and delivery of services has increased, a process augmented by a new level of consumerism and collaboration between service providers and their patients. These developments have paralleled, in some instances, a reorientation in theory—for example, the suggested shift from the "old" transcultural psychiatry to the "new" transcultural psychiatry.

Against this background are a variety of national and international trends, fueling activities in this area. One influential factor is the increasing recognition of the role of cultural factors in the definition of health, disease, help seeking behavior, and utilization of human services. In addition, for a variety of reasons, alternative health care systems are gaining more adherents in both majority and minority populations. This shift appears to be especially common in patients who have chronic illnesses and for whom "scientific" medicine seems to offer little hope.

Another major factor contributing to the burgeoning interest in transcultural psychiatry is the continued volume of human migration, forced or voluntary. There are multiple facets to these social phenomena. The acceptance and adjustment of immigrants even in the United States, a country with a long and unique tradition of immigration, remain problematic and complex. For example, different generations may respond differently to acculturation. The rise of ethnicity and nationalism, in some cases resulting in purulent racism and at times savage wars (such as in Bosnia, Somalia, and Chechnya in the 1990s), is another aspect of this problem. The United States dream for a "melting pot" society is perhaps not realizable. In fact, a more realistic hope is that the country realize and appreciate the potential richness of its cultural diversity.

Issues of transcultural psychiatry are also relevant from an international perspective. Redrawing national boundaries and forming new political entities, as well as trends toward greater globalization of trade industries and technologies, are likely to result in a greater opportunity for individuals to travel, visit, and work in foreign countries.

These trends, combined with a few other factors, motivated me to undertake the project of editing this book. In the last 15 years or so, I have regularly attended scientific meetings of transcultural societies. My unique position as an alien and a minority has enabled me to closely observe the proceedings of these societies in terms of their membership, the patterns of attendance, and the focus of the meetings. My candid opinion is that the efforts and achievements of groups restrictive in membership and narrow in focus pale in comparison to the achievements of the societies open and willing to be more collective. In other words, the latter groups celebrate diversity. Another distinguishing characteristic among the groups is the relevance of their agendas concerning society, culture, and mental illness. The more progressive groups are willing to include minority issues, not just immigrant or refugee issues; they also examine issues of cultural relevance to majority groups. There is participation, inclusion, celebration, and relevance.

In the other groups marked ethnocentrism exists, in spite of the avowed interest in culture and mental health.

My clinical practice often consists of transcultural cases and interactions; these have provided me with challenges and opportunities for reflection and enrichment. I am from Nigeria, was educated in Great Britain, and practice psychiatry in the United States (Nashville, Tennessee). In my experience, I have found that sociocultural identities of patients and therapists are aspects tantamount to the diagnosis and treatment of mental illness. Many years ago, during my last supervisory session in family therapy, my supervisor asked, and I paraphrase, "Is this family different from your family?" I responded, "Not really." With much clinical experience behind me now, I have mulled over that neophyte response. My revised answer is "yes and no," and therein lies the complexity of transcultural psychiatry.

Furthermore, in recent years many health-related professional associations, including the American Psychiatric Association, have emphasized a need to augment and improve the transcultural content of their training programs. This perspective derives partly from a greater recognition of cultural factors in the definition of health and disease and the role of cultural factors in help seeking behavior and utilization of services. However, the attainment of the goal of improving the transcultural content of training and clinical practice is compromised by a relative lack of trained teachers and the unavailability of suitable standard texts necessary for providing a knowledge base.

Thus the goal of this volume is to provide a sufficiently concise and comprehensive text of transcultural psychiatry, using case studies and clinical experience to illuminate the subject. It will familiarize readers with the definitions and principles of transcultural psychiatry. (The majority of psychiatry texts make only cursory references to transcultural psychiatry.) The volume highlights the significance of cultural factors in the causation and meaning of pain, suffering, and healing of mental illness. Its purpose is to illustrate some principles and practices of transcultural psychiatry and to familiarize the average health care professional in training and practicing clinician with a basic foundation of culturally informed psychiatry upon which he or she may build. Our definition of transcultural psychiatry is essentially an encounter between a therapist and a patient within which real or imagined differences may exist. Ethnicity and racial background are not the only sine qua non: educational background, social class, age, gender and gender orientation, and religious practice or orientation are also integral.

To minimize confusion, this volume emphasizes transcultural psychiatry as an entity with a dynamic core in which an attempt is made by the therapist to show empathy and respect for cultural differences. In such a relationship, the therapist remains open and willing to be informed by the patient. The clinical conflicts are defined within the patient's cultural context, and the goals of therapy are predicated on a dynamic and bilateral relationship between therapist and patient. This definitional approach is justified by its simplicity and parsimony. It attempts to reduce the time and energy spent on debating the various meanings of *transcultural,* and it sensitizes the caregiver or therapist to possible subcultural elements among issues concerning the patient.

About the Book

Section 1, "An Overview of Transcultural Psychiatry," consists of three chapters illustrating essential elements in transcultural psychiatry. Leighton confronts perplexing issues of personality and culture and introduces ideas of common sense and pragmatism in clinical practice. Ekblad et al. summarize some essential factors of immigration and mental health.

Section 2, "Cultural Psychiatry and Mental Health Services," deals with some of the epistemological value issues relevant to helping individuals with mental illnesses. Ponce, Lefley et al., and Sachdev provide background examples of model mental health services in multicultural settings. Lipsedge and Dein illustrate the bidirectional dynamics of bicultural psychiatry and incorporate patients' perceptions of their therapists. El-Islam provides the reader who is not familiar with Arabic and Muslim culture with knowledge about the history of the culture and an understanding of how changes influence the behavior and attitudes of the people. Kinzie and Edeki discuss psychopharmacologic problems of ethnicity and caution clinicians to be vigilant about noncompliance with medical prescriptions.

Section 3, "Treatment Approaches," provides an orientation to assessment and treatment of patients whose social and cultural backgrounds are different from their therapists' backgrounds. The relevance of common sense as an essential factor in therapy is discussed, along with settings of therapeutic alliance in individual and family treatment.

In Section 4, "Recent Research and Special Topics," Bartocci et al. draw attention to the roles religious and supernatural beliefs play in individuals' personal cultures, and Van Moffaert highlights the issue of somatization as a mode of communication. In Section 5, "Education and Training," Foulks et al. address educating clinicians in various levels of training on transcultural psychiatry. DiNicola's chapter in Section 6, "Women and Children," concentrates on families in cultural transition. Young addresses an ever-growing problem of the welfare of refugee women and the torture they so often endure. Finally, Naik et al. examine the intricate connection between culture and psychiatry within the subcontinent of India.

References

American Psychiatric Association: Diagnostic and Statistical Manual of Mental Disorders, 4th Edition. Washington, DC, American Psychiatric Association, 1994

Eisenberg D: Unconventional medicine in the United States: prevalence, costs, and patterns of use. N Engl J Med 328:246–252, 1993

Geertz C: Unabsolute truths. The New York Times Magazine, April 9, 1995, p 46

An Overview
of Transcultural Psychiatry

CHAPTER 1

Transcultural Psychiatry
A Note on Origins and Definitions

RAYMOND H. PRINCE, M.D., M.SC.
SAMUEL O. OKPAKU, M.D., PH.D.
LARRY MERKEL, M.D., PH.D.

The view that psychiatric phenomena may vary from one social group to another has existed for approximately 200 years. Early in the nineteenth century, philosophers and physicians argued that the frequency of mental illnesses increased with the development of civilization and decreased with rural, tension-free living. For example, commenting on asylum admission rates in Great Britain and Ireland during the 1820s, Sir Andrew Halliday (1828/1969) referred to the rarity of insanity among "the savage tribes of men," "the contented peasantry of the Welsh mountains," and those dwelling in the "wilds of Ireland" (Rosen 1969, p. 183). And the much-traveled American sea captain Charles Wilkes (1798–1877) was in agreement: "During the whole of my intercourse with the natives of the South Seas, I met no deranged person, and I am satisfied that insanity is a disease incidental alone to civilized life. I am confident that had any instance of mental derangement among the natives occurred it would have been observed by us" (Wilkes 1845, pp. 285–286).

Some early authors implicated political systems in these variations. Thus Amariah Brigham (1798–1849), an American asylum superintendent, indicated, "There is but little insanity in the countries where the government is despotic. The inhabitants of such countries possess but little mental activity compared with those who live in a republic or under a representative government." According to Brigham, it was because of autocratic rule that there was little insanity in

China, Turkey, Spain, or Russia (Hunter and Macalpine 1963, p. 824). Another view was that rates of mental illness varied with social upheavals such as civil wars or revolutions. The eighteenth-century psychiatrist Benjamin Rush (1745–1813) observed that "hysterical women who favoured the [American] revolution were cured of their condition." He also thought that those who remained loyal to England suffered "a hypochondriasis which was popularly called protection fever" because of their excessive concern over their persons and their property (Rosen 1969, pp. 176–177). Rush, of course, espoused the revolutionary cause and was a signatory of the Declaration of Independence in 1776. We have been unable to find clear reference to what we would today call social class or socioeconomic influences upon rates of psychiatric disorders among these early authors (although Halliday's mention of the contented peasantry of Wales may have some relation to these concepts). In the United States today, low social class and poverty are viewed as the clearest group correlates of increased prevalence of psychiatric disorders.

Detailed and systematic reports began to appear in psychiatric journals only when European psychiatrists took up posts in the asylums of overseas colonies in the latter part of the nineteenth century. It should be noted at this point, however, that the use of the expression *culture* (in place of terms such as *savage tribes, primitive, civilized, mode of life,* and so forth) did not appear in psychiatric publications until the early twentieth century. Although T. Duncan Greenlees (1895), for example, was probably groping for a concept approaching our present transcultural psychiatry in his descriptions of psychotic patients in South Africa, a careful reading suggests that he was probably thinking of biological rather than social origins of the differences he observed. Greenlees noted marked "native" versus European differences in rates of melancholia and general paresis in the Grahamstown Asylum, Cape of Good Hope. He examined the diagnoses of 473 consecutive admissions between 1875 and 1894. Acute and chronic mania were by far the most common diagnoses (Kraepelinian diagnostic patterns such as dementia praecox and manic-depressive disorders had not yet reached South Africa). Greenlees noted a remarkable excess of mania over melancholia (222 cases versus 31) and that "examples of melancholia are rare among natives. . . . I have never found this condition so acute as among white patients." He found general paresis to be so rare that "among the pure, uncontaminated natives it may be considered to be practically unknown" (p. 76).

Emil Kraepelin (1856–1926) made more detailed observations a few years later and seemed to be thinking in somewhat more cultural terms than Greenlees. In 1903 Kraepelin spent approximately four months at the Buitenzorg Asylum in Java to collect reliable observations on the occurrence of neurosyphilis in tropical countries. But as he tells us, he considered even more important "the need to determine whether dementia praecox also occurred in [non-European] populations of entirely different origins and under completely different life conditions. . . . I had the idea that the characteristics of a population would be revealed by the frequency as well as the form of different types of mental disorders. A comparative psychiatry, therefore, should provide valuable insights into the minds of peoples and should contribute to our understanding of psychopathological processes" (Boroffka 1990, p. 232). Kraepelin found that the mental illnesses of the European patients in the asylum at the time of his visit were virtually the same as those of the patients in Germany. But there were several interesting differences between the asylum's European and Javanese patients. General paresis was virtually absent among the Javanese, whereas 8 cases occurred among the 50 European male patients. Manic-depressive psychoses were definitely rare among Javanese patients, but epileptiform states were more frequent; dementia praecox was common among Javanese but "less colourful" than among Europeans; catatonic phenomena were less developed, auditory hallucinations less frequent, and coherent delusional ideas were rare or absent; frank depression among Javanese was very rare and, when present, was transitory; and ideas of sinfulness were not manifested (Kraepelin 1904/1974).

Psychoanalytic thinking made its appearance in the field at about the same time. Freud published his much maligned *Totem and Taboo* in 1913 (first translated into English by Brill in 1918), and other analytic writers perused ethnographic descriptions for behaviors and beliefs that were relevant to psychoanalytic theories. Most of these analysts were armchair philosophers, but a few conducted fieldwork. The Hungarian geographer Géza Róheim (1891–1953), who was analyzed by Sandor Ferenczi, made expeditions to such culturally contrasting areas as Somaliland, central Australia, and the Normandy islands. He interpreted myths, rituals, and normal and abnormal behavior in psychoanalytic terms (Morales 1988). The Hungarian-born anthropologist and psycho-analyst George Devereux (1908–1985) also conducted fieldwork with a number of cultural groups, including Amerindians (Hopi and Mohave) and Melanesians (Roro and Karuama). In addition, he was clinically ex-perienced, having conducted a psychoanalytic practice for several years in New York (Bourguignon 1986). Although controversial, psychoanaly-sis has clearly opened important windows upon comparative psychiatric studies (La Barre 1958).

The realization that most cultural groups had well-developed in-digenous psychiatric systems, including etiological theories and treat-ment methods, appeared somewhat later than comparative epidemio-logical observations and identification of non-European syndromes. The German physician and medical historian Erwin Ackerknecht (1971) was one of the pioneers in this field in the 1930s. Unlike most of his medical contemporaries, Ackerknecht argued against the view that indigenous medical systems should be regarded as a kind of embry-onal precursor of scientific medicine. As a student of American anthro-pologist Ruth Benedict (1887–1948), he believed that each cultural system, including its healing systems, was a world unto itself and in-comparable to others, and that each medical system should be exam-ined and understood in its own right. He also thought that there were as many impostors and quacks within scientific medicine as there were in primitive medical systems.

An intelligible and convincing description of such a system of in-digenous psychiatry had to await the detailed fieldwork of Alex and Dorothea Leighton in the late 1930s. They observed that the world view of the Navajo portrayed illness and misfortune as resulting from disharmony between a family and its natural or social world. Navajo healing was a two-step process requiring the determination of the spe-cific cause of the disharmony by a diviner, and then the restoration of harmony through the ministrations of a "singer" who provided the ap-propriate treatment. These treatments, designated "healing ways" by the Navajo, consisted of healing modules comprising an elaborate song cycle, sand drawings, herbal preparations, and distinctive rituals. Each singer knew only 1 or 2 of the approximately 35 healing ways, because each required several years to master. Performance of a healing way called for several weeks of preparation by the patient, family, and singer and could be quite expensive. The performance itself required from two to nine nights. The Leightons concluded that Navajo healers provided "a powerful suggestive psychotherapy which can certainly aid states of anxiousness and render the physically ailing better able to bear his illness" (Leighton and Leighton 1941, p. 522). Since the Leightons' publication, numerous other indigenous psychiatric systems have been described. One of the best collections remains that of Ari Kiev (1964), which includes more or less detailed descriptions of a dozen such indigenous systems.

There were two additional developments before the synthesis known as transcultural psychiatry emerged in the 1950s. The first was the important contribution of several Western psychiatrists who made careers of their involvement with non-Western cultures. Examples include the late Sir Burton G. Burton-Bradley in New Guinea and John Cawte in Australia, who spent a good part of their lives studying and writing about psychiatry in non-Western cultures. It should be noted that Burton-Bradley is the only individual to be knighted for work in transcultural psychiatry. A second and perhaps even more important development was the contributions of non-Western psychiatrists who were able to bring fresh insights into the field through the optic of their own cultures. Examples include Shoma Morita (1874–1938) in Japan, Yap Pow Meng in Hong Kong (1921–1971), Thomas Adeoye Lambo (1923) in Nigeria, and A. Cader Raman (1920) of Mauritius.

Transcultural psychiatry was established as a distinct discipline by psychoanalyst E. D. Wittkower (1899–1983) when he set up his Section of Transcultural Studies at McGill University in Montreal in 1955. Although he had many precursors, Wittkower succeeded in focusing worldwide psychiatric attention upon the importance of taking culture into account both for practitioners and theoreticians. He was the first to set up a specific transcultural section within a university department of psychiatry, and in 1956 he inaugurated the *Transcultural Psychiatric Research Review,* the first journal devoted to the field.

Evolution of the Culture Concept

As already outlined, the concept of culture in the anthropological sense was a late-nineteenth-century invention. But this idea seemed to fill an important niche in twentieth-century thought and rapidly entered everyday parlance; Kroeber and Kluckhohn (1963) claimed that the significance of the idea of culture was "comparable to such categories as gravity in physics, disease in medicine and evolution in biology" (p. 3) in its explanatory importance and generality of application. The word *culture* has had a rich and varied evolution with a web of meanings and connotations reflected in such diverse concepts as cult, colony, couture, and cultivator (Eliot 1948, Williams 1983, Winthrop 1991). Indeed, according to Williams (1983, p. 71), *culture* is "one of the two or three most complicated words in the English language." For our present purposes, however, we need only briefly explore two of these meaning clusters that remain in current usage: culture as high-level artistic and humanistic development and the social anthropologists' version of culture as a group's socially transmitted blueprint for living. The English poet and critic Matthew Arnold (1822–1888) provided an influential didactic view of culture as humanistic excellence in his *Culture and Anarchy* published in 1869. It must be admitted that the manifestations of Arnold's "sweetness and light" seemed to be most highly developed among the well-to-do Victorian English.

The splitting off of something approaching the modern anthropologist's idea of culture seems to have begun in the eighteenth century, notably in the work of the German poet and critic Johann Gottfried von Herder (1744–1803). Herder argued forcefully against the idea that civilization, or *kultur,* was a unilinear process with eighteenth-century Europe as its apex. Herder believed that it was necessary to speak of cultures in the plural, and that human beings had created a multitude of societies, each with its own version of human excellence.

But by the time such ideas as plural manifestations of human excellence passed from the German literary world to the English world of science, Spencer's and Darwin's ideas of evolution had taken firm hold. One early example of an evolution-modified concept of multiple cultures appeared in Sir Edward B. Tylor's (1832–1917) *Primitive Culture* published in 1871 (Winthrop 1991). As is evident by his title, Tylor saw that culture was not restricted to nineteenth-century Europe; it was also a property of primitive social groups. "Culture or civilization," wrote Tylor in his opening paragraph, "is that complex whole which includes knowledge, belief, art, morals, law, custom, and any other capabilities and habits acquired by man as a member of society" (Winthrop 1991, p. 52). But Tylor was also imbued with the evolutionary ideas of his time. Although he saw cultures as plural entities, they were not of equal value and ranged in an evolutionary series from primitive to civilized, with nineteenth-century Europe at the apex.

One further transformation of the concept of culture was of special significance for transcultural psychiatry. This was the elaboration of the idea of cultural relativism, the special focus of Franz Boas (1858–1942) and his American anthropology students. Spurred by the racist implications of the evolutionary theory of cultures, Boas reintroduced some of Herder's views: European cultures were not superior to others; each cultural configuration had its own place in history and occupied a unique historical niche; indeed, each was virtually incomparable to any other. Judgments of cultures are essentially reduced to the idiosyncrasies of the observer's personal taste.

The Problem of Cultural Relativism

Cultural relativism is one of the major controversial areas along the interface between psychiatry and anthropology. As we have noted, the view that cultures were parallel developments of adaptive excellence rather than linear progressions from primitive to civilized was developed by Herder and elaborated by Franz Boas. Of Jewish descent and born in Minden, Germany, Boas had early experience with racism. His family milieu was liberal, antiauthoritarian, and free-thinking (Kardiner and Preble 1961). Although mathematics and physics were the focus of his early education, he later turned to physical, then cultural geography; and after a year among the Inuit of Baffin Island at the age of 25, he became enchanted by ethnography. Through extensive fieldwork, he struggled to free himself from the Eurocentrism of his predecessors.

He used his highly developed critical faculty to good advantage in demolishing the grandiose and unprovable theories of many of his colleagues. The generalizations of psychoanalysis were not exempt; he particularly attacked Freud's suggestion that the primitive mind was like the mind of a child or a psychotic. Boas was also scornful of his student Ruth Benedict's idea that cultures are personalities writ large; the "megalomaniac boasting and acting of the Northwest Coast Indians does not make them act like megalomaniac insane" (Boas 1911/1963, p. 163).

The attitude that each culture is unique and incomparable to any other greatly influenced the work of Boas. He argued that relativism has to do both with ethical matters and with research methods (Winthrop 1991): ethical relativism holds that behavior should be judged good or bad only in terms of the values of a given culture; as a methodological principle, beliefs and customs must be understood in the context of the culture that generated them. For example, Boas noted that employing our Western concept of murder in other contexts is misleading: "The person who slays in revenge for wrongs done, a youth who kills his aged father before he gets decrepit in order to enable him to continue a vigorous life in the world to come, a father who kills his child as a sacrifice for the welfare of his people, acts from such entirely different motives, that psychologically a comparison of their actions does not seem permissible" (Boas 1911/1963, p. 173). Boas saw grave difficulties in interpreting behavior, symbols, and other entities across cultures. He pointed out that although the natural sciences are marked by clear and consistent definitions, the same is not true in anthropology. For example, we know what a family, state, or government is in our own culture, but when we apply these to other cultures, "we do not know in how far these may correspond to equivalent concepts. If we chose to apply our classifications to alien cultures, we may combine forms that do not belong together . . . if it is our serious purpose to understand the thought of people the whole analysis of experience must be based on their concepts, not ours" (Boas 1943, p. 314). Harris (1968, p. 316) has noted that Boas insisted that "two cultural elements are not the same if they mean different things to the people who possess them."

This relativistic incomparability of one culture to another is a mixed blessing, even for anthropologists. On the positive side, the relativist approach enables anthropologists to study other cultures with a minimum of ethnocentric bias, and Boas had great influence in making this attitude a commonplace in anthropology. But problems arise when relativism is taken to the extreme. "It is when he [Boas] carries this cultural relativism to the point where it seems to deny the possibility of making any comparative and general statements about cultures that some students begin to wonder what anthropology can contribute to the knowledge of human behavior. This is a problem which continues to haunt anthropology" (Kardiner and Preble 1961, p. 153).

As far as transcultural psychiatry is concerned, radical relativism virtually precludes cross-cultural comparisons of syndromes or psychiatric epidemiology. Since notions of cause and meanings of illness are highly variable from one culture to another, and if, as Boas claims, "two cultural elements are not the same if they mean different things to the people who possess them," no transcultural psychiatry is possible (Harris 1968, p. 316).

This relativistic difficulty is clear in controversies over culture-bound syndromes (CBS). Cassidy (1982) has proposed a meaning-centered definition of CBS; when considering the CBS status of a given disease, notions of etiology should be included. Using protein-energy malnutrition (*kwashiorkor*) as an example, Cassidy admits that the symptoms of the disease are universal, but since it is attributed to a wide variety of culture-linked causes, *kwashiorkor* should be designated a culture-bound syndrome. Clearly such a definition is not acceptable within scientific medicine. Diseases do not change on the basis of changing notions of their etiology.

In addition, radical relativism precludes cross-cultural epidemiological studies. According to the ideology of cultural relativism, rates of even well-established universal syndromes such as schizophrenia cannot be meaningfully compared because of differing culture-related ideas of cause or meanings. In his radical relativism, Boas created his own grandiose and unprovable dogma. For transcultural psychiatrists, humankind shares many commonalities across cultures; even Boas in his saner moments would probably have concurred.

Transcultural Psychiatry: What's in a Name?

Much more than the designations of similar terms in most other academic disciplines, the label *transcultural psychiatry* has been controversial. Specialists in the field still argue over the appropriateness of the term. Besides *transcultural psychiatry*, other possible labels include *comparative, cross-cultural, ecological, prescientific, intercultural, ethnopsychiatry,* or simply *cultural psychiatry.* Possibly the conflict over designation is at least in part due to the field's multidisciplinary nature. Besides psychiatry and medicine, relevant disciplines include anthropology, medical history, psychology, sociology, social work, and nursing.

Wittkower's choice of the designation *transcultural* was probably unfortunate. The prefix *trans* is burdened with connotations from such words as *transcend,* which suggests overarching or going beyond a limit, and *transcendental,* which even suggests a mystical exceeding of human knowledge. These are all shades of meaning that Wittkower certainly did not intend.

Wittkower himself had worried a good deal about definitions and boundaries. "Cultural psychiatry," Wittkower explained in 1966, "concerns itself with the mentally ill in relation to their cultural environment within the context of a given cultural unit. The Latin prefix 'trans' in the term 'transcultural psychiatry' denotes that the vista of the scientific observer extends beyond the scope of one cultural unit to another, whereas the term 'cross-cultural,' as we use it, has a methodological connotation. It refers to the comparison of psychiatric observations between at least two culture areas." He further clarified his concept of transcultural psychiatry by reference to five objectives: (1) exploration of the similarities and differences in the manifestations of mental illness in different cultures; (2) identification of cultural factors that predispose to mental illness and mental health; (3) assessment of the effect of identified cultural factors on the frequency and nature of mental illness; (4) study of the forms of treatment practiced or preferred in different cultural settings; and (5) comparison of different attitudes toward the mentally ill in different cultures (Wittkower 1966, p. 228).

What about some recent usages? *Transcultural psychiatry* is perhaps the term most commonly used by non-Western psychiatrists; for example, the World Psychiatric Association designates one of its more active subdivisions as the Transcultural Psychiatry Section. However, American psychiatrists seem to favor *cultural psychiatry* (notwithstanding the title of this volume). Social scientists such as anthropologists or sociologists seldom use *transcultural* and lean more toward *cross-cultural*; psychologists publish the *Journal of Cross-Cultural Psychology*, which includes some material that overlaps with what psychiatrists might call transcultural psychiatry or cultural psychiatry. It should be noted that H. B. M. Murphy (1982), Wittkower's long-term associate at McGill, wrote an important textbook in the field using the title *Comparative Psychiatry: The International and Intercultural Distribution of Mental Illness*. Murphy rejected the term *transcultural psychiatry* and returned to Emil Kraepelin's earlier designation. Elsewhere, Murphy commented on the naming problem as follows: "The choice of the term 'transcultural' caused some debate, since 'cultural,' 'ethno-cultural,' and 'comparative' could have been used, each carrying a somewhat different connotation. The 'trans' part of the term even caused some unease, since it appeared to imply that the field would be concerned only with features that transcended cultural boundaries, not those that remained within them; but on the other hand it could be taken as implying intercultural comparison, and that was definitely the intention of some of us" (Murphy 1986, p. 13).

Kleinman (1977) calls for a "new cross-cultural psychiatry" that takes into consideration local meanings and related behaviors in cross-cultural comparisons in order to better achieve the traditional goal of assessing the universality of human psychopathology, while bringing cultural psychiatry in line with medical anthropology. This approach stems from various efforts, including medical history via Foucault, academic psychology focusing on the universality of emotions and cognition, the sociology of knowledge, various critical interdisciplinary developments such as Marxism, semiotics, structuralism, ethnomethodology, deconstructionism, and the philosophies of Wittgenstein and Lacan. All of these emphasize the lack of distinction between theory and observation, fact and value, and objective and subjective. The new cross-cultural psychiatry criticizes psychiatry for failing to deal effectively with the dialectic between biology and society, thus promoting a "shift in emphasis from cross-cultural comparisons of psychiatric categories to examining psychiatric epistemology and clinical practice in all societies" (Littlewood 1990, p.309).

Although Kleinman's work has been generally well received, there are significant criticisms. Prince (1991) has suggested that the concept of the "new" versus the "old" transcultural psychiatry is a false dichotomy. It began with Arthur Kleinman's (1977) accusation that "old" transcultural psychiatrists were intent upon forcing non-Western psychiatric disturbances into the procrustean beds of Western diagnostic categories. This accusation had been triggered by a review of the cross-cultural literature on depression by K. Singer (1975), in which Singer concluded that "[t]here is insufficient evidence to support a prevalent view that depressive illness in primitive and certain other non-Western cultures has outstanding deviant features." For some reason, Kleinman took Singer's views as representative of the "old" transcultural psychiatry. This of course was a straw man. As we have already emphasized, the pioneers of transcultural psychiatry such as Wittkower, Murphy, and perhaps even Kraepelin were all interested in exploring culture-related *differences* in psychiatric phenomena.

Ironically Kleinman's (1977) own well-known research on neurasthenia in Chinese populations has lead him to be accused of foisting Western diagnostic categories on the Chinese (Lin 1989). Kleinman had concluded that cases of neurasthenia, a popular diagnosis in China, were really cases of masked depression and should be labeled as major depressive disorder. Many Chinese psychiatrists disagreed. Yan He-Quin (1989, p. 143), for example, felt that the extent of depression in neurasthenia reported by Kleinman was too large to be believed and stated the following: "It is our view that the diagnosis of neurasthenia is scientifically based. It is very unscientific to discard this diagnostic label according to the fashion of psychiatric practice."

Commenting on this same neurasthenia research by Kleinman, the anthropologist Vieda Skultans (1991, p. 15) is also skeptical: "However much Kleinman may protest his sensitivity to cultural variations he has not dispensed with the intellectual outlook of the Western psychiatrist. It seems that he has retained a stealthy hold of Western nosology whilst publically proclaiming the wrongness of doing so." Skultans (1991) doubts that it is possible for a psychiatrist to enter an alien culture without carrying along his or her preconceived psychiatric formulations. She suggests that the central difficulty in cross-cultural psychiatry is one of "translation," by which she means the "juxtaposition of, or the finding of approximate equivalents between, categories whose roots lie in quite different social contexts." The ghost of Boas is still with us.

But, in any case, whatever the intellectual difficulties, psychiatrists more or less successfully diagnose and treat patients from alien cultures; the name of the field is not nearly as important as a united concern that the understanding and possible alleviation of human suffering can be advanced by taking as wide a view of the field as possible. For today's transcultural psychiatrist, we can suggest the following descriptive definition: Culture is that blueprint-for-living that is nongenetically transmitted from one generation to the next. It is thought to be exclusive to humans. Culture is the totality of habits, ideas, beliefs, attitudes, and values, as well as the behaviors that spring from them (language, styles of art, marriage patterns, eating habits, and so forth). Ashantis, Germans, Koreans, and Crees feel, think, and act differently; culture accounts for a good deal of the variance.

Any attempt to understand human behavior needs to take into account both its variability and its consistency. This is no less true for any effort to understand mental illness and the suffering integral to the human condition. All societies differentiate normal from aberrant behavior, devise systems for explaining abnormal behavior, and institutionalize procedures of response and treatment. These belief and response systems are integral to their larger belief system, which contains understandings of cause, self and others, and the environment. These beliefs are symbolic and thus capable of not only providing meaning and explanation, but also evoking emotional and behavioral responses. Furthermore, these symbolic belief systems and the associated social system and patterning of behavior are highly variable. And yet there is a commonality in the biological and psychological parameters of human existence. Mental illness is ubiquitous and, at a certain level of analysis, highly consistent. "In most human societies, both primitive and civilized, both Western and non-Western the same major symptom clusters can be recognized: schizophrenia, depressions, conversion reaction, obsessions and compulsions, phobias, and psychosomatic ailments," yet societies differ in the style of symptoms, incidence and prevalence, and possibly total census (Wallace 1967, p.196).

In light of the need for improving psychiatric sensitivity toward cultural variation, psychiatric training has increasingly included didactic and clinical experience in this area (Foulks 1980; Lefley and Bestman 1991; Zatzick and Lu 1991). In addition, in 1991 the American Psychiatric Association's Council on Medical Education and Career Development made training in this area mandatory for approved psychiatric training programs.

References

Ackerknecht EH: Medicine and Ethnology: Selected Essays. Stuttgart, Hans Huber, 1971

Boas F: Recent anthropology. Science 98:311–314, 1943

Boas F: The Mind of Primitive Man (1911). New York, Collier Books, 1963

Boroffka A: Emil Kraepelin (1856–1926). Transcultural Psychiatric Research Review 27:228–237, 1990

Bourguignon E: George Devereux (1908–1985). Transcultural Psychiatric Research Review 23:172–174, 1986

Cassidy CM: Protein-energy malnutrition as a culture-bound syndrome. Cult Med Psychiatry 6:325–345, 1982

Eliot TS: Notes towards the definition of culture. London, Faber & Faber, 1948

Foulks EF: The concept of culture in psychiatric residency education. Am J Psychiatry 137:811–816, 1980

Greenlees TD: Insanity among the natives of South Africa. Journal of Mental Science 41:71–82, 1895

Harris M: The Rise of Anthropological Theory. New York, Crowell, 1968

Hunter R, Macalpine I: Three Hundred Years of Psychiatry (1535–1860). London, Oxford University Press, 1963

Kardiner A, Preble E: They Studied Man. London, Secker & Warburg, 1961

Kiev A: Magic, Faith and Healing: Studies in Primitive Psychiatry Today. New York, Free Press, 1964

Kleinman A: Depression, somatization and the "new cross-cultural psychiatry." Soc Sci Med 11:3–10, 1977

Kraepelin E: Vergleichende psychiatria (1904), translated as "Comparative psychiatry" by Wittkower E. Transcultural Psychiatric Research Review 11:108–112, 1974

Kroeber AL, Kluckhohn CK: Culture: A Critical Review of Concepts and Definitions. New York, Vintage Books, 1963

La Barre W: The influence of Freud on anthropology. American Imago 15:275–328, 1958

Lefley HP, Bestman EW: Public-academic linkages for cultural sensitive community mental health. Community Ment Health J 27:473–488, 1991

Leighton A, Leighton D: Elements of psychotherapy in Navaho religion. Psychiatry 4:515–523, 1941

Lin T-Y: Neurasthenia in Asian cultures. Cult Med Psychiatry 13:105–241, 1989.

Littlewood R: From categories to context: a decade of the "new cross-cultural psychiatry." Br J Psychiatry 156:308–327, 1990

Morales SC: Géza Róheim's theory of the dream origin of myth, in Psychoanalytic Study of Society, Vol 13. Edited by Boyer LB, Grolnick SA. Hillsdale, NJ, Analytic Press, 1988, pp 7–27

Murphy HBM: Comparative Psychiatry: The International and Intercultural Distribution of Mental Illness. New York, Springer-Verlag, 1982

Murphy HBM: The historic development of transcultural psychiatry, in Transcultural Psychiatry. Edited by Cox JL. London, Croom-Helm, 1986, pp 7–22

Prince R: Review essay on the "New cross-cultural psychiatry." Transcultural Psychiatric Research Review 28:41–55, 1991

Prince R: Somatic complaint syndromes and depression: the problem of cultural effects on symptomatology. Transcultural Psychiatric Research Review 27:31–36, 1990

Rosen G: Madness in Society: Chapters in the Historical Sociology of Mental Illness. New York, Harper Torchbook, 1969

Singer K: Depressive disorders from a transcultural perspective. Soc Sci Med 9:289–301, 1975

Skultans V: Anthropology and psychiatry: the uneasy alliance. Transcultural Psychiatric Research Review 28:5–24, 1991

Wallace AFC: Anthropology and psychiatry, in Comprehensive Textbook of Psychiatry. Edited by Freedman AM, Kaplan HI. Baltimore, MD, Williams & Wilkins, 1967, pp 195–201

Wilkes C: Letter to the editor. American Journal of Insanity 2:285–286, 1845

Williams RW: Keywords: A Vocabulary of Culture and Society. London, Fontana, 1983

Winthrop RH: Dictionary of Concepts in Cultural Anthropology. Westport, CT, Greenwood Press, 1991

Wittkower E: Perspectives of transcultural psychiatry, in Proceedings of the IV World Congress of Psychiatry, Madrid, September 5–11, 1966, pp 228–234

Yan H-Q: The necessity of retaining the diagnostic concept of neurasthenia. Cult Med Psychiatry 13:139–145, 1989

Zatzick DF, Lu FG: The ethnic/minority focus unit as a training site in transcultural psychiatry. Academic Psychiatry 15:218–225, 1991

CHAPTER 2

Recollections of Culture and Personality

ALEXANDER H. LEIGHTON, M.D.

This chapter is a revision of an invited presentation given before the Society for the Study of Psychiatry and Culture. Ronald Wintrob suggested that I recollect past experiences and report such *impressions* as might be of interest to the members of the Society.

In the present chapter, I have adhered to the goal of transmitting impressions but have also kept in mind that the present book is about clinical methods. The notions put forward in this chapter are not all assumed to be necessarily true, even though they are for the most part based on observation and scientific thinking; rather they are statements about my sense of likelihood. My hope, therefore, is not so much to convince readers that the main points in this chapter are valid as to convince them that they are worth serious consideration.

I have chosen culture and personality as my theme on the basis of two premises: first, this once very promising field has failed to thrive; and second, certain of the major factors in that failure are still adversely affecting not only culture and personality but also advances in both of its parent fields.

The chapter begins with the subject of personality and then expands to a consideration of culture, mainly because this order follows that of my own experience. In dealing with personality, I examine the distinction between large theories that attempt to be comprehensive explanations and theories that are more methodological in orientation by attempting to be guidelines for conducting examinations of people in order to understand their ideas, feelings, and behavior. The latter orientation involves an emphasis on the psychobiology of Adolf Meyer.

In dealing with culture, I distinguish between general theories regarding culture's power to shape personalities and theories more focused on developing methods by means of which the interplay of culture and personality might be studied.

In turning to culture and personality per se, I review a number of impressions. Primarily because of its past inattention to the distinctions just mentioned, the field became paralyzed by the difficulty of reaching a consensus regarding definitions of concepts and phenomena that would make it possible to connect theories of cause to observable events in nature. I suggest that while the scientific need at this point was for systems by which particular events could be described, classified, ordered, and analyzed, professional interest turned toward comprehensive abstractions based on intuitive appeal rather than empirical data. Culture and personality has thus been barred from the kind of incremental growth that is characteristic of scientific disciplines and has become instead largely a realm of metaphysical discussion. At the end of the chapter, I mention what seem to me some opportunities for again moving forward.

Personality

The Department of Psychiatry at Johns Hopkins University, where I received training between 1934 and 1941, was headed by Adolf Meyer. In his teaching, Meyer presented concepts about normal personality as fundamental to the understanding of psychopathology and the practice of clinical psychiatry. This approach was partially modeled on the way the concepts and phenomena of physiology were taught as fundamental to the understanding of pathology.

In time, I became aware that this method was very different from that taught, under the title of *personality,* by most psychologists, psychoanalysts, and other relevant professionals. For these, personality was not so much the study of actual persons as it was a delineation of a theory or theories about the principles and mechanisms of human motivation. Freud was, of course, a main figure, but there were other prominent individuals as well, such as Adler, Erikson, Fromm, H. A. Murray, Jung, and H. S. Sullivan.

At the Johns Hopkins Department of Psychiatry, personality *study—* rather than personality *theory—*was taught, and this meant training in the use of procedures (largely developed by Meyer) that would help us understand the viewpoint and motivations of another person. The aim was to teach doctors-in-training how to learn those things concerning their patients that would promote a practical comprehension of them as persons, rather than simply as a disease in a body. Personality study was a foundation on which the student would build knowledge about how to study people with psychopathology during the last two clinical years in medical school and throughout residency training—if he or she chose psychiatry as a specialty. During all such work, readings in theory were suggested and their usefulness with regard to particular persons suffering from a disorder was discussed at practically every case-conference. The emphasis was, nonetheless, on how to gather and analyze the "facts" about a person that would aid understanding rather than on how to apply any particular system of interpretation to the case. The advantages of learning about persons through observation were emphasized.

Meyer referred to his orientation as psychobiology, which meant that person, or "self," (the unit referred to by the pronoun *he, she,* or *I*) was the focus of study and that, contrary to the Cartesian dichotomy, each such person united both psychological and biological aspects, constituting a psychobiological whole. Further, there was recognition that the life of each such whole had been and was being modified by interaction with societal and cultural factors. Thus this holistic notion of personhood consisted of an ongoing union of three major facets of individual process: biological, psychological, and socioenvironmental. One was expected to take all of these into account in making a personality study and again later in making a diagnosis.

Meyer had a number of reasons for his approach, but the major one in my opinion was his mistrust of "big theory." This attitude was evident in his view of Freud and other psychodynamic leaders, but it was also applied to biologically oriented clinical theories. The central components of his view can perhaps be most economically illustrated in terms of his reaction not to Freud but rather to Kraepelin's dementia praecox. Meyer admired Kraepelin's work as a brilliant piece of clinical observation and inference. At the same time, he did not believe Kraepelin had established the reality of dementia praecox as a disease entity. He thought that if one believed in the existence of the disorder, it was very easy to find examples in populations of severely ill mental patients.

Careful and prolonged observation of individual patients, however, generally revealed that most did not in fact conform to the dementia praecox syndrome over time. In particular, many were able to achieve improved quality of life and, in some instances, recoveries that were contrary to Kraepelin's emphasis on progressive degeneration.

Meyer thought that medical and popular confidence in the notion of dementia praecox had two exceedingly undesirable consequences. First, once the diagnosis had been pronounced and the disease attributed to a patient, it discouraged further interest. Labeling, in other words, deprived the patient of therapeutic effort that otherwise could contribute to a more satisfying level of adjustment and that could help the clinician realize that the negative diagnostic expectations did not fit. Second, such labeling placed premature emphasis on biological theories of etiology and diminished interest in the role of psychological and interpersonal factors among people with severe psychotic disturbances.

Meyer seemed to be concluding that projective mechanisms occur in psychiatrists and other clinicians as well as in patients, and that etiological explanations are an area of high risk in this regard. Meyer emphasized that in the history of medicine, and especially in psychiatry, a practice among professionals that had cost ill people dearly was combining overconfidence in theory with insufficient observation and commonsense thinking about the particular person at hand.

The Study of Personality

Training in the study of normal personality under Meyer's influence was made up of lectures, reading, and "lab," the latter being a fresh and systematic look at oneself and two or three friends or relatives. The procedure involved meeting individually once a week for an hour or more with an instructor who presented an outline of questions that called for observations, reports, and written analyses. The first few meetings were rather awkward, but were then followed by more and more discussion of problems—including personal problems—that were often very absorbing.

A point of departure was choosing a question that the student considered important as the focus for an examination of himself or herself.

"Why am I in medical school?" was, for instance, a common selection. The second step consisted in writing in chronological order the main events of our lives with some evaluation of how they had come about and how they had affected us. This usually required several weeks. It is important to note that the instructor's comments were often directed at apparent omissions in the story or at possible alternatives to the interpretations we had given. It became clear before long that there was a flexible but real organizing principle in the questions. This was not based on any particular theoretical approach but rather on a sense of what experience shows to be the range of things to consider in various characteristic human situations. I felt the questions were often very illuminating but also frequently balance-restoring.

The third step dealt with describing the view of our present situation and our network of people, supports, and tensions. We were encouraged to list and describe the more important current actors on this stage and their particular views and influences on us. In this context, we were often asked to describe our future aspirations and the assets and liabilities of our personality with respect to the chances of fulfillment.

The final part of the study was a synthesizing process in which main themes were identified and their influence summarized. The focal question—"Why am I in medical school?"—was central to this process, supplemented by the question of what we might have learned in the course of making the study. The last question was usually some form of "How will this affect your thinking and action with regard to making a success of the future?"

The personality studies of the other persons served to highlight variations in human experiences and reactions. The studies also brought forward the great conceptual, methodological, and analytic problems that arise in doing personality studies without having direct access to subjective information of the kind available in studying oneself. In this connection, major issues were raised about how far one can trust the validity of intuition and insight.

When we entered clinical work in the third year, we began to learn psychopathology and applied what we learned in the previous two years to the examination of mentally ill patients. The focal question, for instance, was directed at the "complaint and present illness" of the patients; the examination of their mental status was added as a data-gathering tool, usually employed prior to securing their life story. From that time on, we focused on methods of diagnosis and treatment. Meyer rejected attaching a label or a ready-made theory in diagnosis. Rather, he considered diagnosis a formulation of the major events or streams of events that had been involved in the origins of a patient's disorder, with special attention to those that might be modified to improve the patient's quality of life.

While Meyer admired original ideas and spent considerable time in discussing theories and in having invited experts give grand rounds, he consistently expressed mistrust in abstruse systems, preferring to rely on common sense. Indeed, he often said that science was "common sense systematically extended."

A Clinical Example

At this point it may be useful to try to illustrate some of what I have been saying by means of a case. My involvement with this particular one began in the Yupik-speaking Eskimo village of Gambell on St. Lawrence Island. Although part of Alaska, the island is off the coast of Siberia in the North Bering Sea. Shortly after my arrival there in June 1940, I was asked if I would look at a young man, let us call him Robert, who had been paralyzed from the waist down for some years. Although doubtful that I could do any good, I thought I should at least examine him. Robert arrived at the nursing station in the village school on a sled carried like a stretcher by four or five men and was transferred to the examining table with some difficulty, due to his helplessness, pain, and apprehension. Because he spoke little English and I no Yupik, we had to communicate through an interpreter.

In the course of carrying out as complete a physical examination as possible, I asked him to tell all he could about the onset and nature of his paralysis. I explored his life story with particular attention to his medical history. Finally I asked about his current situation and then sat and sorted through what I had learned, while the interpreter and the patient both stared at me, waiting.

What was impressive to me as a neoanthropologist in a strange culture was the amount of seemingly relevant information brought out by the method I had been taught. In combination with the physical examination, it suggested that Robert's condition was of a psychological not an organic basis, an instance of what was at that time called hysterical paralysis. As part of learning all I could in advance about the St. Lawrence Island culture, I had read about *piblokto* and "arctic hysteria," but Robert was not like these descriptions. He resembled a few patients I had seen at Johns Hopkins who had come from remote rural areas on the Eastern Shore of the Chesapeake Bay and who also suffered from a paralysis that did not seem to have an organic basis.

Similarly, Robert had a problem that he could not handle and that filled him with dread. About five years previously, at the time his paralysis began to develop, he had reached the age when young, able-bodied males in Gambell were expected to spend three or four months a year at an isolated trapping camp in the darkness of winter. This custom meant an arduous and dangerous dogsled journey to reach the camp. The males spent each day alone on the trap lines catching white foxes, the main cash-producing resource for the people of Gambell.

Inquiring about these cultural and economic factors and their meanings was a result of my previous training in the psychobiological method. Through it, I learned more about the ideas and feelings of the various participants—the patient, members of his family, others close to him, and the village in general.

The interpreter and Robert knew I was ignorant of their traditions, so when I indicated that I thought that perhaps a cultural element might be important in understanding his condition, they provided a great amount of information. They too thought it necessary that I should understand Robert's life and its context as well as possible if I were to do him any good.

It appeared that the patient had always been timid and especially fearful about his health, a tendency fostered no doubt by his having over the years watched all the other males in his family die from tuberculosis. Robert's immediate family was now a unit of six or seven females who were terribly worried about his health. Opposed to this fear was the sense of what the role of a man in his society should be, an attitude that was shared not only among virtually the whole population of Gambell but also by Robert, his mother, and his sisters.

In the course of inquiring about Robert's resources, capabilities, and interests, I learned that he was a crack shot, one of the best in Gambell, and had been an expert seal hunter along the shores and on the ice near the village. This skill had gained for him prestige and some economic returns, but he had been forced to give it up as the paralysis increased.

It seemed to me, in view of Robert's family history and what I knew of the prevalence and mortality rates of tuberculosis in the village, that he very likely had an active form of the disease and probably would die of it before too long. If that were so, it seemed more than merely possible that the arduous life of a trapping camp would bring the death sooner. Under these circumstances, the question for me was whether I could devise a solution to Robert's predicament that would be less costly to him and his family than the paralysis.

Hypnosis had been found at Johns Hopkins to work with some cases like Robert's, and I wondered if it could work here. I asked him to consider a relaxing kind of treatment that could make him feel better and found that he was willing to try. He passed into a "trance" rather quickly, and I then made the following suggestions to him via the interpreter:

1. Speaking as a doctor, I said trapping would not be healthy for him. Everyone should put that idea out of their minds. And he could quote me on that.
2. Instead, he should develop his talents as a sharp-shooter and seal hunter and he would be very successful at that.
3. His paralysis could be cured, and that was going to begin right this afternoon. This treatment was already relaxing and reviving his muscles and taking the pain out of them. Presently he would get off the examining table and stand on his feet. Then he would walk up and down the corridor—and then walk home.

After the hypnosis he did just that, including walking home unaided while the sled was carried behind him. By this time a considerable crowd had gathered and they followed him, watching and marveling.

Robert had no return of the paralysis during that summer; when I returned to the island 15 years later, he came to see me and asked for another relaxing treatment. He was walking with a cane because of some arthritis but said he had never again been paralyzed. I think he was hoping that a repeat treatment might help his arthritis. His going to a trapping camp was by this time a dead issue.

From the perspective of many people who are strong believers in cultural determinism and cultural relativity, this story is not very credible. In principle, it would be considered extremely unlikely that an outsider to Yupik culture could make a valid psychiatric diagnosis. As for the claim that I had hypnotized a Yupik man through an interpreter, cured him of paralysis, and sent him walking home, that belonged in the category of an Alaskan tall tale.

In fact, of course, I do not know whether the diagnosis was valid or not. All I can say is that the psychobiological approach brought forth clinical information, including relevant cultural factors, that the patient and interpreter could tell me about and whose functional connections I could at least crudely understand. Furthermore, the information seemed to contain a partial explanation of Robert's paralysis and suggested a line of intervention that had results supporting the partial explanation—a therapeutic test, in other words, of the hypothesis. The case is certainly not as good as a controlled experiment, but it does have some value as evidence regarding probabilities. It seemed to me more tethered to reality than a purely theoretical explanation, no matter how logically the latter might stand on its premises.

Discovering Culture

During my resident training in psychiatry, which began in 1937, I started to think with more focus on choosing a field in which I might have a research career. The whys and wherefores of behavior were my central interest. Majoring in biology at Princeton, I had done an undergraduate thesis on the ethology of beavers that had involved living in the woods with them for some four months (Leighton 1932, 1933, 1935). Afterwards, two years at Cambridge University pursuing preclinical studies and a Natural Science Tripos Part II gave me superb experience in neurophysiology. After completing medical training, I received a clinical grounding in one approach to human behavior, namely psychiatry.

For a time I thought I might be able to build on these studies by entering biological psychiatry. When, however, I began looking at this field more closely, it seemed like a desert scattered with the bleached bones of dead careers. Very little of scientific value had taken place over the previous 30 years, and there seemed little reason in 1937 to believe that things would be different in the near future—despite the fact that shock treatment was now coming into use. Research in neurophysiology itself was extremely lively, indeed bursting with promise, but the level of its investigation was as yet very far from being able to contribute to knowledge about human behavior. In addition, the various schools of psychoanalytic psychiatry were extremely engaging because of the wonderful explanations given to clinical narratives, but their predilection for using intuition and the authority of the master's word as tests of validity resulted in very few portals through which scientific inquiry could enter with much hope of success.

The pragmatic and down-to-earth qualities of psychobiology gave it, for a naturalist, the look of a foundation on which one could build systematic research, except for the fact that, as with all the rest of clinical psychiatry, its effort at scientific knowledge was permeated by a major weakness: conceptions of normal mental functioning were almost exclusively made up of inferences based on the study of persons with mental disorders and very little on the study of well persons. So far as I could see, psychiatry was the only major subfield of medicine for which this was true. Cardiology, orthopedics, ophthalmology, and all the rest stood on a corresponding physiology in which the methods of science were applied to the understanding of normal function, which in turn formed the background for identifying and comprehending pathology. Psychiatry had little that could be considered as corresponding to this practice. It did, of course, draw on world philosophies, religions, and ethical systems; but except for a few studies in child development, it was mostly uninformed by scientific investigations into the functioning of normal persons.

It eventually occurred to me that what had appeared as a forbidding weakness might actually be the research opportunity for which I was looking. Would it be possible to assemble a data bank of normal personality studies that could be used to shed light on what distinguishes functionally normal feelings and behavior from those that are psychopathological in outcome? For instance, would it be possible to describe systematic differences between how life stresses are perceived and handled by those who are well and those patients whom we were seeing every day in hospital and outpatient departments? By degrees I formed the notion of studying everyone in a natural community in somewhat the way I had studied the ethology of beavers, utilizing the personality study as the instrument for collecting and organizing data.

At once there arose an array of questions about how one might go about doing this and about what additional conceptual and operational tools would be needed. With Meyer's strong encouragement, I began acquainting myself with the major scientific disciplines that were studying persons from perspectives that were significantly different from those of psychiatry. Gradually narrowing my focus to psychology, sociology, and cultural anthropology, I attempted to grasp, as well as I could, the relevant principles and methods that were distinctive in each of these fields.

To psychology, I already had received considerable introduction and so could begin building on this framework. With regard to sociology, my initial reading and inquiries failed to inspire adequate appreciation, and it was not until some years later, after I had encountered Robert Merton, that I began to give it the attention warranted (Merton 1949). The concept of culture, on the other hand, struck me at once as an orientation that opened a host of potentialities. In this respect, it was a striking contrast to the picture I had of research opportunities in biological psychiatry or psychodynamic psychiatry.

Particularly appealing were Bronislaw Malinowski's ideas about how cultural patterns perform various functions in the preservation of the human species. These patterns not only constitute vehicles by which biological, cognitive, and affective needs of individuals are satisfied but also make possible that coordinating behavior upon which group life and species survival depend. For someone like myself, oriented toward humans as members of the animal kingdom rather than as creatures apart, this perspective had strong appeal. There seemed to be in functional anthropology the beginnings of an empirical and systematic discipline focused on how patterns of socially integrated behavior and thought are transmitted diachronically from one generation to another, and synchronically from one population to another. It seemed possible for this field to have a place within the theory of organic evolution, and to have a position complemental to genetics.

Following the death of Malinowski, anthropologist Ralph Linton's thinking about this discipline became most influential in my cultural education. Through him I began to see a culture—however complex—as a describable set of phenomena rather than as a purely abstract concept dealing with the construction and transmission of meaning. His discussion of classification issues led me to recognize a considerable similarity to many of the problems with which zoologists struggle and with which we were struggling in psychiatric nomenclature. Linton emphasized classification and tabulation but also maintained the ultimate importance of qualitative thinking, as illustrated by his statement that every element of culture must be assessed for four distinct, although mutually interrelated, qualities: form, meaning, use, and function. He held that "[B]efore we can understand its significance to the total configuration of which the element is a part, these [four qualities] must be distinguished and defined. It is further necessary to define the category of elements within the culture to which these qualities may be said to pertain" (Linton 1964, p. 402).

I found out before long that the workmanlike approach of Linton and some others was by no means universal in cultural anthropology. The prevailing picture was one of many competing orientations, all set in a context made up of interpretations, philosophies, and nonstandardized terminologies. The extent and scientifically inhibiting nature of this multiplexity is well shown in Kroeber and Kluckhohn's *Culture: A Critical Review of Concepts and Definitions* (Kroeber and Kluckhohn 1952). This book is famous for having cited 164 "definitions of culture" and for estimating that the actual total was closer to 300. Although published in 1952, the monograph pays close attention to dates and thus gives a picture of the kinds of issues that social scientists were talking about in my early years of cultural anthropology. In the 1930s, some 35 definitions were added to a preexisting set of 27, while in the 11 years between 1940 and 1950, 100 more were included.

The great popular and professional influence of Ruth Benedict and Margaret Mead and their insistence on culture as *the* outstanding determinant of human behavior was rising at this time, and I was among those who became enthusiastic. There can be no doubt that Benedict and Mead became enormously successful in attracting attention to the notion of culture and to the effects of cultural differences. They did this both on the academic scene and in the world at large, but it is now open to question whether they and their followers advanced cultural anthropology as a science. One can argue that since the postwar decades little progress has been made along the lines recommended by Linton, that is, in devising systems of classification and developing analytic categories such as form, meaning, use, and function. Instead, mainstream trends have focused primarily on meaning and its symbolic representation and have let the other three go. One result, I believe, is that many of those interested in culture have moved deeply into problems of a kind that cannot be answered by scientific procedures.

Culture and Personality

In due course, it became evident to me that to study normal personalities, it would be wise to have some understanding of the cultural process in which those personalities had developed and in which they were currently transacting their lives. Malinowski had been the first to point this out, a view that was endorsed by most of the anthropologists I later consulted. He and they said that it was impossible to have an adequate perception of one's own culture without first living close to and systematically studying at least one other. The general idea in this was that all of us are too much a part of the culture in which we have grown up to be able to see it with even approximate objectivity unless we have undergone special education, and that the best such education is to observe a culture in which one is not a member. One must go to the moon, they said, in order to look back on the earth. This principle was, on occasion, also illustrated by quoting an aphorism attributed to Thomas Carlyle: "If you want to know the facts about salt water, don't ask a cod." A major actualization of the principle, furthermore, was cur-

rently under way in the study of a New England town by W. Lloyd
Warner and his colleagues (Warner and Lunt 1942). Warner's major
previous work had been among the aborigines of Australia.

A fellowship for the academic year 1939–1940 allowed me to engage in field study, preceded by about 3 months at Columbia University. With Linton and Kluckhohn as mentors, I envisioned two goals for
my study. One was to see how far one could go in conducting personality studies of normal Navajo and Yupik people, and the second was to
make observations of two cultures that were in considerable contrast
not only to our own culture but to each other as well. In this connection, it was thought that there would be opportunity to pick up a general but actual sense of what kind of phenomena and conceptualizations about them constitute the notion of a culture. It was also thought
that there would be opportunity to observe a few selected "cultural elements" and come to some understanding of them. We realized, of
course, that due to the briefness of the allotted time, observations and
information gathering would be limited; yet the hope was to make them
introductory and preliminary rather than superficial.

In preparation for the personality studies, I simplified the operational outline to start with the life story and let the focal question
emerge from it and from what could be seen of the person's current situation. For example, focal questions might include the following: "Why
is this person a medicine man?" "Why did this man come here from
Siberia?" "Why does this woman not own any sheep?" Thus, whatever
seemed most germane to a person's experiences comprised the basis of
the focal question.

In anticipating the collection and organizing of personality data, I
felt the need for a conceptual unit that would be at a lower level of abstraction than personality-as-a-whole. The desire was for something
closer to observable behavior—including verbal behavior—and con-
nectable by relatively short chains of inference. For this purpose, it
seemed that the concept of sentiment might be useful.

A ballpark understanding of what is meant by sentiment may be
conveyed by the words *opinions, attitudes,* and *aspirations,* and illustrated by such statements as "Virtue is always rewarded in the long
run," "The most important part of a woman's life is having children,"
and "Our team must win." The term *sentiment* and its use in clinical

settings had origins in the nineteenth century but resurfaced at the British Psychological Society's 1922 Symposium on Complex and Sentiment, with contributions from Bernard Hart, W. H. R. Rivers and others (Rivers et al. 1922). Considerable further development was then provided by William McDougall (McDougall 1936).

In psychiatry during the 1930s, sentiment had a moderate amount of currency. In the Department of Psychiatry at Johns Hopkins, each sentiment was regarded as a unit in the stream of a person's mentation, consisting in a fusion of cognitive, affective, and conative processes and representable by symbols, including verbal symbols. Sentiments were conceived as playing an important part in the wholeness or unity of any given personality due to the integrative effect of consistencies and interconnections among them. Conversely, disunity, emotional stress, and malfunction of personality were seen as occurring when incompatible intraperson sentiments were present.

The notion that sentiments contribute to the functioning of a personality at the level of wholeness seemed to provide a potential guide to hypothesis construction and data collection for understanding the relationship of culture and personality. Thus some cultures might play an important role in favoring well-integrated personalities by inculcating mutually compatible sentiments that form a coherent intraperson network. Other cultures might produce intraperson sentiments that are highly conflictual, resulting in personalities with various kinds of malfunction, some of which could turn psychopathological. People undergoing cultural change, for instance, might be more vulnerable than those in a more stable culture. Such reflections led me to decide that, for each individual chosen as the subject of a personality study, it would be useful to describe the person's prevailing sentiments and his or her main compatibilities and incompatibilities (Leighton 1959).

I became aware during or shortly after the fellowship year that there was emerging in cultural anthropology a concept of values that had marked similarities to the concept of sentiments. It seemed, for example, that values were at the heart of the culture concept in many ways, and that linkages and compatibilities among values made it possible to speak of "a culture as a whole," while incompatibilities among values indicated the "disintegration" of a culture.

Thus, while sentiments could serve as an analytic tool for dealing with the integrative-disintegrative functioning of an individual person, values seemed to be playing this role in the analysis of a culture. Sentiment and value had in common the fusion of the subjective processes of ideation and feeling. Furthermore, it seemed likely that most such fusions could serve as a sentiment in a person, a value in a culture, or both, and that this connection could be of considerable significance in trying to understand the relationship between culture and personality. As a consequence, it appeared important to distinguish between sentiments that were widely shared and those that were not.

The state of knowledge at this time further suggested that a systematic, step-by-step, descriptive approach along the lines outlined by Linton might be the best one to take. This inclination was confirmed as I came in time to realize that despite the ground held in common between sentiments and values, this ground did not as yet constitute a bridge between the two. A gulf was evident in that, for most students of culture, values were devoid of the biological implications that were implicit in the psychobiological notion of sentiments. Thus the word *conation* was missing from the definition of values and so too were words like *temperament*; while both *cognition* and *feeling* referred to psychological processes and scarcely, if at all, evoked their relationship to physiology. Most of those interested in personality and culture, whether coming from psychological disciplines or from the anthropological quarter, seemed oriented by a very strong conviction that any admission of biological etiology would be a death blow to both psychological and cultural causation and especially to the idea that different cultures could result in different personality types.

The most interesting exposition of this latter point of view was the seminar series on culturally formed "basic" personality by Abram Kardiner, with anthropological materials supplied by Ralph Linton. These sessions, which I was able to attend the year before the fellowship began, were stimulating to the imagination, highly systematic, and at times elegant, but left me unconvinced regarding the premises upon which Kardiner erected his theoretical structures. To the extent that my task during the fellowship year was to be a beginning for later scientific work, rather than philosophic, it seemed evident that the notions of personality and culture and the operations undertaken would have to be a good deal less speculative and somehow more closely tied to observable phenomena.

My fieldwork began among the Navajo in January 1940. Numbers of men and women were found who enjoyed telling their life stories and who did not seem to mind answering most of the supplemental questions. By May there were data for six personality studies plus several shorter autobiographical sketches. The subsequent 3 months on St. Lawrence Island were similarly successful, even though the culture and the physical environment were, as expected, exceedingly different.

The ethnographic portion of the task taught me the methods and problems involved in trying to arrive at valid generalizations about a culture and led to a deep appreciation of this science and the importance of its contributions to knowledge. At the same time, the personality studies made me aware of how much cultural elements could vary in expression and meaning from one person to another, and in the same person at different times; and thus it revealed how differently members of the same cultural group might have experienced their culture and how incompatible some aspects of their individual feelings and attitudes might be. Furthermore, the way in which the cultures I was exploring appeared to vary when viewed as parceled out among individuals seemed to fit rather well with Linton's four analytic qualities: form, meaning, use, and function. It looked, for example, as if a cultural element such as a Navajo hogan (house) or Blessing Way song could vary little or much in terms of these attributes from one person to another; and the same could be said for a Yupik boat or a ritual suicide.

In later years after additional cross-cultural studies, I became persuaded that this was a significant though largely unrecognized problem in culture and personality studies, which arose from the fact that most descriptions of cultures had been constructed for a purpose that renders them ill-suited to the analysis of culture and personality relationships. This purpose consists of presenting the reader with a *general*—which is to say holistic, abstract, and approximate—description of the lifeways and values characteristic of a particular group of people. To achieve this result, the ethnographer must pull together and make uniform sense out of largely heterogeneous observations he or she has made and out of reports from a variety of members of the culture. The result is a general picture in which much of the actual variation and inconsistency has become smoothed out. Transactions between culture and personality at the level of the individual, and of the day-to-day, are lost from sight. Yet it is here that the actual influences of culture on personalities take place, and what may be equally important, but has been largely unconsidered—the influence of personalities on culture.

The tendency to picture a culture as more coherent and less variable from person to person than it really is has had the effect, it seems to me, of making the impact of culture on personality—and on human behavior more generally—appear far more singular and powerful than is warranted by any existing scientific evidence. This is not to deny the possibility of important relationships, but rather to suggest that we are still rather ignorant of what they are and that it might be better to regard culture not as consisting of a molding force, but as consisting in multiple streams of influence of variable strengths that are not always compatible with each other, that are spread out unevenly across the arcs of individual lives, and that mingle with other shaping influences on personalities, including those implied by such terms as *temperament, cognitive capacity,* and *conation,* which clearly have organic components that are also of varying strengths and durations.

The impression arises, therefore, that the usefulness inherent in the concept of culture has been handicapped not only by lack of consensus with regard to definitions but also by the desire to work at high levels of abstraction. This inclination has been combined with a tendency to reify these abstract ideas and treat them as if they were phenomena in nature. From this propensity comes much wasted effort directed at trying to identify natural phenomena as examples of the reified abstractions, rather than as bases for making inferences.

It is of interest to note now that in 1952 Kroeber and Kluckhohn insisted that culture was not behavior but an abstraction derived from behavior and, therefore, not itself observable. Behavior is what can be observed, and inferences about culture can be made from it; but they warned against making the mistake of thinking that behavior is culture. Like many other great exploratory ideas, culture is at a different level of conceptualization and is by nature invisible. You can see its intimations in the phenomenal world but not the conceptualization itself. Given what has happened in the realms of cultural determinism, it seems to me that Kroeber and Kluckhohn have proved in their warning to be rather good prophets (Kroeber and Kluckhohn 1952, pp. 61–62, 155).

It seems fairly evident that many of the widely credited theories of personality are also based on smoothed-out observations and also involve the reification of highly abstract ideas. Edward Sapir died at the time I was becoming acquainted with cultural concepts and so I never had the privilege of meeting this pioneer in the development of culture and personality. After my initial field experiences in 1940, however, I became acquainted with his ideas, largely through Kluckhohn, and found them exceedingly congruent with my observations. For instance, he says a culture "varies infinitely, not only as to manifest content, but as to the distribution of psychologic emphasis on the elements and implications of this content." Accordingly, "we have to deal with the cultures of groups and the cultures of individuals" (Sapir 1970, p. 157).

The variation that the individual members of a cultural group show in how they look upon and react to the artifacts, symbols, and values of their culture is not easy to illustrate briefly. Let me try, however, to give the flavor by mentioning three of the men I studied who were much involved in Navajo religion. One of these was very uneasy about his identity as a Navajo because he had spent his youth as a shepherd for Hispanic people and had grown up relatively unfamiliar with Navajo ways. He became a type of religious practitioner known as a "hand-trembler" whose role is to tell sick people what sort of healing ceremony they should have. His success in this gave him a prominent position as a Navajo, even though he remained in many ways ignorant of other aspects of the culture (Leighton and Leighton 1949).

The second man was given to gambling and drinking but also to Navajo ceremonials for which he eventually became a singer or medicine man. In a bit of a contrast to the other two, his enjoyment was primarily in the eating, drinking, and other festive aspects of the religion and in the chance of making a little money, which he often spent promptly and unwisely. He was eventually killed during a fight in a bar (Griffen 1992).

The third man was one whose interest in Navajo religion was not only active but also profound. He looked to it for help in solving moral and practical issues, particularly in deciding the right thing to do in order to stay healthy, take care of his family, prosper economically, and provide leadership for other Navajos. He made a careful study of white American culture and became exceedingly skillful in showing how Navajo and white values could be adjusted to each other.

The experience of examining the impact of culture through personality studies did more than make evident the variability of Navajo and Yupik cultures with respect to time, place, and person; it also suggested very strongly that the transaction occurs in two directions. That is to say, not only are there modifying influences flowing from a culture to individuals, but, equally, there are influences flowing from individuals to their cultures. This was evident in many of my personality studies, but especially in that of the third Navajo man. In Lobos, where he lived in McKinley County, New Mexico, in the heart of an off-reservation Navajo population, there is a building bearing his name: The David Skeet Elementary School.

To some extent, a person in a culture may be likened to an iceberg: the temperature and movement of the water are important in shaping the berg, but simultaneously the outflow of fresh water from the berg changes the qualities of the surrounding sea.

It is probably true that the microchanges in cultural elements brought about by individuals cancel each other out (as Ruth Benedict used to insist) at least much of the time, but it seems equally true that under conditions of population stress, such multiple changes can become directional and cumulative. When people find their culture becoming uncomfortable and hindering survival, they are apt to start making alterations in form, meanings, uses, and functions.

I believe there is evidence to suggest that a fruitful and underdeveloped area for empirical investigations into culture and personality is at the microlevel of behavioral intimations of both culture and personality. We have not, however, developed as yet reliable methods for observing, recording, and systematically analyzing such data.

Conclusion

The accumulation of scientific knowledge in the field of culture and personality has been inhibited by factors that have been and are characteristic of both of its parents. One major cluster of these factors may be described as containing too many theories at too high a level of generalization to permit evaluation by empirical methods. Associated difficulties consist of a lack of consensus regarding definitions, technical language, and the nature of scientific procedures when applied to human affairs.

A possible remedy is to throw out all the old theories and try to create a new one from the ground up that would attract more consensus and be more open to validating techniques. History suggests that this is not how robust theories come into existence. When old theories are abandoned, new ones of similar cast are apt to emerge, flourish for a while, and then also vanish, all for reasons that have little to do with scientific criteria and much to do with philosophical fashions in the academic marketplace. All sciences appear to be affected in this way at times, but some are more volatile than others because of their closeness to issues in which human passions and mind-sets rather than reason are the dominant subjective processes.

There is an alternative that at least in the life sciences has considerable historical evidence in its favor. In the present discussion, it would consist of recognizing both culture and personality, not so much as bodies of theory, but as possibly useful general orientations, and then following this step by putting all forms of dogmatic assertion about them on hold. Such a climate of opinion would free investigators to concentrate on small-scale hypotheses, the probability of which has the promise of being ascertainable by the objective and systematic study of definable and classifiable recurrent events in nature. Methodologically, this kind of science demands that we begin with what is presented to our senses and that we return to it again and again either directly or through the use of instruments and mathematics. The approach, therefore, calls not only for a growth in data and their probabilistic interpretation but also for a progressive reformulation of methods in response to the cumulative growth of knowledge. In culture and personality, it seems to me that this is particularly important with regard to procedures for classification.

In advocating concentration on small-scale hypotheses that take objectively definable phenomena as a major part of their perspective, I have in mind the sentiments and values mentioned in the body of this chapter and their potential for the conceptual bridging of culture and personality. Many people will at once protest that sentiments and values are not objective but, on the contrary, highly subjective. This of course is true by definition, but what makes them researchable is that they are expressed and transmitted exclusively by signals and symbols that are objective inasmuch as they are directly apprehensible by the senses. Even though the subjective meaning of a sentiment or value must always be a matter of inference, the systematic and comparative study of its expression in a variety of persons and contexts can give such inferences a very high degree of probability and considerable power as predictors.

Linton's proposal for the study of cultural elements in terms of four qualities is highly apposite in this connection. *Form* would refer to the morphology or patterns of the symbols through which a sentiment or value is expressed; *meaning* would of course be entirely subjective and refer to the interpretation of the person uttering or receiving the symbol; *use* would have to do with recognized practical ends served; and *function* would pertain to effects, which may or may not be recognized, that contribute to the well-being and survival of individuals and/or groups.

In much of this chapter I have occasionally mentioned a scale of conceptualizations that goes from the large and abstract to the small and concrete; and I have been suggesting that culture and personality has been handicapped by trying to operate at a level of abstraction that, from a scientific point of view, is much too high given the knowledge base and methodology so far available in the field.

The abstract end of the scale has the advantage of being able to deal with transcendental meanings that have far-reaching implications extending into many spheres of existence. Theories at this level are abundant but present great difficulty to all efforts aimed at establishing their degree of probability, much less validity.

The concrete end also involves the conceptualization of relationships that are not directly perceptible by the senses, but these are typically only small leaps of inference among numerous objective facts that provide some opportunity for validity testing. Hypotheses with limited scope but multiple testing possibilities are characteristic of what one finds here. Further up the scale come larger networks of inference

based on tested hypotheses and forming conceptualizations of sufficient scope and rigor to warrant the term *theory*. Validation of a theory is
still a matter of central importance, but it is apt to be much more difficult, elaborate, and indirect. As a rule, scientific consensus with regard
to a theory is achieved through vast amounts of work with lower order
hypotheses that cumulatively build evidence.

If one lights on the most abstract end of the scale and attempts to
build a theory on the basis of premises and reasoning alone, such action, albeit one with an enormous and respectable history behind it, belongs in philosophy rather than science. For scientists, the most important characteristic about the scale is what level the field in which they
are working has so far achieved. They must then adjust their concepts,
goals, and methods accordingly. Attempts to take a shortcut by copying
directly the methods of the more advanced sciences have a habit of
turning out to be misplaced effort.

Acknowledgments

The writing of these recollections has been markedly aided by suggestions from my wife, Jane M. Murphy, and by the challenging questions
raised by Dr. Okpaku and his thoughtful reviewers. The fieldwork
among Navajos and Yupik-speaking people of Alaska was carried out on
a fellowship from the Social Science Research Council in 1939 and
1940. The fellowship was shared with Dorothea Cross Leighton, who
was my wife at that time and who contributed very greatly to the cultural studies.

References

Griffen JJ (ed.): Lucky The Navaho Singer. Albuquerque, NM, University of
    New Mexico Press, 1992
Kroeber AL, Kluckhohn CK: Culture: A Critical Review of Concepts and Def-
    initions. Papers of the Peabody Museum of American Archeology and Eth-
    nology, Harvard University XLVII, No 1. Cambridge, MA, Peabody Mu-
    seum, 1952
Leighton AH, Leighton DC: Gregorio the Hand-Trembler: A Psychobiological
    Personality Study of a Navaho Indian. Papers of the Peabody Museum of
    American Archaeology and Ethnology, Harvard University XL, No 1. Cam-
    bridge, MA, Peabody Museum, 1949

Leighton AH: My Name Is Legion: The Stirling County Study of Psychiatric Disorder and Sociocultural Environment, Vol 1. New York, Basic Books, 1959

Leighton AH: Notes on the beaver's individuality and mental characteristics. J Mammalogy 13:117–126, 1932

Leighton AH: Notes on the relations of beavers to one another and to the muskrat. J Mammalogy 14:27–35, 1933

Leighton AH: Notes on the behavior of Norwegian beaver. J Mammalogy 16:189–191, 1935

Linton R: The Study of Man: An Introduction (Student Edition). New York, Appleton, Century Crofts, 1964 (originally published by D. Appleton Century Co, 1936)

McDougall W: An Introduction to Social Psychology, 23rd Edition. London, Methuen, 1936

Merton RK: Social Theory and Social Structure. New York, Free Press, 1949

Rivers WHR, Tansley AG, et al: The relation of complex and sentiment: contributions to the symposium prepared for the meeting of the British Psychological Society in Manchester, July 1922. Br J Psychol 13:107–148, 1922

Sapir E: Culture, Language and Personality. Selected essays edited by Mandelbaum DG. Berkeley and Los Angeles, University of California Press, 1970

Warner WL, Lunt PS: The Social Life of a Modern Community. New Haven, CT, Yale University Press, 1942

CHAPTER 3

Psychological and Clinical Aspects of Immigration and Mental Health

SOLVIG EKBLAD, PH.D.
ROBERT KOHN, M.D.
BENGT JANSSON, M.D.

Migration, both voluntary and forced, has become an increasingly important issue for many countries of the world during the twentieth century. Refugees, émigrés who flee because of war or political or religious persecution, are of particular concern to mental health professionals. These individuals may have additional psychological burdens and potential risk factors for mental illness not encountered in non-refugee immigrants or migrants.

The numbers of refugees have increased yearly worldwide. At least 20 million refugees have fled their own countries, and an additional 20 million displaced persons are "refugees" within the borders of their own countries (Leopold and Harrell-Bond 1994). The burden for hosting refugees falls disproportionately on the poorest countries. In 1990, 3.75% of refugees and asylum seekers sought refuge in Europe, while 32% went to African countries. Many refugees are forced to flee to undemocratic countries with residents who are intolerant, disrespectful of outside cultures, and suspicious of newcomers as economic competitors. As international assistance has declined, so has the ability to meet nutritional, housing, health, and psychological demands (Vernez 1991).

Immigrants, whether refugees or not, often migrate to countries where the language, customs, and culture are foreign to them. Some groups face enormous transitions, such as migrating from rural agrarian communities to technologically advanced urban societies. The immigrant in need of mental health care must negotiate not only the challenges of acculturation but also attitudes toward the mentally ill and mental health systems with which they are unacquainted. Similarly, most mental health professionals do not have knowledge of the immigrant's language, culture, or attitudes about mental illness. Consequently, clinicians should know how to conduct an assessment, derive a psychiatric formulation, and provide treatment for patients culturally diverse from themselves, which requires an understanding of premigration, migration, and postmigration risk factors for mental illness.

Mental Health and Immigration

Whether immigration itself has a causal relationship to mental illness should be examined by asking two central questions: 1) Does immigration increase the risk for poorer mental health and, if so, why? 2) Is the increased psychopathology noted among immigrants a result of the immigration process and the stresses of acculturation, a result of a selection bias, or a reflection of psychopathology in the country of origin? Neither question has been clearly addressed in the migration and mental health literature.

The issue of the mental health of immigrants has been debated since the earliest epidemiological studies. In 1855 Jarvis noted increased psychopathology in the Massachusetts pauper class, which consisted of many Irish immigrants. Pioneering work examining the psychiatric consequences of migration became of interest in the 1930s with the work of Ødegård (1932) and Malzberg (1935). These early studies from treated samples suggested that immigrants had a higher incidence of psychotic disorders than the general population. H. B. M. Murphy (1973) postulated three reasons for the differences noted from the host population: 1) the process of migration and acculturation induces mental disorder at a higher (or lower) rate than the host population; 2) the decision to migrate is made by those who are more (or less) vulnerable to mental disorders; and 3) the migrant population reflects the higher (or lower) morbidity rate of the country of origin.

The earliest mental health and immigration studies examined hospital admission rates and outpatient clinic referrals. Most such studies found higher rates of mental illness among immigrants. However, these treatment studies are open to criticism on the basis of small sample size and insufficient examination of age, social class, and gender influences. Other complications include the inability to account for disorders not resulting in hospital admission or multiple admissions, lack of investigation of the attitudes toward help seeking by both the host and immigrant populations, and reliance on proper documentation of the country of origin retrospectively. Hospital admissions seriously underrepresent the true rates of psychological disorders and consequently may be a reflection of selection factors such as ability to recognize psychiatric disorders and differences in the degree of social support.

Others, in examining differential suicide rates among immigrants and their hosts as a reflection of the mental health of the immigrant community, have noted increased rates for immigrants (Stack 1981). Interpreting these suicide studies to mean that immigrants have worse mental health is problematic. Differential reporting of completed suicide and suicide attempts between groups and countries may occur. Only a select few studies compare the immigrants' suicide rate with that in their country of origin. Suicides are one symptom of psychopathology and are not representative of the entire spectrum of pathology. Some cultures may attach less stigma to suicide, making it a less pejorative alternative and consequently not reflective of increased pathology.

Community surveys. Given the limitations of suicide and hospital admission studies, community studies have recently been utilized to investigate the issue of immigrant mental health. Two types of community studies exist: those that examine psychiatric symptoms or psychological distress and those that evaluate the prevalence of specific psychiatric disorders. Community surveys also have the advantage of including potential risk factors within their study design.

Overall, these cross-sectional examinations of distress within an immigrant community have demonstrated variable results, depending on the immigrant group, their location of migration, and the type of instrument used to measure psychological distress. Not all immigrant groups appear to be at risk for increased psychological distress. These studies appear to indicate that the risk factors that exist, particularly those related to acculturation, may make an immigrant vulnerable to such distress. However, because there is little consistency in the way studies measure psychological distress and risk factors (e.g., acculturation, social support, and life events), comparison of the results is problematic.

Other community surveys have used as their contrast group different generations of the same immigrant group rather than nonimmigrants. Examining generations by such an approach may weaken the effect of selection factors such as the type of person who decides to immigrate or the country of origin's original mental health burden. This approach allows for the differences that are noted to result from the immigration process itself. Unfortunately, such conclusions must rely on a number of unsubstantiated assumptions: that little has changed in the immigration process from the arrival of the original immigrants to the community; that other than the acculturation process, the whole society has not altered since the arrival of the new immigrant and the birth of his or her offspring; and that the second generation is already assimilated to the community at large.

An alternative approach to eliminating a number of confounding factors, such as the potential selection bias of who decides to immigrate and the mental health risk associated with the country of origin, has been carried out by examining a single immigrant group that migrates to two different countries. After controlling for known differences among the individuals who choose one country over another, the resultant differences between the two groups are due to their respective countries of immigration. Such studies provide strong evidence for the influence of the host community on psychological distress but do not address the broader issues of psychiatric disorder and immigration. The differences in the immigrants' mental health may also have been a result of variables that the investigators failed to or could not control for or a reflection of the differences in psychological distress of the host countries' general populations.

These studies measure only psychological distress or symptoms. They do not measure the prevalence of specific disorders encountered and rarely provide rates of psychiatric cases. Examining symptoms can be misleading since symptom presentation may vary among cultures; however, this factor may not necessarily be present for the broad range of psychiatric diagnoses. It appears, at least in examining distress, that certain groups of immigrants may be at risk. However, the literature is far from unambiguous on this issue.

Specific psychiatric disorders. Even fewer community studies have been conducted specifically examining psychiatric diagnosis. Although very few studies using diagnostic instruments have been undertaken, there appears to be little evidence to support the assumption that differences in rates of specific psychiatric disorders exist between immigrants and nonimmigrants. This finding raises the issue of whether mental health professionals should be concerned with discovering specific disorders in the immigrant population as a measurement of their health or whether they should be examining nonspecific psychological distress. Studies of mental health services utilization have found that a sizable proportion of individuals do not meet criteria for specific diagnoses, adding further fuel to the debate about whether distress alone merits clinical attention.

Research that comprehensibly answers the issues raised originally by Murphy has yet to be conducted. Such a study would need to examine the mental health of immigrants in their host country and their country of origin. Thus far two groups have attempted such research. Fichter and colleagues (1988) administered the General Health Questionnaire (GHQ) (Goldberg 1978) to Greek adolescents in their native lands and to a sample of guest workers in Munich. Mavreas and Bebbington (1988) used the Present State Examination (PSE-CATEGO) (Wing et al. 1977) to examine immigrants, individuals in their country of origin, and their hosts. They sampled Greek Cypriot immigrants in Camberwell, an English sample in Camberwell, and a population in Athens. However, not one study conducted to date has been able to fully address the three explanations proposed by Murphy for the frequent finding of higher rates of psychological distress and the suggested increased rate of mental illness among immigrant populations.

Mental Health of Refugees

A review of the recent literature about refugees suggests that migration by itself does not account for an increased risk for poorer mental health (Marsella et al. 1994; National Institute of Mental Health 1991). As suggested by a study of Central American immigrants (Cervantes et al. 1989), refugees are at an increased risk for adverse psychiatric outcomes in comparison with voluntary immigrants because of their high rate of traumatic experiences. Psychiatric symptoms including those of posttraumatic distress were found to be highest among Central American immigrants who migrated as a result of war, followed by other Central American immigrants, then Mexican-American immigrants, and lastly nonimmigrants in the United States. The rates of psychiatric disorders among refugees appear to be correlated to the degree of traumatization and may reach epidemic proportions. In a study using the Structural Clinical Interview for DSM-III-R (SCID) (Spitzer et al. 1990) on a consecutive group of Vietnamese refugees to the United States undergoing mandatory health screening, ethnic Vietnamese immigrants had a significantly higher rate of DSM-III-R (American Psychiatric Association 1987) psychiatric disorders (24.1%) compared with ethnic Chinese immigrants (14.4%). The ethnic Vietnamese group reported much higher rates of traumatic events (Hinton et al. 1993). In a community study of Cambodian Hmong immigrants (Sack et al. 1994), more than half had posttraumatic stress disorder (PTSD) and fewer than 20% were free of any DSM-III-R psychiatric diagnosis.

The refugee's perception of control over his or her destiny may determine individual psychological outcome. The degree of successful adaptation may depend on factors such as motivation, degree of tolerance to stress, amount of time elapsed since immigration, and attitudes of the receiving country. For example, a study of political activists in Turkey showed that survivors of torture had significantly more symptoms of PTSD, anxiety, and depression than nontortured subjects (Basoglu et al. 1994). However, prior knowledge of and preparedness for torture, a strong commitment to a cause, increased social supports, and immunization against traumatic stress as a result of repeated exposure appeared to be protective against PTSD in survivors of torture.

Westermeyer and colleagues (1983, 1984a, 1984b, 1989) have found that the Hmong have increased symptoms at the time of immigration but show improvement over a course of 10 years. They found that symptoms of depression, somatization, phobia, and poor self-esteem improved with time, but little change was noted with paranoia, hostility, and anxiety symptoms. The groups also noted that traditional ties, older age, marital problems, and medical complaints were associated with elevated symptoms. Beiser (1988) has also shown longitudinal improvement with Vietnamese and Laotian refugees. These studies suggest that at least some symptoms noted among refugees may be transient; however, the role of repeated testing is unclear.

Refugee adjustment is a complex process that unfolds across time and can be conceptualized in a multivariate risk/resilience model of trauma experience and refugee adjustment and adaptation (see Table 3–1). The mental health risk and resilience factors are conceptualized according to three time periods in refugees of war: prewar, war, and re-

Table 3–1. **A multivariate risk/resilience model of trauma experience and refugee adjustment and adaptation**

Prewar	War/violence	Resettlement	Mental health outcome
Sociodemographic factors: age, gender, marital status	Witness to war injuries, death	Access to basic needs and services	Somatic complaints and psychosomatic symptoms
History of mental illness	War exposure	Level of arrival distress	Anxiety
Life events of high or low magnitude	Imprisonment	Second traumatization	Pain
Coping strategies	Active combat experience	Loss of resources or separation	Depression
Social support	Experience of bombings, fires, shooting	Coping skills	Posttraumatic stress disorder
	Loss of resources or separation marital cultural social or interpersonal	Social ties and support	Substance abuse
	Cognitive appraisal of violence low control low predictability highly life threatening		Positive outcome

settlement. A wide range of individual and environmental factors may influence the refugee's adjustment and acculturation to the host society; a combination of factors from each of these time periods may lead to varying mental health outcomes.

Adaptation and Acculturation

Acculturation occurs when two cultures in contact come to adopt beliefs, values, and practices from one another, a continuous process of one group learning from the other. Today, however, we view acculturation as a minority society trying to adapt to a majority society. Problems often arise in clinical settings if a clinician and patient of different cultures assume that they possess common values when in fact they do not. The clinician must gain an understanding of the patient's value system. Values are largely unconscious; they are the concepts, moral goods, and desirable ends or goals to which a people attach positive emotional valence. Norms are the guidelines that define socially acceptable behavior. Each culture and ethnic group has its own ideals and norms, and culture and ethnicity forge one's identity. Issues with identity can pose a risk factor for poorer mental health (Flaherty et al. 1988). Cultural competence is the ability of the immigrant to function effectively and efficiently in a culture at a level consistent with his or her own goals and social roles. Language skills and awareness of the host country's cultural norms are necessary for achieving cultural competence.

Anomie refers to the abandonment of cultural norms and values. Durkheim's (1951) studies on suicide suggest a link to social origins in the presentation of psychopathology and found that anomie posed serious social and psychiatric risks. Anomie may be self-imposed but can also result from suppression by the dominant culture, as occurred when the United States government initially did not allow American Indians to perform traditional ceremonies or speak their own languages.

Refugees and immigrants in general, in adjusting to a new culture, may face difficulties that could predispose them to psychopathology. A number of investigators have tried to conceptualize the various styles of immigrant adjustment and the resulting pathology that may arise.

Meszaros (1961) divided the adjustment patterns of immigrants into five categories. The overaccepting immigrant is characterized as being enthusiastic, denying difficulties, struggling to adapt to the new situation, suppressing hostility, and possibly rejecting his or her own former ethnic identity. The actively critical immigrant rejects the new setting, makes unfavorable comparisons, idealizes the former community, frequently exhibits depression, and feels discriminated against. The inhibited immigrant becomes emotionally withdrawn, expresses little feeling toward the past or present environment, and may be insecure or fearful. The hyporeactive immigrant feels perplexed and lost, is unable to undertake readjustment tasks, and exhibits frequent dissatisfaction, bitterness, chronic loneliness, and homesickness. The fifth type of immigrant, the hyperreactive person, is emotionally labile, with alternating behavior patterns, and may become violent or otherwise act out. He or she is at risk for brief psychosis or suicide attempts.

Berry (1976) used a simpler scheme to explain immigrant adjustment styles. He viewed the immigrant's effort to adjust as a conflict that resulted in either adjustment, reaction, or withdrawal. The adjusting immigrant resolves the conflict by trying to make the two cultural or regional backgrounds more similar or integrated. The immigrant who deals with the adjustment process through reaction attempts to reduce the conflict by retaliating against the source of the conflict, the new culture. The immigrant who withdraws abandons the conflict by returning home or entering an ethnic enclave.

Khoa and Van Deusen (1981) described three patterns of immigrant adjustment. They termed the first the old-line pattern, which is characterized by rejection of the new culture and refusal to adapt. This pattern is often found among elderly immigrants. An assimilative pattern is exhibited by one who embraces the new customs by giving up the old, a response seen in very young individuals. For example, the immigrant teenager from a traditional conservative culture may insist on always wearing blue jeans and overusing makeup. The bicultural pattern is seen mainly in young adults and results in their selectively adopting new customs while maintaining some former conventions.

A hypothesis conceptualizing the paths of immigrant adaptation has also been proposed by Lin and colleagues (1982). The neurotically marginal immigrant develops high levels of anxiety while trying to comply with the expectations of both cultures. One who has deviant marginality becomes isolated because he or she ignores the norms of both cultures after being unable to satisfy them simultaneously. Those who adopt a traditionalist form of adapting withdraw into the old culture to escape loss and confusion. The overly acculturated immigrant abandons the former culture, loses traditional supports, and, as a result, becomes more vulnerable. Finally, the immigrant who integrates both cultures with the best possible compromises adjusts through biculturation.

Another way to view the possible outcomes of adjustment to a new culture is through assimilation, integration, separation, or marginalization. Integration results in the least stress and is shown in the bicultural person who takes something from both societies. The assimilated individual or group rejects the previous culture. In separation, the individual or group lives in its own cultural ghetto, rejecting the new society. The path of most stress and greatest risk of pathology is marginalization, in which the individual or group rejects both the old and new cultures.

A number of factors go into determining which of these adjustment styles the immigrant will assume. The immigrant's personality determines his or her attitude toward the change and the course chosen to deal with it. The difference between the community from which the immigrant came and the one he or she has immigrated to is a driving factor. The attitude of the host community toward the immigrant is also important; some communities are accepting, others rejecting. At times the reaction of the host community is open and welcoming, but this is not always the case. Age is also an important consideration in immigrant adjustment. Older individuals frequently lean toward the traditional past, younger individuals often try to leave their past behind, and adults commonly try to assume a bicultural position.

Berry (1991) summarizes this moderating relationship between acculturation and stress into five factors: 1) the mode of acculturation: integration, assimilation, separation, or marginalization; 2) the phase of acculturation: contact, conflict, crisis, or adaptation; 3) the nature of the larger society: multicultural versus assimilationist and the presence of prejudice and discrimination in the host society; 4) the characteristics of the acculturating group including age, status, and social support; and 5) the acculturating individual's traits determining his or her relationship with stress: capacity for appraisal, coping abilities, attitudes, and extent of desire for contact with the host community. Ekblad and colleagues (1994) have further outlined these factors in examining Swedish migrants and refugees.

The adjustment problems that immigrants may encounter are not only with the new society but also within their own families (Wester-meyer 1989a). The children may acculturate more rapidly than their parents, leading to role reversals in which the child assumes adult roles. Families may no longer be intact because of death or incarceration of a parent in the homeland. Gender roles also may be altered upon immigration to accommodate the norms of the new culture. Intergenerational conflicts develop frequently, since the child acculturates faster than the parents and tries to cast away traditional values. Failure of parents to acculturate exacerbates these conflicts, increasing the risk for the child to fail as well.

Family structure also may affect the acculturation process, as in the case of a patriarchal family adapting to a society with more egalitarian family roles. Refugees, such as the Irish immigrants whom Jarvis described, are overrepresented in the socially disadvantaged sectors of their new society. They tend to suffer disproportionately from poor living and working conditions, unemployment, and social prejudice. Physical and psychological trauma may occur not only before and during flight but also after resettlement during the period of adjustment and adaptation (Allodi 1991; Hauff et al. 1989; Kroll et al. 1989; Mollica et al. 1987). Unfortunately, this issue has rarely been examined in individuals over the age of 25. Refugees, particularly those migrating to non-Western countries, frequently face minimal resources, increasing their risk for a poor mental health outcome during all phases of the refugee resettlement process. An international conference in Stockholm, Sweden, in 1991 brought to the forefront a number of these risk factors (Jablensky et al. 1992):

> *Marginalization and minority status:* Migrants and refugees are often identified and perceived as alien, undesirable, and inferior by others and, in some instances, by themselves. As a result, serious problems in self-esteem, self-confidence, and powerlessness develop.
> *Socioeconomic disadvantage:* In absolute and relative terms, migrants and refugees frequently lack the essential economic re-

sources necessary to maintain basic survival needs. Poverty and deprivation are often constant accompaniments of forced migration and refugee status both in transit and in the relocation phases.

Poor physical health: The stress of migration often leads to serious problems in physical health, including unattended chronic illness. These problems are directly or indirectly linked to poor sanitation, poor nutrition, crowding, and the absence of shelter.

Starvation and malnutrition: Starvation and malnutrition are especially serious problems for infants, children, adolescents, and lactating mothers. Stunted growth, mental deficiency, and brain damage are critical problems for the young refugee.

Head trauma and injuries: The stress of migration is greatly exacerbated by the increased risk of head trauma and serious injuries. Because of the absence of medical facilities, head trauma and injuries are often left unattended, resulting in long-term disabilities and handicaps. An added problem is the interaction between head trauma and problems of infection, starvation, and malnutrition.

Collapse of social supports: The breakdown of established and habitual social support networks and structures adds to the stress of refugees. The cultural disintegration results in anomie and alienation and imposes on the experience additional burdens of helplessness and uncertainty.

Mental trauma: Mental traumas are often a constant and continuous part of the migration and refugee experience. The traumas have many sources and forms, including physical assault, rape, robbery, family separation, loss or death of relatives and friends, and so forth. Recognition that the cumulative or additive effects of mental trauma may lead to chronic psychological disorders and disabilities is growing. The symbolic or imprinting effects of trauma (e.g., witnessing violence being inflicted on family members) may be more traumatic to children than suffering injury themselves.

Adaptation to host culture: After resettlement in host countries, refugees face numerous psychological problems, including those related to language differences, unemployment, underemployment, misemployment, poverty, housing, profound acculturation stress, racism, prejudice, social isolation and rejection, and availability and acceptability of health care services and education.

In addition to the risk factors outlined, illegal immigration creates a barrier to acculturation and adaptation to the host community. Asylum seekers who have not obtained official refugee status are at risk for forcible repatriation, a continuous stress. A special risk group is made up of asylum seekers awaiting permanent resettlement, in particular individuals in camps or in detention. Asylum seekers are faced with prolonged periods in restricted and monotonous environments surrounded by others in a similar situation. Mounting despair, suspicion, and frustration characterize their plight. The presence of a language barrier may create feelings of isolation, disorientation, and entrapment.

An Australian study (Silove et al. 1993) found that these refugees frequently have PTSD symptoms and exhibit unresolved grief, depression, helplessness, and hopelessness. Similarly, in a Canadian study (Matas 1992), 70% reported symptoms of tension, anxiety, and depression; 58% stated that their symptoms had worsened since arrival, with only 16% reporting a decrease in psychological distress. Approximately 20% of those living in Canada for 2 years reported suicidal preoccupation; interestingly, a suicide rate of only 3% was found in those who resided in the country for more than 5 years. Illegal immigrants fear repatriation and, in such circumstances, have difficulty in determining whom to trust.

Assessment and Treatment of the Refugee Patient

No specific disorders are associated with immigrants or refugees, perhaps with the exception of PTSD and somatization disorders and some cultural-bound syndromes. PTSD is a common problem in victims of torture, war injury, and other physical mistreatment (Boehnlein et al. 1985; Hauff 1993; Kinzie and Fredrickson 1984; Kroll et al. 1989). Organic brain syndromes secondary to head trauma, as well as other psychiatric disorders such as major depression, may also be present in these individuals. Somatization is a common presentation in immigrants who come from cultures that are not psychologically minded or where expressing psychological distress is unacceptable (Kohn et al. 1989). However, Beiser (1994) cautions against such popular aphorisms. Cultural-bound syndromes should be considered judiciously since the clinician may easily begin to stereotype and look at an individual from a distinct cultural group in terms of culture-specific disorders rather than the broader range of psychopathology. Is it useful for a clinician who is not from the individual's culture to treat a disorder that is foreign to his or her framework? Is it better to frame the presenting pathology in a context more familiar to the clinician, who consequently has more confidence in treating the problem?

How does the mental health professional clinically assess a patient from a culture distinct from his or her own and in particular one who does not speak the same language as the clinician? Before undertaking an assessment, the mental health professional should be mindful that individuals with a mental illness often had the illness before immigration. The immigration process and premigration trauma may accentuate the presentation or result in a relapse of a preexisting disorder.

The first step in conducting an assessment is to discover and understand the presenting complaints. The second step is to obtain a complete history, including past disorders, family history, and medical problems. Refugees frequently have medical problems that impact their psychiatric presentation; for example, a Guatemalan refugee presented with symptoms consistent with major depression, panic attacks, and seizures. She had a parasite, cysticercosis, in her brain, and tuberculosis. The third step is understanding the patient's current strengths and resources. Are family and social supports available? Are there financial barriers to care? What are the patient's understanding of and attitudes toward mental health care?

A migration history should also be obtained. This history includes premigration status, including the social network, social and psychological function, and life events. The clinician should inquire about premigration planning, reasons for migrating, duration and extent of planning, and goals to be realized. The migration experience, its duration, the difficulty and dangers encountered, and the resettlement phase should be explored. Changes in roles and activities abandoned and adopted and the extent of life changes that the individual has undergone should be included in the migration history. Patients may neglect to mention vital information that is pertinent to their histories and presentations unless specifically asked (Westermeyer 1989b). This omission is particularly common in those who have been tortured, raped, or psychologically harmed in other ways. The patient may have feelings of guilt and shame, a desire to forget, emotional distress when recalling events, and fear of reprisal. An inquiry into nightmares and dreams may prove useful. This assessment is not significantly different from that used with psychiatric patients in general; however, it requires more time, effort, and creativity. It is crucial not only to allow enough time to complete such an assessment but also to demonstrate an interest in understanding the patient's point of view.

As with any patient, a mental status evaluation is central to the psychiatric examination. However, its interpretation in immigrant populations requires caution. Traditionally, we include in the mental status examination behavior, cooperation, appearance, speech, affect, thought process, thought content, cognition, insight, and judgment. Ethnicity may affect a distressed individual's presentation. Cultural differences in dress and grooming are wide and varied. Facial expressions and body movements often used in the communication of affect may be more reflective of cultural manifestations than of pathology. If the clinician is unfamiliar with the individual's culture, a reliance on history may be more useful than focusing on the patient's dress and mannerisms.

An interviewer evaluating a nonnative speaker should be careful of interpreting disturbances in speech or thought process. A patient who is unsure of his or her command of the clinician's language may exhibit stuttering, for example, or may appear circumstantial when no such problem actually exists. If using the services of a translator and listening to a language unfamiliar to him or her, the therapist could misinterpret the speech as pressured or the answers as overly long and involved. One should ask the interpreter whether these assumptions are correct. Therapists cannot assume that patients always understand what they mean. The concept of hallucinations, for example, can be easily misinterpreted (Westermeyer 1989b). The cognitive examination may be particularly tricky. Education and literacy have an important and biasing role. A properly conducted psychiatric evaluation allows for facilitation and clarification. The patient needs adequate time to fully express him- or herself and may require repeated or restated questions to fully understand the interviewer's intent. Use of idioms or slang expressions should be avoided; patients and interpreters may translate the terms literally, distorting their meaning and confusing the patient and the clinician.

The bilingual therapist has the opportunity to conduct an assessment in either language. Patients should be given the opportunity to choose which language will be used. Frequently, patients prefer that the session be conducted in the host country's language rather than in their native language. This desire may reflect that individual's acculturation process. Also, a bilingual clinician may speak a dialect different from the patient's.

A translator is often necessary to properly conduct an evaluation and later for continued care. Translation raises special issues in conducting therapy or performing an initial assessment. A translator can create complications that may compromise care; therefore, if the patient speaks enough of the clinician's language, even if it is broken, one should perhaps first try to obtain as much information without the aid of a translator and then later use the translator's services if necessary. Regardless of the translator's skill, an artificial barrier of indirect communication is introduced. Patients may not be as open if a peer or family member is present as translator. Translators who are not accustomed to mental health may be embarrassed to ask certain questions; as a result, they may not ask patients' questions but give their own answers instead or make patients seem normal when they are not. They may only paraphrase what the patient says, preventing the interviewer from accurately assessing the emotional content and affect. The translator may not know how to explain the affect and may not provide this information. Transference and countertransference issues, which the clinician cannot sort out or is unaware of, may exist between the translator and the patient.

Before using the services of an interpreter, the interviewer should give the interpreter clear instructions on how to conduct the translation process. The patient must see that the clinician, not the interpreter, is in command of the session. The therapist is legally and ethically responsible for the interpreter. In addition, particularly for the refugee who has undergone trauma or torture, the interview room should not be threatening, small, dark, or closed in. Neither the interviewer nor the interpreter should come across as interrogating the patient, which may create an unpleasant, frightening atmosphere (Kinzie 1987).

Several models for using an interpreter's services are available (Westermeyer 1989b). The triangle model, which provides a dialogue between the patient and therapist, interpreter and patient, and therapist and interpreter, is the most appropriate, although its six lines of communication complicate the dialogue. Members should be able to see one another. Some therapists choose to keep the translator to the side, giving the therapist more prominence; others position the therapist to the side. However, seating arranged in an equilateral triangle may be most useful. This model facilitates a mutual working relationship between the therapist and interpreter. It also permits the therapist to better observe the interaction between the translator and patient, especially in evaluating nonverbal behaviors. The triangle model allows the translator to provide the therapist more data than merely the spoken words of the patient, in contrast to the two-way model.

In the two-way model the interpreter's role is only that of taking the message and passing it on. This model describes the most common way clinicians and translators interact. Unfortunately, it often does not work because the translator frequently feels demeaned in this role. The junior clinician model is used fairly frequently by psychiatrists in mental health centers. Here, the clinician does not deal with the patient directly but allows the translator to conduct the session and simply report back. This translation model usually involves clinically trained personnel.

When working with a translator, only one person should speak at a time. Realize, then, that interviewers will need twice the normal time to complete a session. Use of simultaneous translation may save time, but it also creates numerous problems that make it disadvantageous. It results in greater stress on all of the parties involved and increases the potential for errors. The translator cannot assume the role of providing education or support to the patient. It is a two-way model of interpretation.

In conducting psychotherapy with individuals of different cultural backgrounds, the therapist needs to recognize cultural transference and countertransference issues (Westermeyer 1993). Cultural transference refers to the feelings and attitudes a patient may have for the clinician's ethnic group. Cultural countertransference relates to the feelings and attitudes of the clinician toward a patient's culture. We all have preconceived notions and stereotypes, though at times we are unaware of them. Supervision may prove useful in uncovering cultural assumptions by the therapist and subsequently improving therapist-patient interaction.

Another factor that may complicate a therapeutic relationship is the patient's family. In many cultural groups, neither the family nor the patient wishes to be left alone with the clinician. This situation may make it difficult for patients to discuss sensitive issues or serve as a means for the family to keep the patient from broaching taboo topics. Therapists must use their own judgment about when to allow the family to join in the sessions. At times it is useful to allow a family member to be part of the sessions until such time as the therapist, patient, and family have established a working relationship.

One needs to take into consideration special cultural issues not only in conducting psychotherapy but also in managing psychopharmacology. The pharmacokinetics of drugs may differ by ethnicity. Pharmacodynamics, such as a flushing response found with alcohol use in some races, also differ by cultural groups. Psychosocial differences in tolerance to the side effects of medications must be taken into account. Inappropriate expectations about the effectiveness of drugs should be explored. Education is important because many patients believe medications will work immediately, which is not true of most psychotherapeutic agents. In some cultures patients may have preconceived notions about the effect of a medication based on its color. Many immigrant groups may use folk remedies in addition to medications prescribed by the psychiatrist or primary care clinician. One should make inquiries and investigate these remedies, since they may complicate the action of the psychopharmacological agent or aggravate the patient's pathology. Often there is no interaction and the patient may safely use the folk medication in conjunction with his or her prescription drugs.

Cultural Formulation and Diagnosis

In diagnosing and making a cultural formulation in the management of the immigrant patient, debate has centered on the applicability of current psychiatric nosology. Diagnostic systems such as DSM or ICD have been accused of "category fallacy" (Twemlow 1995), developing criteria for a particular population and applying it to members of another culture without establishing the validity of the category for that culture.

DSM-IV (American Psychiatric Association 1994), unlike its predecessor, takes culture into account with every diagnostic category and should be considered as a resource in diagnosing and making a formulation in the management of the immigrant patient. The description of each diagnostic category includes a section entitled "Special Cultural Features." DSM-IV also includes a glossary of culture-bound syndromes. DSM-IV, like its predecessors, contains five axes; however, it takes culture into account in each of the five axes (Rogler 1993; Stein 1993).

Axes I and II are the mental disorders. Cultural factors can affect the entire range of symptom formation, experience and communication, normative judgments of emotions and distress, and illness attributions. This influence may lead to amplification of some symptoms and inattention to others. Such factors may affect variations in duration that distinguish normal and abnormal experience, differences in course and prognosis of particular disorders, and even the organization of distinct forms of psychopathology. The influences of one's ethnicity, race, and gender are often important in shaping illness behavior associated with standard diagnostic entities. Cultural factors can affect the conceptualization and listing of Axis I disorders (Mezzich et al. 1993).

Kleinman (1977) highlights the influence of ethnicity, race, and gender on depression. Although we view the symptom of major depression to be the emotion of sadness, in most societies people suffering clinical depressions do not complain mainly of unhappiness. Individuals from other cultures may talk about symptoms of depression as real physical experiences, such as fatigue, headaches, backaches, stomach upset, insomnia, or loss of appetite. Kleinman and Good (1985) further point out that we also describe depression as feelings of being "blue" or "down." Our cultural model may be foreign to an immigrant, who may view the experience of depression as an emptiness.

As for Axis II disorders, special sensitivity to cultural issues may be required. Definitions of "normal" personality structures may vary across society, culture, and ethnic groups. Behaviors considered highly deviant in one context may fall within the norm in another. To date, there is little evidence to support the universality of specific personality disorders (Mezzich et al. 1993).

The general medical disorders are coded on Axis III. Clinicians should be alert to the differential distribution of specific medical disorders across social groups and their complex interactions with psychopathology. For example, we looked for cysticercosis in the Guatemalan patient mentioned earlier because we knew it was highly prevalent where she lived and could result in behavioral complications.

Axis IV disorders describe psychosocial stresses and supports. Individuals who migrate may well have stressors of high frequency. Cultural factors may influence the structure of social supports and the evaluation of their effectiveness. Clinician awareness of variations in family and community interactional patterns is important. Social expectations and cultural styles should be considered in rating Axis V, the patient's level of functioning (Mezzich et al. 1993).

To better organize and facilitate the presentation of the cultural diagnostic formulation, DSM-IV recommends conducting a cultural formulation in addition to the multiaxial diagnostic assessment. The purpose of the cultural formulation is to provide a systematic review of the individual's cultural and ethnic background, the role of the culture in the expression and evaluation of symptoms and dysfunction, and the effect cultural differences may have on the relationship between the individual and the clinician. The cultural formulation should consist of the following components: the cultural identity of the individual, cultural explanations of the individual's illness, cultural factors related to the psychosocial environment (e.g., religion and support network) and levels of functioning, cultural elements of the relationship between the individual and the clinician, and an overall cultural assessment for diagnosis and care.

Unlike DSM-IV, ICD-10 (World Health Organization 1992) does not include the same detail about the role of culture in each diagnosis. ICD-10 has specifically avoided including a section on cultural-bound syndromes. The ICD-10 mental disorders section, unlike in its earlier editions, incorporates data from international field trials at 151 clinical centers in 32 countries, including third world nations (Sartorius et al. 1995), to make it more culturally relevant. Interestingly, ICD-10 provides a diagnostic category under the adjustment disorders that is specific for problems encountered by immigrant populations resulting from acculturation, "culture shock, F43.28."

Conclusions

Because immigrants are from culturally heterogeneous populations, the clinician must be flexible and adaptive in his or her treatment approach to such patients. In addition to the difficulties encountered by all immigrants, refugees may be victims of war and trauma and at increased risk for PTSD; the emotional and physical traumas encountered by the refugee should be addressed. The role of the immigration process itself as a risk factor for mental illness remains unclear. However, the pattern of acculturation used by the immigrant may increase or decrease the psychological burden. As with any patient, a thorough psychiatric assessment with a formal mental status examination is necessary. The use of interpreters alters the traditional patient-clinician relationship to include a third party. Mental health treatment in immigrants may require modification of diagnostic assumptions and treatment approaches. Creating a cultural formulation may assist in developing a multiaxial diagnosis and a culturally specific treatment plan. No one diagnosis is specific to a particular immigrant group. Our knowledge about transcultural psychiatry and various cultural groups is only a guide to developing a treatment approach for an individual patient. In the end we must treat the individual, not his or her culture or immigrant status.

References

Allodi FA: Assessment and treatment of torture victims: a critical review. J Nerv Ment Dis 179:4–11, 1991

American Psychiatric Association: Diagnostic and Statistical Manual of Mental Disorders, 3rd Edition, Revised. Washington, DC, American Psychiatric Association, 1987

American Psychiatric Association: Diagnostic and Statistical Manual of Mental Disorders, 4th Edition. Washington, DC, American Psychiatric Association, 1994

Basoglu M, Paker M, Paker O, et al: Psychological effects of torture: a comparison of tortured with nontortured political activists in Turkey. Am J Psychiatry 151:76–81, 1994

Beiser M: Influences of time, ethnicity, and attachment on depression in Southeast Asian refugees. Am J Psychiatry 145:46–51, 1988

Beiser M, Cargo M, Woodbury MA: A comparison of psychiatric disorder in different cultures: depressive typologies in Southeast Asian refugees and resident Canadians. International Journal of Methods in Psychiatric Research 4:157–172, 1994

Berry JW: Human Ecology and Cognitive Styles: Comparative Studies in Cultural and Psychological Adaptation. New York, Sage, 1976

Berry JW: Managing the process of acculturation for problem prevention, in Mental Health Services for Refugees. Washington, DC, National Institute of Mental Health, 1991, pp 189–204

Boehnlein JK, Kinzie JD, Ben R, et al: One-year follow-up study of post-traumatic stress disorder among survivors of Cambodian concentration camps. Am J Psychiatry 142:8, 956–959, 1985

Cervantes RC, Salgado de Snyder VN, Padilla A: Posttraumatic stress in immigrants from Central America and Mexico. Hospital and Community Psychiatry 40:615–619, 1989

Durkheim E: Anomic suicide, in Suicide: A Study in Sociology. Edited by Simpson G. New York, Free Press, 1951, pp 241–276

Ekblad S, Eliasdotter-Andersson I, Jansson-Aberg MB, et al: Care and rehabilitation of women suffering sexual violence from the war in the Republics of the former Yugoslavia: guidelines for Swedish midwives and nurses working with asylum-seeker women. Paper presented at the Fourth International Conference on Grief and Bereavement in Contemporary Society, Stockholm, June 12–16, 1994a

Ekblad S, Ginsburg B-E, Jansson B, et al: Psychosocial and psychiatric aspects of refugee adaptation and care in Sweden, in Amidst Peril and Pain: The

Mental Health and Well-Being of the World's Refugees. Edited by Marsella AJ, Bornemann T, Ekblad S, et al. Washington, DC, American Psychological Association, 1994b, pp 275–292

Fichter MM, Elton M, Diallina M, et al: Mental illness in Greek and Turkish adolescents. Eur Arch Psychiatry Neurol Sci 237:125–134, 1988

Flaherty J, Kohn R, Levav I, et al: Demoralization in Soviet-Jewish immigrants to the United States and Israel. Compr Psychiatry 29:588–597, 1988

Goldberg DP: Manual of the General Health Questionnnaire. Windsor, Ontario, Nelson, 1978

Hauff E, Vaglum P: Vietnamese boat refugees: the influence of war and flight traumatization on mental health on arrival in the country of resettlement. A community cohort study of Vietnamese refugees in Norway. Acta Psychiatr Scand 88:162–168, 1993

Hauff E, Lavik NJ, Dahl CI, et al: Psykosociale problemer blant flyktninger I Norge. Tidsskr Nor Laegeforen 109:1867–1870, 1989

Hinton WL, Chen YJ, Du N, et al: DSM-III-R disorders in Vietnamese refugees. J Nerv Ment Dis 181:113–122, 1993

Jablensky A, Marsella AJ, Ekblad S, et al: International Conference on the Mental Health and Well-Being of the World's Refugees and Displaced Persons, Stockholm, Sweden, October 6–11, 1991. Journal of Refugee Studies 5:172–183, 1992

Jarvis E: Insanity and idiocy in Massachusetts: report of the commission of lunacy (1855). Cambridge, MA, Harvard University Press, 1971

Khoa LX, Van Duesen JM: Social and cultural customs: their contribution to resettlement. Journal of Refugee Resettlement 1:48–51, 1981

Kinzie JD, Fleck J: Psychotherapy with severely traumatized refugees. Am J Psychother 41:82–94, 1987

Kinzie JD, Fredrickson RH, Ben R, et al: Posttraumatic stress disorder among survivors of Cambodian concentration camps. Am J Psychiatry 141:645–650, 1984

Kleinman A: Depression, somatization, and the "new cross-cultural psychiatry." Soc Sci Med 11:3–10, 1977

Kleinman A, Good B: Introduction: culture and depression, in Culture and Depression: Studies in the Anthropology and Cross-Cultural Psychiatry of Affect and Disorder. Berkeley and Los Angeles, CA, University of California Press, 1985, pp 1–33

Kohn R, Flaherty JA, Levav I: Somatic symptoms among older Soviet immigrants: an exploratory study. Int J Soc Psychiatry 35:350–360, 1989

Kroll J, Habenicht M, Mackenzie T, et al: Depression and posttraumatic stress disorder in Southeast Asian refugees. Am J Psychiatry 146:1592–1597, 1989

Leopold M, Harrell-Bond B: An overview of the world refugee crisis, in Amidst Peril and Pain: The Mental Health and Well-Being of the World's

Refugees. Edited by Marsella AJ, Bornemann T, Ekblad S, et al. Washington, DC, American Psychological Association, 1994, pp 17–31

Lin KM, Masuda M, Tazuma L: Adaptational problems of Vietnamese refugees, III: case studies in clinic and field: adaptive and maladaptive. Psychiatric Journal of the University of Ottawa 7:173–183, 1982

Malzberg B: Mental disease in New York State according to nativity and parentage. Mental Hygiene 19:635–660, 1935

Marsella AJ: Ethnocultural diversity and international refugees: challenges for the global community, in Amidst Peril and Pain: The Mental Health and Well-Being of the World's Refugees. Edited by Marsella AJ, Bornemann T, Ekblad S, et al. Washington, DC, American Psychological Association, 1994, pp 341–364

Marsella AJ, Bornemann T, Ekblad S, et al (eds): Amidst Peril and Pain: The Mental Health and Well-Being of the World's Refugees. Washington, DC, American Psychological Association, 1994

Matas D: Mental health and refugee claimants. Paper presented at the Refugees in the '90s conference, Vancouver, BC, October 1992

Mavreas VG, Bebbington PE: Greeks, British Greek Cypriots, and Londoners: a comparison of morbidity. Psychol Med 18:433–442, 1988

Meszaros AF: Types of displacement reactions among the post revolution Hungarian immigrants. Canadian Psychiatric Association Journal 6:9–19, 1961

Mezzich JE, Kleinman A, Fabrega H, et al: Cultural issues for DSM-IV, in DSM-IV Sourcebook, Vol 3. Edited by Widiger TA, Frances AG, Pincus HA, et al. Washington, DC, American Psychiatric Association, 1997

Mollica RF, Wyshak G, Lavelle J: The psychosocial impact of war trauma and torture on Southeast Asian refugees. Am J Psychiatry 144:1567–1572, 1987

Murphy HBM: Migration and mental disorders: an appraisal, in Uprooting and After. Edited by Zwingmann C, Pfister-Ammende M. New York, Springer-Verlag, 1973

National Institute of Mental Health Refugee Mental Health Program: Mental Health Services for Refugees. Washington, DC, National Institute of Mental Health, 1991

Ødegård Ø: Emigration and insanity: a study of mental disease in Norweagian born population of Minnesota. Acta Psychiatrica et Neurologica Scandinavica Supplementum 4:1–206, 1932

Rogler LH: Culture in psychiatric diagnosis: an issue of scientific accuracy. Psychiatry 56:324–327, 1993

Sack WH, McSharry S, Clarke GN, et al: The Khmer adolescent project, I: epidemiologic findings in two generations of Cambodian refugees. J Nerv Ment Dis 182:387–395, 1994

Sartorius N, Üstün B, Korten A, et al: Progress toward achieving a common language in psychiatry, II: results from the international field trials of the

ICD-10 diagnostic criteria for research for mental and behavioral disorders. Am J Psychiatry 152:1427–1437, 1995

Silove D, McIntosh P, Becker R: Risk of retraumatization of asylum-seekers in Australia. Aust N Z J Psychiatry 27:606–612, 1993

Spitzer RL, Williams JBW, Gibbon M, et al: SCID User's Guide for the Structured Clinical Interview for DSM-III-R. Washington, DC, American Psychiatric Press, 1990

Stack S: Comparative analysis of immigration and suicide. Psychol Rep 49:509–510, 1981

Twemlow SW: DSM-IV from a cross-cultural perspective. Psychiatric Annals 25:46–52, 1995

Vernez G: Current global refugee situation and international public policy. Am Psychol 46:627–631, 1991

Westermeyer J: Mental Health for Refugees and Other Migrants. Springfield, IL, Charles C Thomas, 1989a, pp 99–130

Westermeyer J: Clinical assessment, in Psychiatric Care of Migrants: A Clinical Guide. Washington, DC, American Psychiatric Press, 1989b, pp 63–110

Westermeyer J: Cross-cultural psychiatric assessment, in Culture, Ethnicity, and Mental Illness. Edited by Gaw A. Washington, DC, American Psychiatric Press, 1993, pp 125–144

Westermeyer J, Vang TF, Neider J: Migration and mental health among Hmong refugees: association of pre- and postmigration factors with self-rating scales. J Nerv Ment Dis 171:92–96, 1983

Westermeyer J, Neider J, Vang TF: Acculturation and mental health: a study of Hmong refugees at 1.5 and 3.5 years postmigration. Soc Sci Med 18:87–93, 1984a

Westermeyer J, Vang TF, Neider J: Symptom change over time among Hmong refugees: psychiatric patients versus nonpatients. Psychopathology 17:168–177, 1984b

Westermeyer J, Neider J, Callies A: Psychosocial adjustment of Hmong refugees during their first decade in the United States: a longitudinal study. J Nerv Ment Dis 177:132–139, 1989

Wing JH, Nixon J, Mann SA, et al: Reliability of the PSE (ninth edition) used in population survey. Psychol Med 7:505–516, 1977

World Health Organization: The ICD-10 Classification of Mental and Behavioural Disorders. Geneva, World Health Organization, 1992

Cultural Psychiatry
and Mental Health Services

CHAPTER 4

Cultural Epistemology and Value Orientations
Clinical Applications in Transcultural Psychiatry

DANILO E. PONCE, M.D.

"Who are you?" said the caterpillar. This was not an encouraging opening for a conversation. Alice replied rather shyly, "I—I hardly know, sir,
just at present—at least I know who I *was* when I got up this morning,
but I think I must have been changed several times since then."
—Alice's Adventures in Wonderland *by Lewis Carroll (1974, p. 58)*

Although much internal and external conflict currently exists in the
world of psychiatry, the psychiatric clinician is most concerned
with trying to do a reasonably good job of alleviating psychiatric disorder, pain, and suffering. This clinician is really being confronted, rather
urgently, with the task of integrating not only the tangled biopsychosocial aspects of his or her clinical practice but also that slippery slope of
another dimension of clinical reality called *culture*. For example, the
noble, if quixotic, idea of America being a melting pot (E PLURIBUS
UNUM) is quite simply no longer realistic. Political movers and shakers,
as well as policy and decision makers, now think of America as "The
World's First Multicultural Society" ("New face of America . . ." 1993).
Even if clinicians willfully try to limit their practices, health reform
movements are already in place that, like it or not, will ensure the *multicultural* composition—the so-called "rainbow coalition"—of one's patient population. Therefore, if a psychiatric practitioner is to survive, he
or she must pay attention not only to the biological, psychological, and
social dimensions of a practice but also to that of culture.

The other dimension that the clinician must consider is the *spiritual* dimension. I am, of course, quite aware of the objections some empiricists might have in even discussing this dimension; however, I think it is quite important for any clinician (regardless of his or her beliefs) to be aware of this dimension, especially since nationwide surveys show, for example, that 53% of Americans feel the need "to experience spiritual growth" (Kantrowitz et al. 1994). As a concession to the increasing importance of this dimension, DSM-IV (American Psychiatric Association 1994) includes a new category of "Religious and Spiritual Problems (V62.89)" spurred on no doubt by papers including that by Lukoff and associates (1992) documenting the significance of this dimension in people's lives. It is beyond the scope of this chapter to discuss this particular dimension, and I am mentioning it here simply for the sake of completing a model of human existence that I would like the reader to use in locating the role of *culture* in the overall scheme of things (see Figure 4–1). In using the term *spiritual,* I am not necessarily referring to religion and religious practices. I am referring more to the so-called

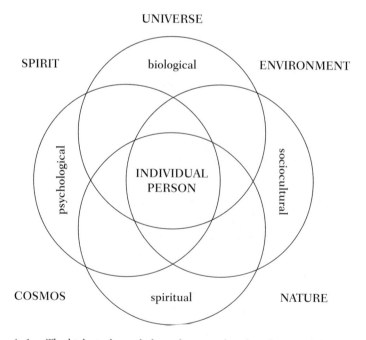

Figure 4–1.   The biological, psychological, sociocultural, and spiritual dimensions of human existence.

invisible and imponderable aspects of human existence: "What is the purpose of my life?" "Is there life after death?" "Why is there evil in this world?" "Why me?" "Why now?" The spiritual dimension provides meaning in and purpose to one's life (Kantrowitz et al. 1994). The biological (organic), psychological (intrapsychic), social (interpersonal), and cultural (group) aspects of a patient should all be amenable to scientific scrutiny and methodology. The spiritual aspect is an intensely personal and subjective experience but nonetheless is very influential on the other four dimensions.

To be sure, the average clinician is without a doubt reasonably competent with the *biological* (i.e., the structural aspects of his or her practice, including the role of genetic endowment, medical or neurological diseases, and endocrine disturbances), the *psychological* (i.e., the functional aspects of his or her practice, such as the role of id, ego, and superego; coping and defense mechanisms vis-à-vis internal and external stressors; cognitive dissonances; and faulty philosophical and worldview assumptions), and the *social* (i.e., the ecological aspects of his or her practice such as the role of poverty, war, class, caste, divorce, immigration, and economic stressors) dimensions. But what about the *cultural* dimension? Considering that respondents offered about 150 different definitions of *culture* the last time such a survey was conducted (Krueber and Kluckhohn 1952), the clinician could very well find himself or herself in the horns of an interesting dilemma. Jay Haley (1977), well-known for his groundbreaking work in family therapy, put his finger on the nature of this dilemma in stating the following: "[R]esearch investigators require complex theories and clinicians need simple ones. Clinicians must choose key variables and act rather than accounting for, and reflecting on innumerable variables" (p. 100). Is there a *simple* model of culture that is valid and that can be used reliably in one's clinical practice?

Paradigm, Epistemology, and Value Orientations

Based on my own clinical practice in a multicultural setting (Hawaii), I can say without hesitation that there is indeed a simple model. However, before I present it, let me lay the groundwork for the rationale and internal logic of the model by first discussing two related and key concepts: paradigm and epistemology. As originally conceived by its progenitor and popularizer, scientific historian Thomas Kuhn, *paradigm* has two meanings in the context of describing the evolution (and the revolution) of sciences: "On one hand, it stands for the entire constellation of beliefs, values, techniques and so on shared by the members of a given community. On the other, it denotes one sort of element in that constellation, the concrete puzzle-solutions which, employed as models or examples can replace explicit rules as a basis for the remaining puzzles of normal science" (Kuhn 1970, p. 175). Kuhn originally used *paradigm* as a useful concept in explaining the discontinuous (as opposed to prevalent notions about the orderly, epigenetic nature of scientific "progress") and revolutionary (as opposed to evolutionary) nature of science.

In this particular text, I shall refer to the dominant paradigm of a culture as signifying "the basic ways of *perceiving, thinking, valuing, and doing* associated with a particular view of reality [emphasis added]" (Harman 1988, p. 10). The Ptolemaic view of reality, the sun revolving around the earth, is an example of a paradigm with very profound and far-reaching psychosocial-religious consequences continuing until the time this paradigm was replaced by the Copernican view of reality, the earth rotating on its axis and orbiting the sun. The consequences of this paradigm shift are incalculable. In the Ptolemaic view, humans are the center of the universe; in the Copernican view, they are just a part of the cosmic scenery. More familiar, and perhaps more relevant to psychiatrists, is the substitution of the paradigm that attributed psychiatric disorders (as we know them today) from demonic possessions or suitable punishments for sinful transgressions to the biopsychosocial factors mentioned elsewhere. Regardless of one's paradigmatic persuasions, the point is that individual or collective paradigms dictate what one looks for (e.g., demonic possession? neurochemical imbalance? irrational beliefs? poverty?), where one looks for it, and what measures one uses to ensure one has found it.

Epistemology, the other concept, owes its popularity to two theoreticians, Gregory Bateson (1972), the late anthropologist and ex-husband of Margaret Mead, who provided the theoretical underpinnings of the family therapy or system theory movement in psychiatry and allied sciences, and the late Jean Piaget, who mapped out the cognitive development of children and who eventually called his studies "genetic epistemology" (Flavell 1968). Similar to the term *paradigm,* *epistemology* has come to have a fecundity of meanings attached to it. I will be using epistemology to mean an individual or group's way of knowing, or, to put it in more formal terms, epistemology is the study of how one knows how one knows.

The pattern that connects (to use a Batesonian phrase) paradigm, epistemology, and culture is the presupposition that an individual or group's values, belief systems, worldviews, perspectives, assumptive worlds, and the like (that is to say, their paradigms and epistemologies) *organize,* if not *determine,* what that individual or group construes as reality. Put another way, the presupposition is that there really is no objective reality in the outside world to be *discovered*: first we construct our realities based on structures (e.g., our sensory organs, central nervous system, or muscles) that are available to us, then we see (i.e., discover) these realities that we have constructed. As the radical constructivists in philosophy (Von Glassersfeld 1984) and the structural determinists in biology (Maturana 1978) would put it, we believe first and then we see. If this fundamental presupposition is correct, then certainly if one has information (or access to such information) regarding an individual or group's key paradigms and epistemologies, it would constitute a uniquely elegant way of understanding that particular individual or group. The value orientations (VO) model (see Table 4–1) is based on this presupposition. Initially developed by Florence Kluckhohn and Fred Strodtbeck (1961) as a tool to provide a frame of reference in understanding and dealing with variations among individuals and groups, it is based on the following explicit assumptions:

1. There are a limited number of common human problems for which people at all times must find solutions.
2. Although there is a variability in solutions of all of the problems, it is neither limitless nor random.
3. All alternatives of all solutions are present in all societies at all times but are preferred differentially.
4. There is a rank ordering of preferences.

With this set of assumptions in mind, Kluckhohn and Strodtbeck isolated five common human problems for which people at all times must find solutions. These problems may be thought of as existential

Table 4–1. **The value orientation model**

Dimension	Value orientation		
Time	Past	Present	Future
Human activity	Being	Being-in-becoming	Doing
Relationship to other people	Lineal	Collateral	Individualistic
Relationship to nature and supernature	Subjugation to nature	Harmony with nature	Mastery over nature
Innate human nature	Evil	Neutral or mixture of good and evil	Good
	(mutable or immutable)	(mutable or immutable)	(mutable or immutable)

questions. That is to say, they are not only ubiquitous but must be faced on a moment-to-moment basis by the individual or group from birth to death as part and parcel of being human. The five problems together with three possible responses (solutions or answers) to each of the five problems are configured in the form of philosophical conundrums:

1. What is humanity's orientation to *time* (i.e., past, present, and future)?
2. What is humanity's orientation to *activity* (i.e., being, being-in-becoming, and doing)?
3. What is a person's *relationship* to other people (i.e., lineal or hierarchical, collateral or affiliative, or individualistic)?
4. What is humanity's relationship to *nature* or *supernature* (i.e., subjugation to nature, harmony with nature, or mastery over nature)?
5. What is the nature of *humanity* (i.e., good [fixed or changeable], neutral or a mixture of good and evil [fixed or changeable], or evil [fixed or changeable])?

Common and shared preferred responses by a particular group of people may be construed as that group's VO profile. Culture could then be defined as a particular group of people held together by similarly preferred VOs. It is important but not necessary that this group live in close proximity with one other. Together with their common VOs, however, they should have a shared history and some kind of assurance of continuity in the future. In this context, institutions and systems such as the military, health, education, justice, legislative, and corrections; organizations (e.g., American Medical Association and National Football League); and corporations (e.g., IBM and GM) can be construed as cultures, aside from our commonly understood notion of culture as involving ethnic, racial, and geopolitical enclaves.

The instrument designed by Kluckhohn and Strodtbeck to elicit the preferred response to each of the five problems described a hypothetical "generalized life situation" and three possible responses that would then reveal the individual or group's preferences. The following examples in the time modality show three people's approaches to rearing children.

> *Past:* Some people say that children should always be taught the traditions of the past (the ways of the old people). They believe the old ways are best, and that it is when children do not follow them that things go wrong.
>
> *Present:* Some people say that children should be taught some of the old traditions (ways of the old people), but it is wrong to insist that they stick to these ways. These people believe that it is necessary for children to learn about and take on whatever new ways will best help them to get along in the world of today.
>
> *Future:* Some people do not believe children should be taught (future) much about past traditions (the ways of the old people) except as interesting stories of what has gone before. These people believe that the world goes along best when children are taught the things that will make them want to find out for themselves new ways of doing things to replace the old.
>
> Which of these people has the best idea about how children should be taught? Which of the other two people has the better idea? Considering again all three ideas, which would most other persons in _____ say had the better idea? (Kluckhohn and Strodtbeck 1961, p. 81)

The last two questions in the survey instrument are designed to tap leanings and perceived congruence with the cultural mainstream.

Kluckhohn and Strodtbeck believe that the model has not only a descriptive but also an evaluative aspect. As such, it contains *cognitive, affective,* and *directive* elements, so that the VOs substantially influence an individual or group's predisposition to act in certain predictable and patterned ways. For example, an individual or culture strongly wedded to the past orientation in the time modality would be expected to plan, make decisions, and in general organize their lives around traditions and their ancestors and elders' beliefs about important issues in their lives. This outlook is so ingrained that conceivably it permeates even such quotidian activities as their choice of furniture, their preference for art, and the music they listen to. It is a rearview mirror perspective of life. In contrast, an individual or a group preferring the future orientation will predictably choose future goals and outcomes as a basis for running their lives. The group oriented to the present is grounded in the demands of the here and now, with scant attention to the "dead and irrelevant past" or the "illusory and unpredictable future." The homeless, refugees, survivors of disaster, students, and the like would be expected to function primarily in the present orientation.

An individual's orientation during his or her lifetime may shift often (evolution or devolution), but the VOs of the culture remain stable. The teenage years might predispose one to preferring and acting within the present, "doing," mastery, individualistic, or neutral or changeable orientations, whereas the same individual in senior years might subtly and effortlessly have shifted to past, "being," harmony, collateral, or neutral or fixed orientations. For example, we are all aware of employees who, while on staff, rabidly espouse democratic or affiliative (collateral) orientation but who, when promoted to chief or chairperson, do an almost miraculous Jekyll-Hyde transformation, championing the virtues of linear or hierarchical modes.

Individual changes and the vicissitudes of flux notwithstanding, the culture's continued existence is dependent on a kind of internal homeostasis that manages to stabilize these fluctuations and perturbations. Only when there is a wrenching and more or less enduring assault on the integrity of established VOs is there danger of collapse and even demise of the culture in question. Examples of these sustained and intense assaults are prolonged war, famine, natural catastrophes (e.g., earthquakes, firestorms, or flooding), and permanent contacts of previously isolated cultures (e.g., isolated tribes in the Amazons) with the modern world. *Culture shock* (Jank 1977), with its accompanying signs and symptoms of confusion, disorientation, anxiety, depression, and numbness, is the initial indicator of a transition, that, if not acknowledged, could very well lead to culture demise. The collapse of cultures (e.g., the collapse of communist cultures in Europe and of a dominant culture in America) and the transition period before a stable set of VOs are established once again account for many of the negative symptoms in that particular culture (e.g., increase in crimes, violence, and psychopathology). What we are seeing may not be so much the downward spiral deplored by hand-wringing politicians and clinicians (pundits have been complaining of these very same things since antiquity) as cultures in rapid and intense transitions.

Facilitating the collapse of traditional cultures as we know them are the tremendous technological advances that are transforming the world into a literal (not just figurative) *global village* (Iyer 1993) in the McLuhanesque sense (McLuhan and Fiore 1967; McLuhan 1968). John Naisbitt (1984) rightly points out that McLuhan, as radical and as mind-boggling as his ideas might have been in the 1960s, was wrong when he identified television as the medium that would accelerate the demise of semiautonomous, isolated cultures. McLuhan, of course, did not live long enough to see the proliferation of technical marvels like communication satellites, fax machines, interactive television, cellular phones, videophones, supercomputers, modems, and so forth that have already transformed the world into one gigantic information superhighway. The latter has very definitely replaced and made obsolete the image of the world as a global village. To repeat a theme expressed earlier, but this time on a more urgent and encompassing note, anyone living in the twenty-first century, regardless of title or profession, will need to be a multicultural "expert," like it or not. In psychiatry and allied sciences, there simply is no choice.

Clinical Applications of Value Orientations

I use the VO model in the remainder of this chapter to describe in detail its usefulness in a variety of clinical and ancillary work. In all fairness, it must be stated once again that Kluckhohn and Strodtbeck came up with VO model primarily to identify and explain *variations* in the VOs of societies, subgroups within societies, and even the individuals within the groups of people—much like variations in physical and biological phenomena. As anthropologists, Kluckhohn and Strodtbeck aimed their work toward a more universal and expansive scope. I certainly am not aware that they envisioned the model being used for conflict resolution on a clinical basis. Hence, any methodologic objections must not be leveled at their model per se but to clinicians (like me) who have extrapolated from their model useful principles in clinical work (Ponce 1995). In addition, it must be pointed out that the VO model is only one among many competing models that might be useful in cross-cultural work with patients (for a brief but useful introduction to these models, see Robert Kohl's chapter "Models for Comparing and Contrasting Cultures" in Reid 1988). All of these caveats aside, I have used the VO model in my cross-cultural clinical work because, by enabling the clinician to access the individual patient and possibly his or her significant other's VO, the model lends itself more fully to diagnostic, treatment, management, and quality assurance processes than any other model. Since the focus is on *organizing principles* of behavior rather than the behaviors themselves, the clinician is not saddled with the well-nigh impossible task of having to memorize thousands of behavioral units and their meanings.

Individual psychotherapy. The most obvious application of VO in one-to-one clinical situations such as psychoanalysis, psychotherapy, behavioral management, and counseling is to enhance the therapeutic alliance by ensuring a therapeutic match or fit (deShazer 1984). A *match* implies that the caregiver approximates the patient's VOs. In a match, the therapeutic relationship is *symmetrical* in that both protagonists are, for all intents and purposes, members of the same culture, working together on the well-known principle of *similia similibus curantur* ("like cures like"). Not all beneficial therapeutic liaisons work in this way, however. As a matter of fact, in most clinical situations, it is *difference that makes a difference,* oftentimes resulting in dramatic and lasting positive therapeutic outcomes. In this instance, the therapeutic alliance is *complementary,* and the caregiver-patient relationship is a fit, instead of a match; a pair of shoes is a match, a lock and a key is a fit. Bandler and

Grinder (1975/1976), founders of the Neuro-Linguistic Programming (NLP) approach to psychotherapy, are generally acknowledged to have done the most work in applying the principles of match and fit as a major cornerstone of their theory on how to effect therapeutic changes.

From a VO perspective, a patient who is stuck in pathological mourning because of an orientation to the past could benefit by being assisted to shift to the future orientation, thereby operating on the therapeutic principle of fit. On the other hand, a similar patient who is grieving pathologically may be doing so because well-meaning relatives and friends are pressuring him or her to "forget the past and think about the future." In this case, allowing the patient to process the past in the past VO mode may be more appropriate, thereby effecting a match. Value orientation will *not* dictate to the clinician the "right" decision—that is still a matter of the clinician's skill and sensitivity—but will assist in identifying the key and relevant VOs with which the patient is dealing.

In addition to identifying the nature of therapeutic matches or fits, VO can be used quite effectively in pinpointing origins of therapeutic impasses, resistance, refractoriness to treatment, and treatment failures. Quite frequently, all of these treatment problems can be traced to therapeutic mismatching or lack of therapeutic fit. Carol Gilligan (1982), for example, spoke of the fundamental differences among men and women in the way they view relationships and make moral judgments—differences that, if they go unrecognized, could lead to any one of the previously mentioned problems in a therapy situation. These differences are quite evident, according to Tannen (1986), even in such a basic process as the way men and women communicate with each other. Interestingly, it is not only the way people communicate with each other but also *languages* themselves that have differing VO preferences (Ortuno 1991). By providing a reliable tool in identifying the nature of these unrecognized and undeclared differences, many of the hitherto perplexing problems in therapy could be presented and resolved if not mediated.

Another fruitful and perhaps rather unique way of using VO in therapy is the intriguing notion that schools of psychotherapy, and by fiat their practitioners, are cultures unto themselves, having clearly identifiable VO profiles (Remer and Remer 1982). Knowing the VOs of a given therapeutic approach (e.g., behavioral, existential, Gestalt, humanistic, client-centered, rational-emotive, psychoanalytic, and transpersonal) makes it more amenable to be matched (i.e., make it compatible) with a particular patient's orientations. As a corollary, it could prevent costly mismatching or at least provide some kind of explanation as to why a certain therapeutic approach may not be working with a given patient or client.

Marital or conjoint therapy. As VO reveals potential matches or fits between caregivers and patients, it reveals just as easily matches or fits (or lack thereof) between husbands and wives or between partners, more so when the marriage or partnership is an intercultural one (Ponce 1977). Value orientation is particularly useful in this type of therapy, because it provides the couple with a frame of reference that they can use in understanding, explaining, and processing their problems or conflicts (much like therapists and their patients) in a way that *does not* lead to blame or attribution of malicious intents and instead defines problems as "mere differences in perceiving things."

Therapist: Bill (a Caucasian male), were you aware that Lydia (Bill's wife, of Japanese ancestry) is more inclined to try to get along with others (harmony), whereas you tend to see relationships more in terms of winning and losing and what you could get out of it (mastery)?

Bill: Now that you mentioned it, no. I thought that was just her humility, you know, not wanting to stick out like a sore thumb. As a matter of fact, that was what attracted me to her initially . . . but then, as time went on, I got more and more "pissed off," because I saw people treating her badly, and she wouldn't do a damn thing about it. She would just smile that stupid smile of hers. I wish she would tell them off, or at least stop being such a hypocrite.

Lydia: I guess like him, I too was initially attracted to him because he had a direct way of getting things done. But then I began to see it more and more as rude and crass behavior.

Therapist: And the two of you are ready to get a divorce because you see things differently?

Family therapy. Value orientation is extremely helpful in making concrete what intuitive clinicians who work with families have called generation gaps. By going beyond the average, expectable, and predictable differences in preferences for clothing, music, food, activities, and so on and providing access to deeper and more meaningful value clashes, the clinician, as in marital or conjoint therapy, supplies nuclear and extended family members with tools to understand and possibly bridge their gaps.

Mr. McDonald (father):   I don't give a damn what she does when she turns 18, but so long as she is in my house, she will live by my rules (lineal). That means I don't want her boyfriend in my house when nobody is home, and especially not in her room!

Kristen (daughter):   But dad, we're not doing anything wrong. Would you rather we go somewhere else? Besides, don't you think I'm old enough to know what's right and wrong and make my own decisions (individual)? How will I learn to make my own decisions if you don't give me the opportunity to do that?

Therapist: You know Jim (Mr. McDonald), it sounds to me like we need to find out a way in which your values are acknowledged by Kristen, while at the same time giving her the opportunity to make responsible decisions. Is there a middle ground somewhere?

Mr. McDonald: Well, I guess we could talk things over (collateral).

Group therapy.   Value orientation profiles of group therapy members and the therapist provide the therapist with an individual as well as collective *weltbild* (worldview), which could then be used as a map to understand group process and dynamics. For example, a member who believes that human beings are primarily evil or fixed will be expected to consistently view the other members and the process with suspicion. The natural tendency is to try to convince the member that the group can be trusted, which ironically usually results in more mistrust. The therapist who has an insight into this member's orientation could, instead of fighting his or her view, reframe the orientation to the following: "[Y]ou are being quite cautious, and that is good. You should look before you leap."

Value orientation is also particularly useful in support groups (e.g., cancer and AIDS groups), because it enables the leader to structure the group's composition (i.e., match and fit), the group's communication styles (e.g., lineal, collateral, or individualistic), and the group's relational preferences (i.e., being, being-in-becoming, or doing). It also helps the leader to understand individual members' coping styles vis-à-vis their illness (i.e., some will give up [subjugation], some will fight [mastery], and some will live and let live [harmony with their illness]).

Psychopharmacology. Even in what appears to be a relatively straight-forward matter—taking medications—successful compliance often depends on a host of nondrug factors such as the patient and his or her significant other's ingrained beliefs about illness, the role of drugs in the treatment of illnesses, and the doctor-patient relationship. Put in VO terms, a patient whose orientation is lineal will rely heavily on the force of authority and will probably have no difficulties complying with taking medications; however, the opposite may be true of someone who is individualistic. Someone in the collateral mode will probably need much to-and-fro dialogue regarding pros and cons about taking the medications. Even in someone who is compliant, the manner in which the medication's effects and side effects are explained is value oriented. For instance, in explaining methylphenidate's (Ritalin's) effects on a child to his or her mother who is "being" oriented, it is probably wise to tell her that because Ritalin will increase her child's attention span, concentration, and frustration tolerance, it will probably make her child feel better about himself or herself, increase his or her self-esteem, and therefore help him or her to get along better with other children. To a parent who is more "doing" oriented, the emphasis should probably focus more on the child's being able to do more and better work, enhance his or her grades, and have more friends.

Ancillary Uses of Value Orientations

Because clinics, departments, service-delivery systems, organizations, and institutions are made up of groups of people with missions, goals, objectives, and methods of accomplishing them, they are, by definition, cultures unto themselves and therefore have identifiable VOs. Their VOs in turn are usually shaped by the nature of their missions, the target population they serve or product they produce, and the service they provide. As a culture, these systems themselves qua systems (regardless of their varying nature and goals) are usually hierarchical (i.e., chain of command), grounded in the past (i.e., policies, procedures, and practices), mastery oriented (i.e., raison d'être based on the premise of fixing something), doing (i.e., continued existence based on tangible and measurable results), and mixed or changeable (i.e., reward for the "good," punishment for the "bad").

Mental health professionals routinely work with systems, and to understand and work effectively with systems is to understand their VOs. Conversely, failure to appreciate or understand the potency of the VO of a given system is to ensure failure or conflicts in working with that particular system.

Consultation and liaison.   Knowing a system's VO enhances a consultant's effectiveness, but VO is also quite helpful in patient-centered, consultee-centered, and program-centered consultation-liaison work. For instance, VO could be used to analyze a particular program's relevance and effectiveness with its target population. Furthermore, it could be used to see whether the staff matches the program's explicit VOs. Vague feelings of frustration and demoralization are often symptomatic of unrecognized mismatching or VO clashes among staff, between staff and the population they serve, or between staff and the values of the program or institution that employs them.

Supervision.   Value orientation is an effective, easy-to-grasp, easy-to-apply tool in diagnosing incompatibilities, problems, conflicts, and impasses or, conversely, effective work between caregivers and patients. As explained earlier, the mechanics of therapeutic match and fit could be the basis of a supervisory model to discuss and analyze cases presented by students, trainees, or staff.

Mediation and facilitation.   Value orientation has been used in understanding and facilitating the mediation of conflicts among interracial and interethnic groups (Carter 1990) and ethnic groups and institutions (Florence R. Kluckhohn Center 1988, 1991, 1993). As in using VO in a clinical context, the basic principle in mediating conflicts or facilitating positive group processes is the axiomatic acceptance of the notion that no one value is superior or right and that understanding another group's perspective is a necessary first step in the mediation process.

Interreligious dialogues.   It should not come as a surprise that most destructive and enduring wars are religious in nature. Like the microcosm of two individuals of varying VOs who are unable to get along with each other but do not understand why, the macrocosm of interreligious holy wars are fed by a vicious lack of appreciation of differences of values or the virulent wish to establish one's values as the only or at least the dominant force, exerting a hegemony over the religious values of others. Somewhat analogous to mediating conflicts between husbands and wives or between conflicted groups, an important first step is taken if the key values of a religion are known, and, based on the appreciation of these values, meaningful interchanges are effected.

Conclusions

Understanding VOs is a valuable tool that enables a clinical practitioner to integrate cultural factors meaningfully with the biopsychosocial matrix. The underlying principles behind the model are quite simple (but certainly not simplistic or reductionistic), easy to grasp, and very helpful in the clinical processes of diagnostic evaluations and treatment and management. Aside from using it in one's clinical work, there are also numerous ancillary ways the interested clinician could put the model to use. Because use of the VO model could have a potentially powerful impact on one's clinical practice, it would be prudent to remember a number of caveats (Ponce 1995): 1) VO does not establish pathology or normalcy but merely variations and differences among individuals and groups (no one orientation is superior or more adaptive than others in the absolute sense); 2) VOs should not be used either wittingly or unwittingly as the basis for cultural stereotyping; and 3) VOs should not be used coercively to enforce unwelcomed or unwanted changes. Bearing these caveats in mind, we can, however, raise questions that may have potential heuristic implications. For instance, are some VOs more adaptive, in the sense of being more effective and efficient, in dealing with a specific problematic situation? I mentioned earlier that VOs could change on an individual level in response to changes in developmental ages or stages, professional career status, and the like and on a collective level as a result of intense, sustained, and enduring assault on a group's VO (e.g., war, natural catastrophes, or prolonged contact with other groups as a result of technological advances). Could we identify which VO seems to be more adaptive to which situation? In clinical work, for example, which VOs are more adaptive in depressed individuals? In anxious individuals? I have found in my own clinical practice that regardless of a particular culture or family's VO, those involved seemed to respond more positively when I acted in lineal, future-oriented, and "doing" modes during crisis times and times of ambiguities or transitions (e.g., death or relocation). Patients were very appreciative of my "decisiveness" and my "competence" in "telling them what to do." In quieter times, however, even in the same patient or family, I was criticized as being "too bossy" and "dictatorial." It seems to me that these and other similar questions could lead to fruitful research answers for those inclined to investigate the issue.

References

American Psychiatric Association: Diagnostic and Statistical Manual of Mental Disorders, 4th Edition. Washington, DC, American Psychiatric Association, 1994

Bandler R, Grinder J: The Structure of Magic, Vols 1 and 2. Palo Alto, CA, Science & Behaviour Books, 1975, 1976

Bateson G: Steps to an Ecology of Mind. New York, Ballantine Books, 1972

Carroll L: Alice's Adventures in Wonderland. Cleveland, OH, Wm. Collins & World Publishing, 1974, p 58

Carter RT: Cultural value differences between African Americans and white Americans. Journal of College Student Development 31:71–79, 1990

deShazer S: FIT. Journal of Strategic and Systemic Therapies 3:34–37, 1984

Flavell JH: The Developmental Psychology of Jean Piaget. Princeton, NJ, Van Nostrand Reinhold, 1968, pp 249–266

Florence R. Kluckhohn Center: Lummi Indian Nation and the Washington Department of Natural Resources. Bellingham, WA, Florence R. Kluckhohn Center, 1988

Florence R. Kluckhohn Center: Lummi Indian Nation and Tacoma City Light. Bellingham, WA, Florence R. Kluckhohn Center, 1991

Florence R. Kluckhohn Center: Lummi Indian Nation and Pacific International Terminals. Bellingham, WA, Florence R. Kluckhohn Center, 1993

Gilligan C: In a Different Voice: Psychological Theory and Women's Development. Cambridge, MA, Harvard University Press, 1982

Haley J: Problem Solving Therapy. San Francisco, CA, Jossey-Bass, 1977, p 100

Harman W: Global Mind Change. Indianapolis, IN, Knowledge Systems, 1988, p 10

Iyer P: The global village finally arrives. Time 142:86–87, 1993

Jank M: Culture Shock. Chicago, IL, Moody Press, 1977

Kantrowitz B, King B, Rosenberg D, et al: The search for the sacred: America's quest for spiritual meaning. Newsweek, November 28, 1994, pp 52–65

Kluckhohn F, Strodtbeck F: Variations in Value Orientations. New York, Peterson & Row, 1961

Kohl R: Models for comparing and contrasting cultures, in Building the Professional Dimension of Educational Exchange. Edited by Reid J. Yarmouth, ME, Intercultural Press, 1988

Krueber A, Kluckhohn F: Culture: A Critical Review of Concepts and Definitions. Cambridge, MA, Peabody Museum, 1952

Kuhn T: The Structure of Scientific Revolutions, 2nd Edition. Chicago, IL, University of Chicago Press, 1970, p 175

Lukoff D, Lu F, Turner R: Toward a more culturally sensitive DSM-IV: psychoreligious and psychospiritual problems. J Nerv Ment Dis 80:673–682, 1992

Maturana H: Biology of language: the epistemology of reality, in Psychology and Biology of Language and Thought. Edited by Miller GA, Lennenberg E. New York, Academic Press, 1978

McLuhan M: War and Peace in the Global Village. New York, McGraw-Hill, 1968

McLuhan M, Fiore Q: The Medium Is the Message. New York, Bantam, 1967

Naisbitt J: Megatrends. New York, Warner, 1984, p 3

New face of America: how immigrants are shaping the world's first multicultural society. Time Special Issue, Fall 1993, pp 3–87

Ortuno M: Cross cultural awareness in the foreign language class: the Kluckhohn model. Modern Language Journal 75:449–459, 1991

Ponce DE: Intercultural perspectives in mate selection, in Adjustment in Intercultural Marriage. Edited by Tseng WS, McDermott JF. Honolulu, HI, University Press of Hawaii, 1977, pp 22–32

Ponce DE: Value orientation: clinical applications in a multi-cultural residential treatment center for children and youth. Journal of Residential Treatment for Children and Youth 12:29–42, 1995

Reid J (ed): Building the Professional Dimension of Educational Exchange. Yarmouth, ME, Intercultural Press, 1988

Remer R, Remer P: A study of the discrepancies among the value orderings of 12 counseling theories: the quantification of value differences. Counseling and Values. 10:12–16, 1982

Tannen D: That's Not What I Meant: How Conversational Style Makes or Breaks Relationships. New York, Ballantine, 1986

Von Glassersfeld E: An introduction to radical constructivism, in The Invented Reality. Edited by Watzlawick P. New York, WW Norton, 1984, pp 17–40

CHAPTER 5

Traditional Healing Systems in a Multicultural Setting

Harriet P. Lefley, Ph.D.
Mercedes Cros Sandoval, Ph.D.
Claude Charles, M.A.

Traditional, or folk, healing systems are embedded in a psychocultural context in which human behavior is mediated by multiple forces, both natural and supernatural. Healers' skills range from knowledge of appropriate medicinal herbs to modes of negotiation with powerful spirits. Although some folk systems clearly distinguish the roles of medicinal herb doctors and priest-healers, most models of traditional healing, whether for somatic, psychological, social, or spiritual ailments, incorporate a supernatural or religious element. Diagnostic and treatment paradigms are anchored to etiological concepts that typically involve some imbalance in life forces, an imbalance that can be corrected only by invoking appropriate counterforces or by ritualistic fulfillment of religious obligations.

In the treatment of mental disorders, these paradigms are applied for the resolution of presenting complaints that may range from culturally acknowledged aberrant behavior to existential problems of living. The theater of intervention includes not only the therapist and patient—or more typically the therapist, patient, and family group—but also one or more supernatural forces that are inextricably involved in etiology and cure. In treating mental or emotional problems, most traditional healing systems require the intercession of supernatural powers, either directly or through the mediumship of the healer. The therapeutic alliance literally binds all of these elements together in a battle for the patient's mental health.

To begin this chapter we deal first with clinicians' attitudes toward traditional healing systems. Many clinicians perceive these systems as a primitive and harmful alternative to scientific care. Others may view them as an ancillary resource in the alleviation of emotional distress, a mechanism for conveying a sense of control, hope, and social support to the believer. We discuss the treatment domains typically differentiated by the healers themselves—that is, their distinctions between culturally recognized mental illness that is best treated by psychiatrists and spiritual or emotional disorders or problems in living that are considered within their province of cure. An overview of several supernatural belief systems incorporates traditional healing modalities and a comparison of the common conceptual and therapeutic paradigms of folk healing with those of Western psychiatry. Empirical examples of various roles that mental health professionals have fulfilled in dealing with the beliefs of their patients and in utilizing alternative healing systems are given. These include roles as knowledgeable interpreters, brokers, collaborators, or even practitioners.

We end with the changing functions of alternative healing systems and their value dimensions as systems of care in the evolving acculturative process of immigrant populations. Included is an evaluation of the problems of chicanery and exploitation inherent in unregulated treatment systems; the real danger of rejection of appropriate psychiatric interventions; negative aspects of sorcery and witchcraft; and, on the positive side, the potential for integrating folk healing as an adjunctive resource for a more holistic approach to patient care.

Mental Health Professionals' Attitudes Toward Traditional Healing

Clinicians often find it difficult to deal conceptually with the salience and personal meaning of the religious beliefs of their patients. Many clinicians are uncomfortable with beliefs based on a conviction of external locus of control and divine intermediaries. In mainstream religions such beliefs may include faith in an all-powerful deity whose will determines everything that happens in a person's life, with relief of stress more dependent on prayer than on personal actions. In marginal religions or supernatural belief systems, the patient may believe in many gods or spirits, some of whom must be propitiated in ritually defined ways to alleviate psychological distress. A patient's firm conviction of supernatural agency and design seems to militate against basic therapeutic goals of helping people take personal control of their lives and become the architects of their own destinies.

Therapists can usually accommodate the beliefs of patients who practice the major religions in the United States, particularly those who accept the explanatory models of modern psychiatry. Far greater difficulty is encountered in dealing with more marginal belief systems and their healing methods, such as those of Mexican *curanderismo,* Puerto Rican *espiritismo,* Afrocuban *santeria,* Brazilian *umbanda,* Haitian *vodou,* Caribbean *obeah,* and Southern black rootwork. These systems are generally considered to be based on primitive superstitions, their healing rituals countertherapeutic substitutions of magic for free will.

However, many established churches also have healing rituals for mental and emotional problems. There are Christian and Jewish rituals for exorcism of the symptoms of severe disorders such as schizophrenia when the behaviors are ascribed to demonic possession (Bilu and Witztum 1993; Csordas 1992) or even severe obsessive-compulsive disorders (Rapoport 1990). Favazza (1982) has described modern Christian healing rituals reflecting a shift from suffering and self-mortification to divine healing as practiced by Jesus in the gospels. Csordas (1992) has noted three active traditions of healing within contemporary Catholicism: healing through prayer to the saints, who already have given evidence of posthumous miracles; healing by the Virgin Mary, typically at shrines; and healing of one believer by another, typically through the laying on of hands. The latter method, in which the healer is a medium for God-given curative powers, is practiced in many Protestant sects as well.

Many clinicians actively oppose the use of traditional healing practices in mental health treatment. Weiss (1992) has noted that psychiatric patients and their families who utilize folk healing, often because orthodox aftercare treatment has failed them, have good reason to conceal their involvement with these practices because of clinicians' disapproval.

Clinicians' willingness to accept traditional healing as a component of an intervention is also related to their basic theoretical orientations. Practitioners are generally placed along a universalistic-eclectic continuum. A large number subscribe to universalistic theories of human behavior and interpersonal transactions with correlative treatment models. In their practice, sensitive clinicians use cultural input as an additive rather than a transformative clinical tool, superimposing cultural knowledge on an existing technology (Lefley 1991). Cultural information is used in the service of understanding linguistic and behavioral cues, behavioral anomalies, belief systems, normative family transactions, and diagnostic profiles, which sensitive clinicians realize they may misinterpret. Regardless of whether these clinicians subscribe to psychodynamic, interpersonal, behavioral, cognitive, or traditional family systems models, their basic diagnostic and therapeutic approach is considered appropriate for accommodating all varieties of human problems, provided they do not misinterpret cultural cues.

On the other extreme are clinicians whose diagnostic assessments go well beyond all five DSM-III axes (American Psychiatric Association 1980), incorporating quality of life, social support networks, rehabilitative potential, and spiritual needs. Treatment modalities are eclectic, tailored to specific problems and contingencies. Eclectic practitioners may opt for brief supportive psychotherapy or directive counseling. They may elect to work with families, using psychoeducational interventions and social network designs in lieu of or together with psychodynamic, structural, or strategic therapies. They may apply the latter techniques pragmatically, without necessarily accepting their underlying theoretical paradigms or generalizability across cultures. This model has been used by various community mental health centers throughout the United States, particularly those serving low-income, multicultural populations (Lefley and Bestman 1991).

Eclectic clinicians are cognizant of the high dropout rate of ethnic minority patients and recognize that their first mandate is to retain the patient and family in treatment. Persons from culturally diverse backgrounds are often bewildered by the mental health system, have different expectations of what will be offered, cannot see the potential benefits of psychotherapy, and feel alienated by institutional settings that they do not understand. Many patients expect brief, directive counseling focused on the presenting complaint, anticipate speedy resolution, and are wary of follow-up appointments (Chien and Yamamoto 1982). The therapist must be viewed as a valuable resource in motivating the patient to return.

Sue and Zane (1987) have pointed out that a therapist's cultural expertise is valuable only when it is linked with two factors: credibility and giving. A therapist's use of cultural knowledge, such as being more directive and structured in interactions with patients from traditional cultures, correctly interpreting psycholinguistic cues, or conveying an understanding of supernatural beliefs, is not in itself therapeutic. Rather, these behaviors increase the therapist's credibility as a helping resource: "Credibility refers to the client's perception of the therapist as an effective and trustworthy helper. Giving is the client's perception that something was received from the therapeutic encounter" (Sue and Zane 1987, p. 40). Coincidentally, the importance of this factor was verified in our own work in Miami. In an analysis of a videotaped cross-cultural therapeutic session rated by tri-ethnic samples of clinicians and almost 1,000 community college students, credibility and giving emerged as a unitary factor. These were clearly the most salient variables in the raters' assessment of a therapist's effectiveness and prediction of the client's return (Lefley 1986).

The eclectic mental health professional has a broad metaclinical view of true therapeutic effectiveness, and appropriate interventions may require far more than the individual clinical encounter. Cultural diversity often interacts with ethnic minority and low socioeconomic status. In many cases, environmental interventions are needed to resolve reality problems that sap energy, generate reactive depression, and contaminate clinical efficacy. In the multifaceted community mental health program developed by the University of Miami–Jackson Memorial Medical Center, based on seven ethnic community teams, environmental interventions included linking clients with a host of needed resources, ranging from community development projects to finding medical treatment for a sick child (Lefley and Bestman 1991). Research data have indicated that successful environmental interventions are significant predictors of the effectiveness of individual psychotherapy (Lefley 1979).

In some cases, environmental interventions have also included linking patients with traditional healers. These cases were too few to be studied empirically for long-range outcome. To our knowledge, no controlled studies of adequate samples of patient populations in Western countries have been undertaken to determine the comparative effectiveness of professional and traditional healing modalities. The closest is Koss's (1987) study of patients receiving either mental health care or spiritist healing in Puerto Rico. A total of 56 patients completed pre- and postintervention ratings of expected and reported symptom alleviation or problem resolution by their healers or therapists. Koss reported that the outcome ratings of spiritists' patients were significantly better than those of therapists but felt that the difference could be accounted for by the higher expectations of spiritists' patients.

Koss also reported that spiritist patients who were dissatisfied with medical or mental health personnel were the most hopeful, because they viewed the traditional healer as a last resort. However, most anthropological reports suggest that patients tend to use both systems simultaneously (Sandoval 1979, 1983; Weiss 1992). Some of the case histories that follow illustrate short-term effects, which tended to free immobilized patients so that they could benefit from continuing psychiatric treatment.

Conceptual Bases of Alternative Healing Systems: Commonalities and Differences

The anthropologist George Murdock and his associates (1978) have categorized all healing systems in terms of four major etiological belief systems. Natural causation underlies any theory that accounts for illness as the physiological consequence of conditions that might include infection, stress, organic deterioration, accident, or war. Mystical causation accounts for illness as an impersonal consequence of fate, without direct human or supernatural agency. Animistic causation ascribes illness to the behavior of some personalized supernatural agent, such as a wandering soul, a ghost, or a god. Magical causation relates illness to the covert activities of an affronted, envious, or malicious human who uses magical means to injure his or her victim. The latter theory underlies sorcery and witchcraft.

Ness and Wintrob (1981) point out that although natural causation is the theoretical cornerstone of scientific medicine, beliefs about mystical, animistic, and magical causation abound in both non-Western societies and many religious and ethnic communities in Western cultures. Foster (1976) stresses two dimensions in culturally constructed theories of illness. In personalistic models, the illness is part of a more comprehensive theory of misfortune linked to magic and religion. The curer must specify the agent, the reason, and the instrument to effect a cure. Naturalistic theories of etiology are restricted to the illness. The patient is presumed to have caused the disorder through commission or omission of a particular set of behaviors.

Young (1976) has suggested a different twofold classification schema for medical systems. Internalizing systems emphasize physiological explanations. Etiology is linked to a sequence of physical symptoms. Events are ordered within the body in a linear fashion from the onset of symptoms through the course of the illness. Externalizing systems emphasize etiological explanations. The patient provides narratives in which some relevant events take place outside of the patient's body. Causes and effects are identified by precipitating events that occurred in a given sequence of time.

Eisenbruch (1990) used some of these classificatory schemata in developing a Mental Distress Explanatory Model Questionnaire to explore how people from different cultures explain mental distress. A 45-item instrument tapped classification of natural and supernatural causes with items derived from the categories of Murdock et al. (1978). Multidimensional scaling analysis showed four clusters of mental distress: 1) stress, 2) Western physiological, 3) non-Western physiological, and 4) supernatural (mystical, magical, and animistic).

Cervantes and Ramirez (1992) present a four-point conceptual model of Mexican *curanderismo* that seems to apply to most folk healing systems. First is the notion of purpose and balance, mediated by a divine or supernatural power. Failure to follow the prescribed rules of one's belief system upsets this balance, leading to physical or emotional sickness and other ill fortune. Second, illness occurs within a social-interpersonal matrix. Psychological issues have a strong interpersonal base and are directly related to family life cycle and social events as well as to supernatural forces. Third, supernatural causes play a major role, and communication with the spirit world (gods, demons, guardian angels, and the deceased) is required for healing and maintenance of balance. Finally, health is viewed as a naturalistic process "maintained through the balancing of biological needs and social-interpersonal experiences, physical and spiritual harmony, and individual and cultural-familial attachments" (p. 115).

Diagnosis and Treatment

Table 5–1 summarizes some of the major schematic differences between Western mental health treatment and most traditional healing systems in etiological concepts, diagnostic techniques, and treatment modalities. In her study of spiritist healing in Puerto Rico, Koss (1987) reports that causes of illness are viewed as either "material" or "spiritual." Material, or somatic, complaints are initially referred to physicians, whereas emotional problems are thought to be in the spiritual domain. After she developed a collaborative dialogue between mental health professionals and spiritists in the Therapist-Spiritist Training Project (Koss 1980), Koss observed that some of the healers began to identify causation as "psychic" and refer patients to mental health programs.

With respect to Afrocuban *santeria,* Sandoval (1983) points out that *santeros* not only refer patients with organic ailments to physicians but also frequently strengthen the medical intervention with facilitative rituals. In lieu of using their own medicinal potions, "santeros have become content with their new role of assisting physicians in dealing with the physical ailments of their clients by intervening with gods and spirits to enhance the physician's ability to diagnose and treat these ailments" (p. 627). Many healers can also distinguish between major psychiatric illness and problems in living and thus direct the patient toward the mental health system when psychiatric care is indicated. They have collaborated with mental health professionals and advised patients to take their medications and keep follow-up appointments (Sandoval 1979).

What defines a person's behavior as truly pathological and requiring psychiatric intervention or as simply an ephemeral artifact of a religious

Table 5–1. **Comparison of modern and traditional mental health treatment**

Dimension	Modern mental health system	Traditional healing
Etiology		
Source	Biogenetic, psychosocial, and interactive	Supernatural, interpersonal, and interactive
Time frame	Typically historical	Typically ahistorical
Precipitating factors	Psychosocial → interpersonal → intrapsychic	Supernatural → interpersonal
Diagnosis		
Techniques	Observation, interview, anamnesis, and tests	Observation, interview, divination, and mediumship
Symptomatology	Manifest (may or may not specify) → latent (intrapsychic)	Manifest (specifies) → latent (supernatural)
Treatment		
Techniques	Psychodynamic, interpersonal, and systemic: may ignore presenting complaint; focus on understanding underlying psychodynamics, and family and interpersonal relations	Therapeutic regime specific to presenting complaint; focus on counteracting etiologic agent through required behaviors, sometimes changing contingencies of reinforcement to avoid recurrence; alteration of cognitive schemata through appropriate rituals
	Behaviorist and cognitive: specific to presenting complaint; focus on changing contingencies of reinforcement and cognitive schemata	
Mode of interaction	Therapist-patient communication	Communication with supernatural agents
Patient involvement	Primarily verbal or behavioral	Primarily ritualistic performance
Pharmacotherapy	Present as needed	Present as needed
Instrumentality	Insight, abreaction, catharsis, positive human relationship, transference, reinforcement, and corrective behavior	Cleansing, possession, catharsis, corrective behavior (ritualistic), propitiation, and exorcism
Involvement of others	Family or group involvement purposive; dynamic or systems approach	Family or group involvement customary; social support, group cohesion
Major therapeutic goals	Termination of undesirable response: reconstruction and growth	Termination of undesirable stimulus: homeostasis and balance
Therapeutic value orientation	Mastery	Harmony

belief system? How does one differentiate, for example, trance possession behavior that is appropriate in ritual context from behavior that
may be psychotic? Griffith and Ruiz (1977) reported on a hospitalized
practitioner of *espiritismo* and interviewed the patient's family to determine its criteria for psychopathology in cases of spirit possession. They
suggested that possession becomes abnormal when 1) it lasts too long,
since it is typically a quick and transitory experience; 2) there is no per-
ceivable stimulus or condition (i.e., a ceremony, thunder or lightning,
or accidents); and 3) it has a negative orientation. Positive orientation
is ritual possession, whereas negative orientation is sickness possession. In a similar vein, Weidman (1979) suggests that among African-
American and Caribbean groups, fainting as a heightened emotional
response is considered appropriate in ritual context (in church or at fu-
nerals) but is diagnostically differentiated as falling-out, a psychopathological fainting disorder, in extraritual context.

At the therapeutic level, all folk systems may invoke specific herbal
cures; perfumes and potions for cleansing; purification remedies; ritual
prescriptions; sacred words and incantations; and other mechanisms to
resolve problems, achieve desired goals, or undo the malevolent influence of others. Some systems utilize trance possession to effect merger
with the power of a patron saint or god, as in Haitian *vodou,* Afrocuban
santeria, and Brazilian *umbanda.* As Sandoval (1983) has pointed out,
participants gain access to control of the supernatural through magical
manipulation and know-how, conferring a sense of mastery to people
with a history of subjugation and powerlessness.

Integration of Traditional Healing Rituals With Mental Health Treatment

There is considerable debate about whether two basically different conceptual systems may be merged in a psychotherapeutic intervention. In
most cases, we feel that it is inappropriate for nonbelieving mental
health professionals to get into the magical system. Some practitioners
have reported using simulated rituals to attain therapeutic objectives
with difficult patients (Kreisman 1975), and a few have incorporated or

have even performed full exorcisms for "rooted" patients (Lefley 1984). More typical, however, is the use of knowledge of folk beliefs to confirm the clinician's expertise, satisfying Sue and Zane's (1987) paradigm of the culturally sensitive mental health professional perceived as a credible helper.

Applying Cultural Knowledge in Clinical Practice

Cultural knowledge may be essential not only to convey therapeutic credibility but also to avoid potential harm. An example is given by Kinzie et al. (1988) from their work with Southeast Asian Mien refugees. As a stress-reducing exercise in group therapy, they tried to teach the patients relaxation techniques. This procedure was accompanied by dimmed lighting and lower voice tone levels to convey a soothing ambience. The clinicians found that instead of relaxation, the procedures evoked anxiety and apprehension. They later learned that dim light and low voices are associated with a Mien shamanistic ritual to exorcise spirits.

A more positive example of the virtues of attaining cultural knowledge is found in the following case study, in which a therapist went to considerable lengths to become culturally educated in order to unravel what he perceived as a clinical mystery. This case also illustrates that in any culture, traditional healing may apply across all levels of education and socioeconomic status.

A member of a prominent Thai family, Mr. Y, who was working in the United States, was referred to a psychiatrist by his primary physician. The physician could find no basis for Mr. Y's somatic complaints and believed he was clinically depressed, which the patient readily acknowledged. Mr. Y also felt that he was losing his concentration and skills and feared an ignominious return to Thailand that would bring shame to him and his family. Mr. Y's therapy proceeded on the premise of anxiety about meeting the demanding requirements of his job and fear of being unable to fulfill familial expectations. Mr. Y was well educated, knowledgeable about Freudian theory, and a willing candidate for psychodynamic therapy. Historical materials were elicited. However, the patient continued to be depressed and showed at least one symptom that seemed to border on the psychotic. He kept saying that he was afraid of losing his "soul stuff"—that his soul stuff might leave his body and could not be called back.

The psychiatrist questioned Mr. Y about why his soul would leave his body but received no satisfactory answer. The therapist asked about other times that Mr. Y might have thought that he had lost his soul and the precipitating events, but the patient made a gesture of hopelessness, as if he could not explain or the therapist did not understand. At the end of the session, the therapist had the feeling that he had failed in some critical interpretation and that the patient might not return. He sensed massive miscommunication rather than resistance. He had the impression that Mr. Y viewed him (the therapist) as incompetent in some important area of understanding.

The therapist then called the anthropology department of the local university, requested the name of an expert in Thai culture, and was referred to a professor at a university in another city. He set up a formal telephone consultation, told his story, and asked: "Is my patient delusional? Would it be abnormal for an educated Thai to believe that someone is capable of losing his "soul stuff"? The anthropologist replied: "It would probably be abnormal if he did not believe it."

The anthropologist explained that *khwaan nii,* or "my soul stuff flees," is the Thai version of a universal concept in Southeast Asia. It is not synonymous with the Western concept of loss of soul. The *khwaan* is internal spirit, a part of the self, and appears to be essential for ego integration. According to Phillips (1965), "The khwaan has four crucial attributes: (1) although he is of the self, he does not have an independent existence of his own; (2) he is that part of the self that gives the self stability, and, from an analytic point of view, he is really an objectification of human stability; (3) he is recognized to be capricious; and (4) his departure from the body is both cause and effect of the loss of one's wits, steadiness, and equilibrium. If the khwaan stays away too long, the individual may become deranged and may die" (pp. 181–182).

This psychotherapist was quite willing to modify his psychoanalytic stance when he realized that he had failed the patient through his own misinterpretation. Assured that the patient was nondelusional, he called Mr. Y back to treatment after the patient failed, as expected, to keep his next appointment. The therapist discussed with Mr. Y the meaning of the *khwaan nii,* encouraging the patient to educate him on Thai belief systems. He reinforced a plan of action to have a shaman recall the *khwaan* and then was able to disentangle the antecedent and consequent aspects of the patient's anxieties about his role functioning. Many of Mr. Y's anxieties had indeed come about because of the move from Thailand to an unfamiliar culture without familial supports and his fears of not performing adequately in his new job. The reactive threat of losing the *khwaan* could not be dealt with in psychotherapy until the internal spirit had been recalled ritually. Only then could the *khwaan* be recalled psychodynamically.

Sandoval (1977, 1979) has used her knowledge of *santeria* to communicate to patients her understanding of their belief system and their attributions of causality, appropriate remedies, and acceptable and unacceptable behaviors. This knowledge is used to 1) establish trust and rapport, 2) reinforce credibility, 3) legitimate the therapist's authority to set limits on antisocial behavior, and 4) use the patient's own symbolic system in interpretation. However, a clinician's actual performance of folk healing rituals can cause role ambiguity and may result in unwarranted patient expectations.

Ruiz and Langrod (1976) described their involvement with *espiritistas* as follows: 1) identification of mediums; 2) visits to spiritual centers and observations of their modus operandi; 3) exchange of views with mediums; 4) reciprocal referrals; 5) research for training non-Hispanic staff; and 6) plans for sharing training workshops. In the Therapist-Spiritist Training Project in Puerto Rico (Koss 1980, 1987), spiritist healers, mental health workers, and medical and other health professionals met on neutral academic ground over three 10-month periods to exchange ideas and discuss cases, a collaboration resulting in mutual referrals.

Much depends, however, on the patient's type and level of psychopathology. Alonso and Jeffrey (1988) have suggested that a patient's belief in possession may complicate the diagnosis and treatment of psychotic disorders. They state that clinicians need to know about their patients' belief systems (in this case, *santeria*) to understand whether participation in their rituals may be countertherapeutic. Alonso and Jeffrey feel that it is important that some patients avoid rituals involving altered states of consciousness. Indeed, despite the supportive aspects of rituals and cult houses for some persons with schizophrenia (Garrison 1978), it is doubtful whether the highly stimulating ambience of possession rituals, or the altered states themselves, are salutary for persons who are so vulnerable to psychophysiological arousal. In some cases, however, removal of a malevolent spirit or curse may be necessary for the patient to benefit from medications. Examples from our own experience are given in the following section, which briefly describes some major alternative healing systems of African-American, Caribbean, Haitian, and Hispanic heritage.

Applications of Traditional Healing in Miami, Florida

According to Haitian *vodou,* the universe is an interaction of forces emanating from a single almighty power, Gran Met, who shares his power with lesser deities called *loas.* Humans must satisfy their individual *loas's* requirements in order to control most events of their lives, including healing physical and emotional disorders. *Houngans* (males) or *mambos* (females) are *vodou* priest-healers who negotiate with the *loas* on a person's behalf. Their techniques generally involve three modalities. Spiritual reshaping (for depression and anxiety) focuses on counteracting bad luck and reinforces the self-confidence and coping strength of patients by providing them with a greater sense of personal protection. Supernatural strengthening (for phobias, hysterias, and delusions of persecution) appeases spirits, who have been offended by taboo violations, through mechanisms of tribute and reconciliation. Exorcism, the "heaviest" technique, is used for patients presenting with violent hallucinations, unremitting paranoid hostility, and concomitant assaultive behaviors, all believed to be caused by malevolent spirits. These techniques are further described by Charles (1986).

The Afrocuban religion *santeria* also has a pantheon of Yoruba gods (essentially similar to the gods of Brazilian *umbanda*), which in Cuba become syncretized with Catholic saints. Through an initiation process, followers gain access to the power of divine beings, *santos.* The *santo* is a new divinity born of the syncretism between the Yoruba god, or *oricha,* and the Catholic saint. *Santeria* practitioners are called *santeros* (males) or *santeras* (females). Diseases are viewed as products of causes that are both natural (e.g., microbes) and supernatural (e.g., sorcery and witchcraft). Supernatural causes include object intrusion, imitative or contagious magic, loss of one's soul, spirit intrusion, anger of the gods, and the evil eye. *Santeros* use divination systems to identify the causes of disease and their appropriate treatment modalities. Emotional disorders are treated basically by magical rituals (prayers and sacrifices), whereby the authoritarian performance of the *santero* addresses the patient's conflict by inducing catharsis and in some instances suggesting rationalizations and projections that ameliorate ambivalence, fear, and guilt. *Santeros* and *santeras* feel they have considerable ability to deal with depressive, obsessive, hypochondriacal, and phobic reactions (Sandoval 1983). To counter disease or emotional disorder, individuals' *santos* must be appeased and enlisted to work on their behalf. Thus, empowered by the *santero's* authority and knowledge of appropriate rituals, this belief system functionally permits mastery of disorder through manipulation of the powerful gods (Sandoval 1977, 1979, 1983).

Rootwork and *obeah* are essentially medicinal-magical systems without the elaborate infrastructure of the deities of the religious belief systems. Rootwork combines a model of magical causation, involving cures by sorcery with an empiric tradition of natural causation and herbal or medicinal cures of physical disorders. Both sorcery and herbal remedies may be used in the treatment of psychosocial or emotional disorders (Mathews 1987). *Obeah* similarly lacks a pantheon of gods and specific remedies through spirit possession. Both systems essentially have a one-to-one relationship of healer and patient, although the family may be brought in for support.

Spiritism, or *espiritismo,* is a syncretic religious and philosophical healing system developed by a nineteenth-century scholar writing under the pseudonym of Alan Kardec. Kardec developed a means of communication with the spirit world, which, according to Weiss (1992), was for secular rather than religious healing purposes. In this philosophy there are wise and benevolent spirits and troublesome spirits called *causas.* "Causas afflicting an individual can be identified and often 'worked' to some resolution by a medium. Working the causas for others, and developing one's own spiritual 'faculties' (for protection against causas and communication with more benign spirits) helps the individual to surmount his or her own problems" (Weiss 1992, p. 244). Koss (1987, p. 56) describes the healing ambience as follows: "A spiritist healing takes place most frequently in a group setting, and no fees are charged by those healers considered legitimate. Mediums receive spirit messages or become possessed by either good or molesting spirits in order to diagnose, counsel, prescribe herbal and ritual remedies, and prognosticate." Spiritism is one of the most pervasive alternative belief systems, crossing many cultural boundaries. As Koss (1987) notes, Kardec's writings had been widely disseminated throughout Spain, Eastern Europe, and Latin America by the end of the nineteenth century.

Mental Health Professionals' Roles: Some Case Examples

We have previously described the role of the culturally educated clinician whose understanding conveys both credibility and rapport. Such clinicians are able to perceive the discrete gains of their patients' use of dual healing systems without themselves participating in the magical system (Sandoval 1977, 1979). The following two cases describe other roles. Both cases involve removal of a barrier to optimal psychiatric care for nonresponsive hospitalized patients. The first case exemplifies a merged brokerage and alternative healing role by mental health staff.

After 10 days of hospitalization, a Haitian schizophrenic patient could not be stabilized on neuroleptics because he believed he was under a curse that required an exorcism of malevolent spirits. The patient was released overnight to Haitian mental health staff for this purpose. Performed by a *vodou* priest with the participation of Haitian mental health technicians, the syncretic ceremony merged masonic rites with those of *vodou*. After the ceremony the patient was observably calmed, responded to medications, and was soon discharged for outpatient care to the Haitian team.

The second case involves a brokerage function alone on the part of staff. This case exemplifies the interesting crossover ritual, in which a patient from one cultural belief system utilizes a syntonic healing system from another culture because it is perceived as conveying more power.

A medical center anthropologist was called for consultation by inpatient staff for an African-American woman who could not be stabilized on medications. The patient believed that a Hispanic woman in her office was jealous and had hexed her. She felt that African-American rootwork could not help her, because the curse was of Hispanic origin. Both patient and ward staff requested a spiritual intervention. The anthropologist took the patient to a Puerto Rican *espiritista,* who communicated with spirits and then told the patient to take flowers to a cemetery. She was also instructed to throw four coconuts, hard, into the middle of an intersection and to leave without looking back to get rid of the curse. After completing the required tasks, the patient responded well and was soon discharged.

Since both of these cases involved excursions from the hospital, as well as active efforts by the patients, alternative explanations for the improvement are readily apparent.

Working With Haitian Acquired Immunodeficiency Syndrome Patients: Collaboration With *Vodou* Priests

Increasingly we are seeing patients with the human immunodeficiency virus (HIV) in the populations of persons with major mental illnesses. In Miami, Hispanic and Haitian patients with acquired immunodeficiency syndrome (AIDS) are often referred to the few remaining programs for Cuban and Haitian entrants. This situation presents problems for the other patients and adds a new dimension to caregiving for persons with mental illness.

Denial of illness has long been a feature of Haitian culture, because in a poor economy, sickness is equated with loss of productivity, dependency, and ultimately death (Charles 1986). However, AIDS has had a particular stigma ever since the Centers for Disease Control singled out Haitians as a high-risk group, with powerfully adverse political and economic consequences for the Haitian community as a whole.

Working with Haitian AIDS patients in Miami often involves collaboration with *vodou* priests, who are able to keep patients involved in their own healing until the very end. The techniques of applying potions, making deals with the supernatural, and conducting other rituals serve to maintain hope and prevent depression in terminal AIDS patients. *Vodou* practices tend to give these patients more stability and assurance; they offer a way of mastering problems and controlling destiny. Combined with the medical and psychosocial interventions of the mental health system, the *houngan*'s assurance rallied a particular patient and indeed may have prolonged his life.

In our experience at the New Horizons Community Mental Health Center, we found that a collaborative relationship with a *houngan* or *mambo* helps Haitian AIDS patients cope more effectively and accept treatment more readily. Some HIV-positive patients referred to the program quit after a few months. However, those who are treated and linked with traditional healers remain for 2 and sometimes 3 years. Azidothymidine (AZT) has side effects, and patients report that the healers' potions of leaves, roots, and fruits seem to make the side effects less troublesome.

Different Explanatory Models, Positive Outcomes

We end this section with a case sample that may exemplify the different conceptual models used by psychiatrists and traditional healers in addressing etiology, diagnosis, and treatment. The patient was treated by C. Charles and represents crossover cases of African-American women who sought the more powerful magic of a Haitian healer. In discussing this case, we note also that although psychiatry and traditional healing proceed through different conceptual channels, both systems have the final goal of returning competency and control to the patient.

Mrs. Z, an African-American woman of Bahamian descent, presented with symptoms of clinical depression. She believed her lover had another girlfriend who had placed a love curse or hex on her. The hex was causing problems with her children and job and cooling the interest of her lover. Mrs. Z perceived her "blues" as caused by the curse itself rather than as a reaction to her situation. She believed the girlfriend had gone to a Bahamian *obeah* man to provide the hex, so Mrs. Z herself went to an even more powerful Haitian healer to counteract the malevolence. The healer cleansed her with special perfumes, oils, and herbs and gave her special tasks to perform that would align her with the benign forces of the universe. To finalize the therapeutic intervention, the healer took Mrs. Z to a cemetery at midnight, lowered her into an unfilled grave, and covered most of her body with grave dirt. After the ritual "burial," Mrs. Z was euphoric. In a short period of time she reported that her children were acting better. She also issued an ultimatum to her boyfriend to stop seeing the other woman and later ended the relationship herself. Mrs. Z was then able to form a therapeutic alliance and proceed with her counseling at the community mental health center.

The clinician would conceptualize this case in terms of psychodynamics, whereas the traditional healer would view it in terms of exchange. In the therapist's perception, the symbolic burial enabled Mrs. Z to shed her ineffectual self, weakness, and vulnerability and to take control of her life through symbolic rebirth. In the conceptual system of the healer, this control is achieved through removal of spiritual obstacles. In this model, purification and burial are a reordering or rebalancing of universal forces. Mrs. Z is under the influence of a malevolent spirit evoked by the girlfriend's curse. All bad spirits belong to the cemetery, so the healer goes directly to that forcefield and puts the person in the ground. By burying the carrier, one buries the evil spirit. When the person is taken out of the grave, the malevolent influence remains in the ground and the person is free.

In reviewing Mrs. Z's case, it should be noted that both psychodynamic and spiritual healing are oriented toward an outcome of informed personal control. To achieve this goal, psychotherapy typically focuses on insight and abreaction, on cognitive or emotional restructuring, or on behavioral change to effect a more healthy, productive, and satisfying way of life. Patients are led toward recognizing obstacles to change and shedding maladaptive behaviors. In spiritual healing, the ultimate goal is to move patients toward personal control by reassurance that external and internal spiritual obstacles have been removed. Ritualistic performance ensures that the patient is an active participant in removing these obstacles. Each ritual, ranging from lighting a candle to trance possession, represents an alliance with and often an introjection of supernatural power. The spiritual healer conveys the message that because of fulfillment of appropriate behaviors, the patient now has the assistance of spiritual forces; the way was dark, but the pathway is now light, and the person can go forward to engineer his or her own destiny. Both psychotherapy and traditional healing may have short- or long-term goals targeted toward episodic problem resolution or developing internalized skills for coping and mastery. The conceptual and treatment processes of the two systems are vastly different, but important therapeutic objectives seem to be comparable.

Conclusions

A contemporary islandwide study of Puerto Rico found that almost one-fifth of the population had utilized spiritists, often in conjunction with mental health practitioners (Hohmann et al. 1990). In South Florida and other areas with large immigrant populations, both research and clinical experience suggest that many of our patients use multiple systems of care. The use of scientific and alternative healing systems, each serving different needs, in many cases leads to the patient's perception of a more holistic intervention and a more satisfactory outcome.

Traditional beliefs and their healing systems are anchors of security for people undergoing the stresses of uprooting, translocation, and adaptation to the changed values and new reference points of a bewildering new society. However, most belief systems also change, syncretizing with other models and evolving organically into new patterns, and their practitioners change accordingly. In the country of origin, healers were viewed as endowed with special powers for accessing the supernatural. The professional and economic components of the role were separate, so they rarely requested payment. Any reimbursement was up to the patient and family. In their new adaptations in the United States, some healers ask for large sums of money before they will perform. Many practitioners of alternative healing are expanding their base, becoming entrepreneurs, and selling their services to the highest bidders. Although they are not unlike many Western colleagues in this regard, traditional healers function on the basis of spiritual as well as technological skills, and their special powers may become contaminated. Since traditional healing systems are nonstandardized and unregulated, there are new opportunities for mercenaries and charlatans, many of whom may deflect patients from needed medical or mental health resources.

Rappaport and Rappaport (1981) have suggested that since traditional and Western scientific healing systems operate with a different disease model and a different worldview, they are best viewed as complementary rather than integrated systems. In this chapter, we have discussed the complementary roles that the two systems may play, each serving a different vital need of the individual believer. The role of the mental health professional, whether as opponent, knowledgeable observer, or actual linkage agent, depends on personal viewpoint, cultural sophistication, institutional circumstances, available alternative resources, and the needs of the specific patient.

References

Alonso L, Jeffrey WD: Mental illness complicated by the santeria belief in spirit possession. Hosp Community Psychiatry 39:1188–1191, 1988

American Psychiatric Association: Diagnostic and Statistical Manual of Mental Disorders, 3rd Edition. Washington, DC, American Psychiatric Association, 1980

Bilu Y, Witztum E: Working with Jewish ultra-orthodox patients: guidelines for culturally sensitive therapy. Cult Med Psychiatry 17:197–233, 1993

Cervantes JM, Ramirez O: Spirituality and family dynamics in psychotherapy with Latino children, in Working With Culture. Edited by Vargas LA, Koss-Chioino JD. San Francisco, CA, Jossey-Bass, 1992, pp 103–128

Charles C: Mental health services for Haitians, in Cross-Cultural Training for Mental Health Professionals. Edited by Lefley HP, Pedersen PB. Springfield, IL, Charles C Thomas, 1986, pp 183–198

Chien CP, Yamamoto J: Asian-American and Pacific-Islander patients, in Effective Psychotherapy for Low-Income and Minority Patients. Edited by Acosta FX, Yamamoto J, Evans LA. New York, Plenum, 1982, pp 117–145

Csordas TJ: The affliction of Martin: religious, clinical, and phenomenological meaning in a case of demonic possession, in Ethnopsychiatry. Edited by Gaines AD. Albany, NY, State University of New York Press, 1992, pp 125–170

Eisenbruch M: Classification of natural and supernatural causes of mental distress: development of a Mental Distress Explanatory Model Questionnaire. J Nerv Ment Dis 178:712–719, 1990

Favazza A: Modern Christian healing of mental illness. Am J Psychiatry 139:728–735, 1982

Foster GM: Disease etiologies in non-Western medical systems. American Anthropologist 78:773–776, 1976

Garrison V: Support systems of schizophrenic and nonschizophrenic Puerto Rican migrant women in New York City. Schizophr Bull 4:561–596, 1978

Griffith EEH, Ruiz P: Cultural factors in the training of psychiatry residents in an Hispanic urban community. Psychiatr Q 49:29–37, 1977

Hohmann AA, Richeport M, Marriott BM, et al: Spiritism in Puerto Rico: results of an island-wide community study. Br J Psychiatry 156:328–335, 1990

Kinzie JD, Leung P, Bui A, et al: Group therapy with Southeast Asian refugees. Community Ment Health J 24:157–166, 1988

Koss JD: Therapist-Spiritist Training Project in Puerto Rico: an experiment to relate the traditional healing system to the public health system. Soc Sci Med 14B:255–266, 1980

Koss JD: Expectations and outcomes for patients given mental health care or spiritist healing in Puerto Rico. Am J Psychiatry 144:56–61, 1987

Kreisman JJ: The curandero's apprentice: a therapeutic integration of folk and medical healing. Am J Psychiatry 132:81–83, 1975

Lefley HP: Environmental interventions and therapeutic outcome. Hosp Community Psychiatry 30:341–344, 1979

Lefley HP: Delivering mental health services across cultures, in Mental Health Services: The Cross-Cultural Context. Edited by Pedersen PB, Sartorius N, Marsella A. Beverly Hills, CA, Sage, 1984, pp 135–171

Lefley HP: Evaluating the effects of cross-cultural training: some research results, in Cross-Cultural Training for Mental Health Professionals. Edited by Lefley HP, Pedersen PB. Springfield, IL, Charles C Thomas, 1986, pp 265–307

Lefley HP: Dealing with cross-cultural issues in clinical settings, in Innovations in Clinical Practice: A Sourcebook, Vol 10. Edited by Keller P. Sarasota, FL, Professional Resource Exchange, 1991, pp 99–115

Lefley HP, Bestman EW: Public-academic linkages for culturally sensitive community mental health. Community Ment Health J 27:473–488, 1991

Mathews HF: Rootwork: description of an ethnomedical system in the American South. South Med J 80:885–891, 1987

Murdock GP, Wilson S, Frederick V: World distribution of theories of illness. Ethnology 17:449–470, 1978

Ness RC, Wintrob RM: Folk healing: a description and synthesis. Am J Psychiatry 138:1477–1481, 1981

Phillips HP: Thai Peasant Personality. Berkeley and Los Angeles, CA, University of California Press, 1965

Rapoport JL: The Boy Who Couldn't Stop Washing: The Experience and Treatment of Obsessive-Compulsive Disorder. New York, New American Library, 1990

Rappaport H, Rappaport M: The integration of scientific and traditional healing. Am Psychol 36:774–781, 1981

Ruiz P, Langrod J: The role of folk healers in community health services. Community Ment Health J 12:392–398, 1976

Sandoval M: Santeria: Afrocuban concepts of disease and its treatment in Miami. Journal of Operational Psychiatry 8:52–63, 1977

Sandoval M: Santeria as a mental health care system: an historical overview. Soc Sci Med 13B:137–151, 1979

Sandoval M: Santeria. J Fla Med Assoc 70:620–628, 1983

Sue S, Zane N: The role of culture and cultural techniques in psychotherapy. Am Psychol 42:37–45, 1987

Weidman HH: Falling-out: a diagnostic and treatment problem viewed from a transcultural perspective. Soc Sci Med B13:95–112, 1979

Weiss CI: Controlling domestic life and mental illness: spiritual and aftercare resources used by Dominican New Yorkers. Cult Med Psychiatry 16:237–271, 1992

Young A: Internalizing and externalizing medical belief systems: an Ethiopian example. Soc Sci Med 19:147–156, 1976

CHAPTER 6

The New Zealand Maori and the Contemporary Health System

Response of an Indigenous People to Mainstream Medicine

PERMINDER SACHDEV, M.D., PH.D., F.R.A.N.Z.C.P.

Te maatauranga o te Pakeha	The knowledge of the Pakeha (European)
He mea whakatoo hei tinanatanga	is propagated
Moo wai ra? . . .	For whom? . . .
Hei patu tikanga	To kill customs
Patu mahara	To kill memory
Mauri e	To kill our sacred powers.

—*Tuini Ngawai, Ngaati Porou composer, circa 1950*

In this chapter, I discuss the interaction of the indigenous Maori people of New Zealand with the contemporary health system in that country. I highlight the difficulties that the Maori face in their interaction with health professionals from a predominately Western culture and medical tradition and their problems in utilizing the mainstream health system. Relevant socioeconomic and political factors that influence the transactions are discussed briefly. The latter part of the chapter details the attempts to bridge the gap between the community and the health services, with particular emphasis on the response of the Maori community itself and its empowerment to bring about change.

The Maori of New Zealand

The Maori,[1] the indigenous Polynesian people of New Zealand, attribute their presence in *Aotearoa* ("the land of the long white cloud") to waves of migration in the early part of this millennium. Europeans first contacted the Maori in the late eighteenth century when the country was explored by the British naval officer James Cook, paving the way for colonization.[2] The Maori of this period were agriculturists and had reached a high point in the arts of warfare, canoe construction, weaving, and building. The Maori society was divided into groups called *iwi* (tribes),[3] politically and militarily coordinated, with the members of each group tracing their descent to a common ancestor. The *iwi* consisted of a number of *hapu* (subtribes), groups numbering a few hundred, made up of families who married within their group. The *hapu,* in turn, consisted of a number of *whanau* (extended families), which were the units of social life. A comprehensive account of Maori society before and since colonization can be obtained from standard works by Best (1924), Buck (1950), Firth (1959), and Metge (1976).

James Cook estimated the Maori population to be between 100,000 and 300,000 near the end of the eighteenth century (Schwimmer 1974). The numbers dropped sharply during the first century of European settlement but have risen again in the latter twentieth century. At the 1986 Census, 12.4% (404,778) of New Zealand's population identified itself as being of Maori descent, with the majority of the 3.2 million inhabitants being of European extraction (called *Pakeha* by the Maori). The Maori population is youthful: 71% are under 30 years of age, and only 2% are over 65 years of age.

Maori life was profoundly affected by colonization. The unfamiliar capitalist economy of the Europeans changed the whole material basis of life. Christianity cut across sanctions and prohibitions, thus altering the social fabric, which was modified by new beliefs and pursuits.

---

1. The word *Maori,* like many other Maori nouns, is currently used as both singular and plural.

2. The first documented European to arrive in New Zealand was Abel Tasman, a Dutch sailor, in 1642.

3. Williams's (1975) *A Dictionary of the Maori Language* is used as the standard reference for the Maori words used.

After the British formally assumed control of the country following the Treaty of Waitangi[4] in 1840, the Maori waged a series of wars against the colonists that resulted in the loss of enormous tracts of Maori territory and a further disruption of Maori society. Then began a process of readjustment that is still continuing. Massive urbanization of the Maori occurred in the 1950s to 1970s and resulted in increased participation of the Maori in the industrialized economy, as well as increased cultural contact with the Pakeha. This contact led to intermarriage and disruption of the extended family networks traditional for the Maori.

A majority of the Maori remain in the lower strata of New Zealand's social hierarchy, although a dispersion can be seen at all levels. The educational achievement of most Maori children is below that of the non-Maori (62% of Maori leave secondary school without passing at least one subject of School Certificate, compared with 28% of non-Maori; only 9.5% qualify for university entrance compared with 34% of non-Maori). The unemployment rate of Maori youth is more than twice that of the non-Maori. Physical and psychological health indicators again suggest that the Maori are at a disadvantage, as do indicators of social instability such as domestic violence, broken marriages, court appearances, and dependence on social welfare.

General Comments on Methodology

The information presented in this chapter is drawn in part from studies conducted by me between 1983 and 1989 in Auckland (1983–1985), Dunedin (1985–1987), and Sydney (1987–1989); field visits to Tokanui Hospital and Te Awamutu (1984 and 1989) and Rotorua (1985 and 1989); and repeat visits to the psychiatric hospitals in Auckland and

---

4. The Treaty of Waitangi was negotiated between Britain's designated consul and lieutenant governor William Hobson and many North Island chiefs. It was signed at the northern settlement of Waitangi on February 5–6, 1840. The treaty purportedly transferred sovereignty over the Maori people to the British Crown (Kawharu 1989). The motives behind the treaty, the manner of its execution, the adherence to it by later governments, and its current status are all shrouded in controversy, and the treaty has often been a rallying point for activism by the Maori, who accuse the British government of fraud.

Wellington in 1989. I was assisted in my studies by a number of Maori patients, their relatives and friends, Maori and Pakeha scholars, Maori participants in *hui* (ceremonial gatherings), and Maori elders (*kaumatua* and *kuia*).

It became clear early in the investigations that research on the Maori had to be handled with sensitivity and caution. Many Maori people resent ethnographic research that has seemingly misrepresented them in the past or appeared removed from the reality of their existence. In many quarters, there is a suspicion of Pakeha researchers and an expression of the need for Maori researchers who would be more sensitive to the Maori point of view (Awatere et al. 1984; Pomare and de Boer 1988). It was possible to overcome this attitude by showing genuine interest and concern for the Maori people and by persistence. My non-European background and my status as a doctor to many psychiatrically ill Maori patients helped the process, but the initial data gathering was slow. In general, the Maori are a proud people who are quite willing to share their culture with an outsider once trust has been established.

Physical Health of the Maori

Although the health status of the Maori people has improved significantly during the last four decades (Pomare 1980; Pomare and de Boer 1988), it continues to lag behind the non-Maori on most indices of health, with higher rates of many common disorders.

While many causes have been identified for the excess morbidity and mortality in the Maori, several reviews (Pomare 1980; Sachdev 1990; A. H. Smith and Pearce 1984) have implicated behavioral factors, including adverse lifestyle factors such as smoking, alcohol abuse, overnutrition, and accidents, to a major extent. According to the 1974–1978 analysis by A. H. Smith and Pearce (1984), the following behavioral factors could be identified as contributing to the excess mortality of Maori between the ages of 15 and 64 years of age: obesity, 5% for both sexes; smoking, 15% for males and 16% for females; alcohol abuse (excluding alcohol-related accidents), 10% for males and 2% for females; and accidents, 17% for males and 8% for females. A. H. Smith and Pearce also reported that rheumatic and hypertensive heart disease, nephritis, bronchiectasis, diabetes, and tuberculosis, all diseases for which there are effective treatments, were at least five times more likely to prove fatal among Maori than among non-Maori. This finding suggests either a poor delivery of health care services to the Maori or an ineffective use of these services by the Maori (Hyslop et al. 1983).

Psychiatric Illness in the Maori

The data on psychiatric morbidity are from secondary sources, since no population-based survey of the Maori has been conducted. These data suggest that the Maori have a slightly greater risk of psychiatric hospitalization than the non-Maori. First admission and readmission rates for schizophrenia are higher among the Maori. First admission rates for major affective illnesses are roughly comparable with those of the non-Maori, and those for neuroses and neurotic depression are lower in the Maori. Rates of admission for alcohol abuse, alcohol dependence, and personality disorders are much higher for the Maori male aged 20–40 years, the group at greatest risk of psychiatric hospitalization. A larger proportion of Maori are admitted involuntarily, especially under the Criminal Justice Act. The Maori have shown an increase in first psychiatric admission rates since the 1950s, with rapid increases in the early 1960s and the 1980s. The rates for psychotic disorders have been relatively constant, and the most significant changes have been for alcohol abuse, alcohol dependence, and personality disorders. These changes relate to socioeconomic and politicocultural factors, in particular the stress of rapid urbanization (Sachdev 1989b).

The Medical Establishment in New Zealand

The medical establishment in New Zealand is part of the Western scientific tradition. This tradition can be traced back to the early postcontact years when the European settlers brought the Western medical system with them to the colony. Social security was introduced between 1938 and 1940, thus creating a free public health system accessible to everyone. What has emerged since then is called the dual system, which is comprised of both state-funded public provisions and state-subsidized private or voluntary provisions. General practice and other primary care entities belong to the latter category. General (or family) physicians provide initial medical contact, except in emergency situations. Consultation with a general physician is highly subsidized by the state, but the patient still has to pay a small amount, which may be significant for families with low income. Of the total number of hospitals, 80% are state hospitals and free; the remaining 20% are subsidized by the state. Psychiatric patients occupy 42% of all hospital beds, although this situation is changing because of a move toward deinstitutionalization. The country spends approximately 8% of the gross national product (GNP) on health. A few other systems of medicine (e.g., naturopathy, osteopathy, and acupuncture) complement the main system to a small extent but do not compete with it.

How Do the Maori Interact With Modern Doctors and the Contemporary Health System?

Before contact with the Europeans, the Maori consulted the *tohunga* (skilled person) in cases of illness. Illness was generally attributed to violation of *tapu* (supernatural influence or restriction) or the presence of *makutu* (curse). The *tohunga* acted as the intermediary between humans and the *atua* (gods) and performed atonement rites or elaborate rituals to redress lapses or imbalances of supernatural power. A detailed description of *tapu* is provided elsewhere (Sachdev 1989a). Colonization brought with it a number of diseases to which the Maori had not been exposed and against which they had little resistance. The Maori *tohunga* had a limited repertoire of therapies, and "the disease spirits of the white man would not obey his exhortations to leave" (Buck 1950, p. 409).[5] A number of factors led to the adoption of Western medicine

---

5. There were evidently no endemic or epidemic diseases in New Zealand in the pre-European days. Typhoid, tuberculosis, measles, and venereal diseases were all introduced by

by the Maori. One of these factors was the rapid decline in the Maori population to an estimated 37,520 in 1871, to which both wars and Pakeha diseases contributed. The other was the realization that in many cases Pakeha medicine was the only effective cure for certain disorders. Contact with the Pakeha and the adoption of Christianity weakened the hold of *tapu* and *makutu* on the populace, making a scientific explanation of disease more acceptable to them. The accessibility of medical attention to the Maori was another factor in the Maori adoption of Western medicine.

Although significant differences exist in health indicators between the Maori and the Pakeha, as indicated previously, the acceptance of the Pakeha health system by the Maori is generally taken for granted by health planners. Consultation with the *tohunga* is minimal, especially in the urban Maori, who constitute three-quarters of the total Maori population. If the Maori have the same access to the health system as the Pakeha and yet perform poorly on most health indicators, is it possible that their help seeking behavior is different, leading to a suboptimal usage of the facilities? This question has been partially addressed by empirical research. At the primary care level, studies suggest a higher rate of medical contact for the Maori compared with the non-Maori (Davis 1986; West and Harris 1980), although this rate may still fall short of the estimates based on the illness burden (Davis 1986). The hospital data lead to a similar conclusion (Mitchell and Borman 1986). In the case of psychiatric illness, for the years 1981–1983, the patient or his or her relative was the source of referral for admission to psychiatric treatment in 12.5% of Maori, compared with 10.3% in non-Maori psychiatric admissions. These data suggest that the Maori are not particularly averse to seeking Western medical treatment for psychiatric problems and that the Maori use the Pakeha health system.

The more difficult question to address in a research study is whether the Maori use the system effectively. Informed comments suggest that the Maori do not often seek help voluntarily for problems such as obesity (Murchie 1984) or alcoholism (Awatere et al. 1984). Other commentators have outlined various reasons for the Maori's discomfort with Pakeha hospitals and doctors (Marsden 1986; Walker 1982). The

---

the Europeans (Buck 1950). Since the natives lacked immunity to these diseases, the effect was devastating.

major factor identified is the monocultural nature of these institutions that dismisses the obvious, and certainly the subtle, cultural differences and expectations that the Maori bring with them. These cultural differences impact on the interaction of the Maori patient with both the Pakeha doctor and the hospital. Furthermore, Maori commentators have stressed that the Maori concept of health is different from that of the Pakeha, with an emphasis on the spiritual and family components in addition to the physical and psychological ones (Durie 1985). What a Pakeha may view as unhealthy may not be so in Maori eyes and vice versa. Neglect of one aspect of health by the health care system may well lead to the neglect of other aspects as well.

Some Possible Reasons for the Ineffective Usage of the Health System by the Maori

The problems in the interaction of the Maori with the mainstream health system have attracted considerable scholarly interest and comment (Broughton 1984; Durie 1977; *Hui Whakaoranga* 1984; Jacobsen 1983; Older 1978; Pomare 1986) from both Maori (i.e., Durie and Pomare) and non-Maori (i.e., Older and Jacobsen). However, this interest has led to little anthropological investigation. The discussion therefore lacks the credibility of quantifiable data. The following is an attempt to collate observations on which there is a great deal of consensus, especially within Maori society and among those familiar with the culture. Maori attitudes toward Western medicine, problems in the communication between Pakeha health professionals and Maori patients, the inflexibility of the health system to accommodate the cultural differences of the Maori, and relics of traditional Maori beliefs and practices have all contributed to the current problems in the attempt to integrate the Maori into New Zealand's Western medical system. The power equation must not be ignored. The health system is controlled by the Pakeha, and the Maori population is not only an underrepresented minority but a socioeconomically disadvantaged one as well. It is certainly likely that some Maori will see the Pakeha insistence on the Maori utilization of the system as another instance of control by a dominant group whose values are sometimes unacceptable and in conflict with Maori values. This resentment has historical roots and is expressed openly in Maori forums (*Hui Whakaoranga* 1984; Walker 1982); thus, it may explain some of the reported Maori reluctance to use hospitals (Mackay 1985) but cannot be the only reason.

Pakeha-Maori Communication in Medical Practice

Effective communication between the doctor and the patient is a fundamental prerequisite of much of medical diagnostics and management. Maori patients and the Pakeha health professionals treating them have often commented on the difficulties of communication across cultures and the not infrequent misunderstandings that result. Previous cross-cultural studies have demonstrated ethnic differences in illness and help seeking behavior (Kleinman 1980; Landy 1977; Pilowsky and Spence 1977), which would make a study of Maori-Pakeha differences instructive in this context. Since health professionals are predominantly Pakeha (J. Older and D. Jensen, unpublished observation, June 1976), the situation of concern is one of a Maori patient meeting a Pakeha doctor, nurse, or other professional. The following reasons can be identified for the failure in communication:

1. Use of language. English is the common language of communication, and all Maori, except perhaps a rare elderly person in a rural area, speak English. Their command of the language and their use of metaphor and sophisticated nuance has often been demonstrated to be more limited than that of the Pakeha (Bray and Hill 1974). Few Pakeha speak any Maori at all, and, moreover, a large number of urban Maori have little or no knowledge of the Maori language. These factors combine to lead to a situation in which the Maori patient generally has to communicate in limited English, often hesitantly and incompletely. Durie (1984), a Maori psychiatrist, reported that about half of his general psychiatric Maori patients reported feeling inadequate in their usage of English, although staff members assumed them fluent. About half of this group welcomed a chance to discuss their problems in Maori. The emphasis on precise verbal communication in Western culture can often make the Pakeha doctor insensitive to the patient's difficulty in explaining and can lead to a patronizing attitude in the physician and frustration in the patient (Metge and Kinloch 1979). This disruption of doctor-patient rapport is likely to have a detrimental effect on diagnostic precision, especially for psychiatric illness and patient compliance. One further aspect of doctor-patient communication to consider is the positive effect on the relationship if the Pakeha professional has some knowledge of Maori, pronounces the patient's name correctly, and uses the common Maori greetings (Jacobsen 1983).

2. Use of nonverbal communication. The Maori emphasize body language more and verbalization less than the Pakeha (Metge and Kinloch 1979). It is not uncommon to hear the Maori complain about the Pakeha who is "forever talking" but "deaf to what others have to say" (mostly nonverbally). In addition to this emphasis on nonverbal language, a cross-cultural difference in the interpretation of some signs can create difficulties. The Maori patient tends not to look the professional in the eye in deference to the latter's authority but instead looks to the side or at the floor or ceiling. Direct eye contact is often considered threatening (Metge and Kinloch 1979) and is thus avoided.

The Maori may also use different signs to indicate agreement or disagreement. They recognize the nod and headshake as meaning "yes" and "no" but may use other indicators, such as an upward movement of the head and/or eyebrows to indicate "yes" and an unresponsive stare straight ahead or down at the feet to indicate "no." The hunching up of the shoulders often means "I don't know" rather than "I don't care" (Jacobsen 1983). A frown may indicate not only disapproval but also puzzlement or a plea for help (Metge and Kinloch 1979). Sniffing by a Maori often signifies admission of a mistake and an apology rather than rejection. A further difference is in the use of silence. Silence in response to a question indicates either rejection of the idea or that the Maori patient needs more time to think about it. In a busy clinic or hospital, interpretation of silence as affirmation is likely and must be expressly avoided with the Maori patient. These differences aside, the Maori use a number of nonverbal signals in a manner very similar to the Pakeha (Jacobsen 1983).

3. Attitude toward authority. A number of authors have commented on the Maori's deference to the authority of the health professional, especially the doctor (Durie 1984; Mackay 1985). This deference has been traced to the early relationship of the common person with the *tohunga,* who was a man imbued with great *mana* (power, prestige) and therefore worthy of great respect and awe. It may also be explained on the basis of the *mana* associated with age and achievement in Maori society (Buck 1950). A doctor is therefore approached only warily, and few demands are made on him or her. This attitude may also extend to nurses, physiotherapists, and the like (Rostenburg 1981). A Maori patient visiting a busy clinic may hesitate to present all of the facts of the case and may underemphasize his or her problems (Durie 1984). The patient may not challenge the doctor even if he or she disagrees, often leading a Maori patient to discontinue the use of medicines rather than report unacceptable side effects (Tipene-Leach 1978). This attitude may sometimes create problems in examination as well. While being examined for tenderness during palpation of the abdomen, the patient may repeatedly respond, "No, doctor, it doesn't hurt," when in fact the area of the abdomen does hurt (M. J. Beagley, unpublished observation, March 1984) but the patient does not want to indict the doctor for causing pain.

4. The use of touch. The Maori characterize themselves as very "touching people" (Metge and Kinloch 1979). "A hand laid on the hand, arm, or shoulder of another or a generous hug is variously used to convey sympathy, support, gratitude, apology, and a desire for friendship as well as recognition of an established relationship" (Metge and Kinloch 1979, p. 12). This factor can be useful in the clinical setting. On the other hand, the Maori are "shy" of their bodies and reluctant to submit to physical examination, especially of the intimate kind (Jacobsen 1983).

5. Decision making and responsibility. A modern medical practitioner, in communicating with a patient, expects the latter to make a number of choices and to take a degree of responsibility for these choices (Mechanic 1978). It is also generally accepted that Parsons's (1951) description of the submissive, passive, and dependent patient is not applicable to most patients (Segall 1976) and particularly to psychiatric patients (Sobell and Ingalls 1964), who are expected to be active participants in the treatment process. Because these role expectations vary with culture (Segall 1976), they are likely to be different for the Maori. The Maori are reportedly more passive in the therapeutic encounter (Durie 1984). Moreover, they tend to deliberate a great deal on any issue and seek the opinion of others before finalizing any decision (Metge and Kinloch 1979). They are likely to appear indecisive in a busy clinical setting, thus creating the danger that doctors or nurses may make decisions concerning treatment without allowing the patient sufficient time to consider options. In addition, the Maori are generally unlikely to express themselves freely until a personal affective rapport has been established (Ritchie 1963), a trait that carries over to their interaction with health professionals (Walker 1982). In seeking medical advice, they are likely to leave decisions to the "expert" rather than participate in a one-on-one interchange (Tipene-Leach 1978). This kind of behavior toward medical experts has also been described in other cultures that emphasize kinship and affiliation rather than individuality and differentiation (Neki 1976).

6. Involvement of family. The Maori culture greatly emphasizes the involvement of the *whanau* (family group) with the ill person. This characteristic is particularly apparent in the tendency for a large number of family members to stay with the patient during the illness in order to prevent the ailing family member from feeling that he or she has been forsaken. The family is involved in decisions about treatment in practical help to the patient's immediate dependents and in the rehabilitation process.

Traditional Maori Customs Affecting the Utilization of the Modern Health System

Although the long contact with the Pakeha has greatly altered Maori culture, a number of Maori traditions have persisted and continue to influence, consciously or unconsciously, the daily life of the Maori (Dansey 1978). Some of these traditions affecting the interaction between the Maori and the health system follow.

1. Laws of *tapu*.   The concept of *tapu* (supernatural influence or sacred restriction) is pervasive in traditional Maori society. Disease, death, and healing are intensely *tapu* for the Maori, and the etiology of disease is often related to the breach of *tapu* laws. It is for this reason that the Maori relate to illness, doctors, and hospitals with some anxiety and awe. Considering the modern health institutions' secularization and professed egalitarianism, it is not surprising to find that the Maori often complains of lack of "spirituality" in the modern hospital (Pomare 1986). Thus, while accepting Western treatment, it is common for the Maori to simultaneously explore his or her personal and familial circumstances to find "the real cause" (Durie 1977, p. 484), which usually involves breach of some *tapu* law.

Other *tapu* rules may make some of the practices in hospitals unacceptable to the Maori. One of these rules prohibits the mixing of *tapu* and *noa* (not being under supernatural influence) things. For example, things connected with food or cooking (*noa*) are not to be mixed with things connected with the body, especially the head (*tapu*) (Dansey 1978).

2. Use of *tohunga*.   Since a number of Maori patients have an "unspoken and unconscious fear" (Durie 1977, p. 484) of some infringement of *tapu*, families may seek the services of a *tohunga* in their search for the *hara* (infringement), while at the same time participating in Pakeha medicine. This approach is particularly common if the Pakeha treatment is ineffective. Since there are only a few *tohunga* today, a Maori elder (*kaumatua*) with knowledge of *Maoritanga* (Maori cultural values) often takes on this role. Most often, the *tohunga* does not replace the doctor but only complements him or her. Maori leaders have argued for a degree of cooperation between the two systems, suggesting that they be understood as serving different but complementary functions (*Hui Whakaoranga* 1984). Some Pakeha doctors sensitive to cross-cultural issues have advocated a respect for use of the *tohunga* except in life-threatening emergencies, where such wishes may be overruled (Jacobsen 1983).

3. Childbirth. Because childbirth occurs primarily in hospitals, and because the Maori have some special practices (and mythology) related to it, it deserves special mention here. The traditional Maori view birth as a transit into this world from the realm of the gods (J. Smith 1974), the place to which the *wairua* (spirit or soul) will return after death. All customs associated with childbirth are *tapu* and occur either in the open or in a specially constructed *whare kohanga* (nest house) (Heuer 1972). The traditional rituals associated with childbirth, particularly for women of rank, have been described by a number of authors (see Heuer 1972 for bibliography) but do not concern us here because of their minimal contemporary importance. One concern of the modern Maori, however, is the disposal of the placenta. Since the baby brings the afterbirth with it, the placenta is associated with the *atuas* (gods) and is *tapu*, thus the need to dispose the *whenua* (placenta) by burying it in a place where it cannot be tread upon (Buck 1950). The expressed purpose of the burial is to unite the *wairua* of the placenta with the land from which the people come (Durie 1984). The word *whenua* is common for both "land" and the "placenta or afterbirth" (Williams 1975). The family of the Maori woman who has given birth in a hospital often demands the placenta and the umbilical cord, a practice that is prevalent even in urban areas (M. J. Beagley, unpublished observation, March 1984). Hospital staff are expected to cooperate in this demand (Rostenburg 1981).

4. Death. The customs concerning death *(tangihanga)* are some of the most important Maori traditions. These customs demand that the body of the deceased be placed on the *marae*[6] (the Maori community meeting place) as soon as possible, because, when the visitors arrive,

---

6. The *marae,* or the Maori meeting place, has been the focal point of the Maori community for centuries. Almost every Maori community has its own *marae,* and *marae kawa* (protocol) varies from one to another. The *marae* is considered by the Maori to be *waahi rangatira mana* (place of greatest manna), *waahi rangatira iwi* (place that heightens people's dignity), and *waahi rangatira tikanga Maori* (place in which Maori customs are given ultimate expression). For a modern description of the *marae* functions, see Tauroa and Tauroa (1986).

the absence of the body may be viewed as a sign of negligence on the part of the family. The Maori believe that the *wairua* does not depart from the body at the moments of death but rather hovers around the body for some time. Thus the body is addressed by the mourners and watched over until the time of the burial. A delay by hospital authorities in handing over the body to the family, such as in cases requiring a post-mortem examination, can cause considerable anxiety in the family (Durie 1977).

The Maori Response

Maori leaders during the early part of this century realized the value of many aspects of Western medicine and made efforts to increase its acceptance among their people, but they met considerable resistance and prejudice (Buck 1950). Leaders such as Pomare and Buck comment on the value of medical officers with Maori blood and familiarity with *Maoritanga* who could interpret Western medicine to the Maori in their own idiom. The efforts resulted in significant strides in Maori health; thus the Maori race, once considered to be under the threat of extinction, is again thriving in numbers. Modern Maori leaders believe that the improvement of health within the Maori community requires a response from the community itself, so that Western medical technology can be adapted to Maori cultural needs (*Hui Whakaoranga* 1984). In the last few years, a number of efforts have been made in this direction. The main approaches consist of educating health care professionals in *Maoritanga,* training and employment of more Maori in the health professions, and use of bicultural intermediaries and *marae*-based health programs.

Educating Health Care Professionals in *Maoritanga*

An effort has been made to educate Pakeha doctors and other health professionals in those aspects of *Maoritanga* likely to impact on their diagnosis and management of Maori patients. Efforts have also been made to include aspects of *Maoritanga* in the behavioral science courses and projects in the two New Zealand medical schools (J. Older, personal communication, October 1985). Auckland medical students are instructed in *taha Maori* (Maori cultural values and practices) for about 7 hours in their preclinical years and a further 18.5 hours in the clinical program. The school established a *marae* on its premises in 1977 in response to the *Te Rawara* and *Te Aupori* people. There are weekend exchange visits during which issues of medical importance to Maori people are discussed at *hui* (gathering held on *marae* according to protocol). A voluntary tutoring program for Maori and Pacific Island children has been established by the medical students. A voluntary roster system, whereby graduates assist with medical services to community houses, has been developed. Similar programs have been developed at the Otago Medical School and the clinical schools in Christchurch and Wellington. Unfortunately, much of this interaction has been a part of psychiatry and behavioral science programs only and has not penetrated the largely monocultural institutions of medicine and surgery, thereby diluting its impact.

A number of nurse training courses include a Maori cultural awareness training aspect (Mackay 1985), with visits to Maori *hui* and lectures by Maori elders often included. Similar efforts have been made by other health-related disciplines (e.g., psychology, occupational therapy, and physiotherapy). At least two major psychiatric hospitals catering to large Maori patient populations—the Tokanui Hospital near Hamilton and the Carrington Hospital in Auckland—have organized meetings *(wananga)* focusing on the psychiatric health of the Maori with both Maori and Pakeha participation.

Training and Employment of More Maori as Health Professionals and Planners

Currently, the Maori are underrepresented in most health care professions, as well as in other professions (Older 1978). The Division of Nursing of the Department of Health estimated in 1984 that 3.6% of the total nursing workforce was Maori (and 1% other Polynesian) (Department of Health 1987). Efforts to increase this percentage include encouraging more Maori enrollment in technical institutes, establishing prenursing courses for Maori secondary school students, sponsoring a greater percentage of nursing trainees, and establishing more scholarships. The Otago Medical School has maintained a preferential entry plan for Maori (and other Polynesian) students that, until 1974, allocated two places each year for this purpose. In 1974 this number was increased to six (out of 150–200 total matriculants), although a considerable proportion of the openings remain vacant each year (J. Older and D. Jensen, unpublished data, June 1976). The failure or noncompletion rate for Maori medical students is higher than that for non-Maori students. Few Maori work in the mental health profession in positions such as psychiatric social workers or professional counselors, and there are no Maori child psychotherapists (Durie 1985). Although an appeal has been made for greater recruitment of Maori, the results of the efforts to increase participation have been slow. J. Older and D. Jensen (unpublished data, June 1976) trace this underrepresentation to a generally poorer performance by the Maori population in higher education and the lack of a flexible and accommodating response on the part of the educational institutions in the country.

Bicultural Intermediaries

An attempt has been made to enlist the services of Maori individuals with stature in the Maori community who are also versed in Pakeha culture to act as cultural interpreters for the Pakeha health professionals and the Maori patients. In addition, some have tried to train Maori medical paraprofessionals who could then take Western medical practices to their people, either in the hospitals or the community. For example, a number of psychiatric hospitals have enlisted the support of Maori *kaumatua* or *pukenga* (those steeped in Maori culture) to act as counselors for Maori patients and to assist and advise the staff in regard to management. Maori ministers, especially those from the Ratana Church, have been particularly involved. The four psychiatric hospitals in Auckland have lists of local *tohunga* who can be contacted for consultation and referral. They take patient histories, act as liaisons to the families, assist with hostile or noncompliant patients, provide culturally relevant patient counseling, offer a link between the hospitals and the Maori community, and organize bicultural social events.

Additionally, the Department of Health in Wellington has supported the appointment of Maori health liaison officers or Maori health coordinators to general hospitals. About 30 such officers had been appointed by the end of 1989. These individuals are selected from the local Maori community and usually have a background in social work, although formal training is not always necessary. They participate in a short introductory course, followed by periodic 2-day workshops held for ongoing training and the sharing of experiences. I observed the functioning of one such coordinator in a general hospital in Rotorua in the North Island, and the multiple functions she was called upon to perform were readily apparent.

Marae-Based Health Programs

The *marae* has a central role in Maori culture: it is a place to which the Maori belongs, a place he or she visits regularly and feels at home in, and a place that has high *mana*. For this reason, the proposal that health clinics and other activities be based at the *marae* was well received. It was considered the best way to combine the Maori and Western traditions (i.e., to take the best from Western medicine and deliver it to the Maori in a manner that would be readily accepted). The New Zealand government supports the development of *marae* health clinics as part of the distribution of the health resources into Maori hands. The clinic is usually set up with a grant from the Department of Health (about $100,000 in some cases) and distributed by the Area Health Board. The purpose of the clinic is to complement the community health services already in place. The Tumahaurangi *marae* clinic was set up in January 1988 by the Te Arawa Trust. It employs one full-time community health worker and a number of part-time volunteers from the community. Domiciliary nurses and social workers from the area hospital are occasionally on staff. They give advice to workers and volunteers, conduct groups, and deliver educational lectures. A day program, coordinated by the health worker, includes a number of *marae*-based activities. The main purpose of the clinic has been the promotion of good health practices and follow-up care for patients after discharge from a hospital.

Waiora Program in Otara, Auckland

Health programs emphasize activities that have an appeal for the Maori clientele, but stress on physical health is not paramount. For example, the Waiora Program in Auckland was started in 1977 by the Catholic Maori Society of Otara and Otahuhu, two suburbs in the south of Auckland with large Maori populations. The efforts were renewed in 1984. A number of *marae*-based programs attempt to educate and enrich young people, particularly those with a history of psychiatric disorder. Programs include bone carving, wood carving, jewelry making, calligraphy, sewing, catering, hospitality, building, and hairdressing. Participation in Maori cultural activities is common, and *kaumatua* visit regularly, providing job training while enhancing Maori pride. Polynesian and occasionally Pakeha youth also attend.

Bicultural Maori Psychiatric Units

The trend of increasing psychiatric hospitalization and rehospitalization of the Maori led to the development of special bicultural psychiatric units following the Maori *kaupapa* (value systems) and employing bilingual Maori staff but providing Western psychiatric care.

The first such unit, called *Whai Ora* (Maori health unit), was set up in Tokanui Hospital situated in Te Awamutu, about 30 kilometers from Hamilton in the heart of the rich dairy country of Waikato. A 20-bed ward was staffed by workers steeped in *Maoritanga* and involved with the Maori community, and a nurse with high *mana* was appointed as the unit manager. The daily routine was run strictly according to Maori *kawa*. There was a *Karakia* (ritual incantation) before each meal and at bedtime. The ward meetings followed the protocol of the *hui*. Visitors were accorded a formal Maori welcome. Each patient was encouraged to become familiar with his or her Maori roots and identify himself or herself in reference to the ancestors. Instruction was imparted in the Maori language. Egalitarianism was identified as a strong guiding principle, in part as a reaction to the perceived hierarchical structure of the usual psychiatric ward. At the time the unit was set up, the medical superintendent of the hospital was a Maori, an extremely unusual appointment.

Other Health Initiatives

The *Hui Whakaoranga* (1984) argued for the training of *Ringa Awhina* (cultural interpreters). Walker (1982) advocated the adoption of the "barefoot doctor" concept from China. A number of forums (see Mackay 1985) have recommended the training of Maori community health workers. One of the models offered is the Aboriginal Health Worker Training Program (Cawte 1987), successfully used in Australia, but other models are available. The Maori Women's Welfare League advocated a certificate and a salary for the training of Maori community health assistants. A community-based health education scheme in Auckland, called *Te Koputu Taonga,* trains community health workers to educate Maori families on health matters. Groups such as the *Te Ropu Rapu Oranga* (group holding out good health) have sprung up all over the country. And an attempt to deal with the problem of street kids and solvent abuse was made by setting up *whare manaaki* (houses of caring), often run by a caring couple with community support. The success of many of these ventures, along with sociocultural and educational projects such as *Rapu Mahi, Kokiri, Kohanga Reo, Matua Whangai,* and the like, has been acclaimed (see New Zealand Official Year Book 1986–87).

Administrative Changes

Most of the preceding proposals could not have occurred if New Zealand's health bureaucracy was totally inflexible. In the last decade, many changes have taken place or have been proposed at both the national and local levels.

In the Partnership Response 1984 policy statement (*Te Urupare Rangapu*), the government reaffirmed its major objectives with regard to the interests of the Maori to honor the principles of the Treaty of Waitangi; to eliminate the gaps existing between the educational, social, economic, and cultural well-being of Maori people; to provide for Maori language and culture to receive an equitable allocation of resources and a fair opportunity to develop; and to promote decision making in the machinery of government in areas of importance to Maori communities.

A number of proposals were also made: 1) to restore and strengthen the operational base of *iwi* (tribe) by moving toward the development of the Iwi Authorities by 1994 based on Maori self-reliance on their own terms, 2) to develop a new Ministry of Maori Affairs (in 1989) with a similar role and status to that of Treasury and the State Services Commission, 3) to transfer the Maori Land Court's servicing to the Department of Justice (1989), 4) to help develop an Iwi Transition Agency, 5) to conduct an independent review of the Maori Trust Office, and 6) to disband the Maori Affairs Board.

The fifth annual Maori Health *Waananga* (1985) affirmed the idea that a Regional Maori Health Board (RMHB) should be established in each area. It should adopt a broad Maori view of "health" and should be composed primarily of the representatives of Maori health initiative groups active in the area. The final name, composition, and *kawa* of each RHMB should be determined by the Maori people in each area. Legislation to this effect is under consideration.

The mentioned proposals are revolutionary in that the government gave a great deal of power to the Maori to determine their own strategies in dealing with their own problems, as well as incorporating the Maori perspective into legislative activities. It will be several years until the success or failure of these initiatives can be judged.

Resurgence of Other Maori Health Institutions

Maori leaders traditionally recognize three principal institutions as critical determinants of good mental health: *whenua* (land), *whanau* (family), and *reo* (language) (Durie 1985).

From the end of the nineteenth century, the Maori language suffered a gradual decline, primarily due to the educational policy of using English exclusively in schools, as well as the neglect of Maori by the government. The Maori people recognize their language as one of their *taonga* (treasures) that needs to be preserved. Maintaining an oral history is necessary, because it embodies the particular spiritual and mental concepts unique to the Maori people. There is a movement to make Maori an official language, so that it would be taught in all schools, be mandatory in administration, and be utilized in the courts. Television New Zealand broadcasts a Maori language teaching program. The most important attempt made by the Maori themselves to save their language is embodied in the *Kohanga Reo* movement. This movement established a number of preschool day-care centers that use the Maori language exclusively. The intention is to create truly bilingual people who retain a pride in their own language.

Conclusions

The Maori experience highlights the larger issue of the interaction of a minority ethnic group with mainstream medicine. Like many other ethnic groups, the Maori have their own particular concepts of disease and illness, including the presentation, classification, and etiology of symptoms, as well as general beliefs and attitudes toward health and illness. Since their experience of illness is also somewhat different from the predominantly Anglo-Saxon community, the needs of the Maori have to be specially defined. Furthermore, their interaction with mainstream health professionals and organizations is different, and their utilization patterns of hospitals and clinics are determined accordingly. The Maori share these aspects with most ethnic minorities expected to obtain medical care from a mainstream health system that is national yet monocultural. What makes the situation special for the Maori is their specific historical and cultural background. Until recently the majority of the Maori population was isolated from the mainstream culture and institutions of New Zealand. The situation changed dramatically with the urbanization of the Maori. The health institutions of the country were developed on the models imported from the colonizing culture with little input from the Maori population. Maori health practices were either actively discouraged or otherwise allowed to become impoverished. Furthermore, the current health statistics are seen by the Maori as signifying a failure of the Pakeha health system to meet the needs of the Maori and another indicator of their powerlessness and subjugation in the face of Western colonization.

At the same time, the Maori leaders recognize that they cannot return to a precolonial conceptualization of illness and modes of treatment. They understand the benefits of modern medicine and know that they can be utilized within Maori culture. The emphasis in the past has been on the first part of this equation, but this approach has not produced the desired results. Acculturating the Maori to Western medicine has led to Maori resentment. However, change may occur in the following ways: the health institutions must become bicultural without necessarily compromising on the scientific basis of the practice of medicine; the health professionals must become more aware of the cultural and behavioral aspects of the Maori patient, including the general styles of interaction, attitudes toward authority figures, ways of expressing emotion, illness attribution, health concepts, sex-role allocation, and help seeking behavior; more Maori individuals must be trained as health professionals; and key individuals who can mediate between the two cultures must be identified and appointed such that the less acculturated Maori or Pakeha can interact with individuals from the other culture.

These developments could not have occurred in the absence of political will for change. A unique set of circumstances, including the following, was therefore necessary: an awareness of the health status of the population, a political leadership in the country that has been receptive to calls for change, and the presence of leaders in the Maori community and a process of discussion that has produced viable alternatives. Politically, the change has indeed become necessary because of a significant and visible Maori population that now lives in New Zealand's cities. This growing segment of the population has been vocal in its demands and cannot be ignored from a political perspective. Issues of land rights and equal opportunity in employment provide the backdrop for action in the health sector. The change is economically rational, since the Maori can use the health services and receive the expected results. None of the measures introduced is particularly expensive, and their cost-effectiveness can easily be established and maintained. It was therefore a major effort at acculturation by the majority system that has reversed the direction of what has been traditionally practiced, recognizing that the system must change to accommodate Maori culture rather than demanding that the Maori meet the Pakeha expectations or suffer the consequences.

The Maori experience has relevance for minority ethnic communities elsewhere, especially those from prescientific cultures that have encountered similar colonial powers. Considerable literature exists on the encounters of Australian Aboriginals (Cawte 1987; Cawte et al. 1976), Navajo Indians (Kunitz and Levy 1981), and other ethnic groups with mainstream Western medicine. The Maori response to their special problems may be useful as a model in other settings. The major lesson from the Maori experience is that the primary initiative must come from the minority community itself and that dialogic sociopolitical conditions have to be created for the change to occur. The disadvantaged community has to be given a sense of empowerment to bring about change, and the mainstream health system must see such a change as adaptive, rational, and even cost-effective. It will soon be possible to study whether the New Zealand experiment has worked and whether this little nation of pioneers has once again led the world in providing a model of a fair system for its people.

References

Awatere D, Casswell S, Cullen H (eds): Alcohol and the Maori People. Auckland, Alcohol Research Unit, School of Medicine, University of Auckland, 1984

Best E: The Maori, Vols 1–2. Wellington, Board of Ethnological Research, 1924

Bray DH, Hill CGN: Polynesian and Pakeha in New Zealand Education. Auckland, Heinemann Educational Books, 1974

Broughton HR: A viewpoint on Maori health. N Z Med J 97:290–291, 1984

Buck P (Te Rangi Hiroa): The Coming of the Maori. Wellington, Maori Purposes Fund Board, 1950

Cawte J: Aboriginal mental health. Australian Aboriginal Studies 1:100–109, 1987

Cawte J, Kahn MV, Henry J: Mental health services by and for Australian Aborigines. Aust N Z J Psychiatry 10:221–228, 1976

Census 1986. New Zealand Census of Populations and Dwellings. Wellington, Department of Statistics, 1986

Dansey H: Maori Custom Today. Auckland, Shortland Publications, 1978

Davis PB: Office encounters in general practice in the Hamilton health district, II: ethnic group patterns among employed, 15–64. N Z Med J 99:265–268, 1986

Department of Health. Maori Health: *Orango Maori*. Wellington, Department of Health, 1987

Durie M: Maori attitudes to sickness, doctors, and hospitals. N Z Med J 86:483–485, 1977

Durie M: Maori referrals to a general hospital psychiatric unit. Paper presented at the RANZCP 9th Annual Symposium, Social and Cultural Section, Royal Australian and New Zealand College of Psychiatrists, Rotorua, New Zealand, February 1984

Durie M: A Maori perspective on health. Soc Sci Med 20:483–486, 1985

Firth R: Economics of the New Zealand Maori, 2nd Edition. Wellington, Government Printer, 1959

Heuer B: Maori Women. Wellington, Reed, 1972

Hui Whakaoranga: Maori Health Planning Workshop. Wellington, Department of Health, 1984

Hyslop J, Dowland J, Hickling J: Health Facts New Zealand. Wellington, Management Survey and Research Unit, Department of Health, 1983

Jacobsen CT: Family medicine in a Maori community. New Zealand Family Physician 10:182–185, 1983

Kleinman A: Patients and healers in the context of culture. Berkeley and Los Angeles, CA, University of California Press, 1980

Kunitz SJ, Levy JE: Navajos, in Ethnicity and Medical Care. Edited by Harwood A. Cambridge, MA, Harvard University Press, 1981, pp 337–396

Landy D: Culture, Disease, and Healing. New York, Macmillan, 1977

Mackay P: The Health of the Maori People. Whangarei, New Zealand, Northland Community College, 1985

Marsden M: Maori illness and healing. Seminar on mental health: a case for reform. Paper presented at the Legal Research Foundation Seminar, Auckland, September 1986 (reprints available from the Mental Health Foundation, Box 37438, Parnell, Auckland, New Zealand)

Mechanic D: Medical Sociology: A Selective View, 2nd Edition. New York, Free Press, 1978

Metge J: The Maoris of New Zealand: Rautahi. London, Routledge & Kegan Paul, 1976

Metge J, Kinloch P: Talking Past Each Other. Wellington, Victoria University Press, 1979

Mitchell EA, Borman B: Demographic characteristics of asthmatic admissions to hospital. N Z Med J 99:576–579, 1986

Murchie E (ed): *Rapuora*: Health and Maori Women. Wellington, Maori Women's Welfare League, 1984

Neki JS: An examination of the cultural relativism of dependence as a dynamic of social and therapeutic relationships. Br J Med Psychol 49:1–10, 1976

New Zealand Official Year Book 1986–87. Wellington, Department of Statistics, 1987

Older J: The Pakeha Papers. Dunedin, John McIndoe, 1978

Parsons T: The Social System. New York, Free Press, 1951

Partnership Response: *Te Urupare Rangapu*. Wellington, Government Printer, 1988

Pilowsky I, Spence ND: Ethnicity and illness behaviour. Psychol Med 7:447–452, 1977

Pomare EW: Maori standards of health: a study of the 20 year period 1955–1975 (Medical Research Council of NZ Special Report Series No 7). Auckland, Medical Research Council of New Zealand, 1980

Pomare EW: Maori health: new concepts and initiatives. N Z Med J 99:410–411, 1986

Pomare EW, de Boer GM: *Hauora*: Maori standards of health (Special Report Series No 78). Wellington, Department of Health, 1988

Ritchie J: The Making of a Maori. Wellington, Reed, 1963

Rostenburg M: Aspects of the Maori patient. New Zealand Journal of Physiotherapy 9:7–9, 1981

Sachdev P: *Mana, Tapu, Noa*: Maori cultural constructs with medical and psychosocial relevance. Psychol Med 19:959–970, 1989a

Sachdev P: Psychiatric illness in the New Zealand Maori. Aust N Z J Psychiatry 23:529–541, 1989b

Sachdev P: Behavioural factors affecting physical health of the Maori. Soc Sci Med 30:431–440, 1990

Schwimmer E: The World of the Maori. Wellington, Reed, 1974

Segall A: The sick role concept: understanding illness behaviour. J Health Soc Behav 17:162–169, 1976

Smith AH, Pearce NE: Determinants of differences in mortality between New Zealand Maoris and non-Maoris aged 15–64. N Z Med J 97:101–108, 1984

Smith J: *Tapu* removal in Maori religion (Polynesian Society Memoir No 40). Wellington, Polynesian Society, 1974

Sobell R, Ingalls A: Resistance to treatment: explorations of the patient's sick role. Am J Psychother 18:562–573, 1964

Tauroa H, Tauroa P: *Te Marae*: a guide to customs and protocol. Auckland, Heinemann Reed, 1981

Tipene-Leach D: Maoris: their feelings about the medical profession. Auckland, Community Forum, November 1978

Walker RJ: Social implications of medical practice among the Maoris. Tu Tangata 7:31–32, 1982

West SR, Harris BJ: Health need and primary care. N Z Med J 91:264–267, 1980

Williams HW: A Dictionary of the Maori People. Wellington, Government Printer, 1975

CHAPTER 7

Negotiating Across Class, Culture, and Religion
Psychiatry in the English Inner City

SIMON DEIN, M.R.C.PSYCH.
MAURICE LIPSEDGE, F.R.C.PSYCH.

To place into context this account of psychiatry in the English inner city, we start with some biographical data. We, the authors, are Jewish and descendants of immigrants. Dein's grandparents came from Krakow to London in the early 1900s and worked as tailors. Dein's father was a waiter in a famous Jewish restaurant in the East End. Dein obtained a scholarship to a grammar school, where he was one of the few Jewish boys in his year. After medical school, he worked in general practice for 1 year before entering psychiatry. Concurrently, he studied social anthropology and is now doing fieldwork among the Lubavitch Hasidim of Stamford Hill. Lipsedge's grandparents on one side came from Galicia and on the other from Lithuania. The Lithuanian grandparents emigrated to South Africa; their son, Lipsedge's father, graduated in medicine and then settled in England as a general practitioner. We suffered from relatively minor anti-Semitism as children (playground accusations of killing Christ, fights, Gentile parents warning their children not to play with Jews, and the like) but nothing worse.

We both work at the Speedwell Mental Health Center in Deptford. In our professional lives anti-Semitism has never been an issue, so we were profoundly shocked recently when a patient yelled anti-Semitic slogans in the facility's waiting room, warned the other patients to avoid "contamination" by us, and made other "Sturmer"-like comments.

This episode made us wonder how our own ethnic and class background influences our practice of psychiatry. On a fairly banal level, our knowledge of the Old Testament enhances our rapport with our fundamentalist Christian and Rastafarian patients. Our own immigrant provenance means that we espouse self-help and upward social mobility via education. Our experience of anti-Semitism renders us more sensitive to racism and discrimination.

Deptford is an inner-city area in southeast London. It has a population of 30,000 and is characterized by high levels of deprivation. In some areas, unemployment is as high as 22%, and ethnic minorities comprise 40% of the population, with 33% of these being African-Caribbean and 25% being African (National Census 1991). Patients attending Speedwell Mental Health Center derive from social classes IV and V. A very small minority have jobs, unemployment is exceptionally high, and many clients have never had a job. This situation is likely to continue, considering recurrent recessions. Other indices of deprivation such as homelessness and poverty (number of people receiving welfare) are also very high. Many of the patients' homes are overcrowded and lacking in basic amenities. About 50% of the patients are from ethnic minorities, who can be divided into African-Caribbean, Africans, Turks, Cypriots, and Vietnamese. Only two Jews attend as outpatients. The majority of the patients are practicing or nominal Christians, and many others are Muslim. Among the Christians, a large proportion belong to various Pentecostal groups, and some are Rastafarians. A minority of the patients are transient, staying in Deptford for short periods and then moving on. At Speedwell, a large proportion of patients suffer from schizophrenia. This prevalence is typical of other deprived areas of London. Many studies of deprivation and mental illness have focused on social class, since it is readily quantifiable, but this variable neglects individual differences, so we consider separately more specific factors such as poverty, unemployment, and homelessness.

Poverty is a relative concept but can be said to exist when individuals, families, and groups in the population lack the resources to obtain the types of diet, to participate in the activities, and to have the living conditions and amenities customary or at least widely encouraged or regarded as socially desirable (Townsend 1979). In addition to lack of financial resources, a number of environmental stresses, such as poor inner-city housing, increased pollution, lack of play facilities for children, and limited personal and interpersonal space, also exist. A number of psychological effects are associated with the "culture of poverty" (Allen 1970), including a strong feeling of fatalism and belief in chance, strong present-time orientation and short-term perspectives, impulsiveness, feelings of inferiority, and concrete rather than abstract thinking processes (restricted linguistic code) (Bernstein and Henderson 1969). These observations are in accordance with our own experience of many of the patients, and some of these factors relate to problems in communication in therapy. A major difficulty arises in fostering the belief that social mobility is possible where a fatalistic attitude is very strong.

The psychological sequelae of unemployment have been demonstrated by a number of researchers (Brenner and Bartell 1983; Frese and Mohr 1987; Jahoda et al. 1972; Rueth and Heller 1981). These factors include unhappiness; high rates of stress, depression, hypochondriasis, and anxiety; loss of prestige and self-esteem; and increased suicide rates. Unemployment has profound effects on young school dropouts who have no job opportunities. Children of families whose parents are unemployed have been shown to have poor scholastic performance and disturbed behavior (Fagin 1981). At Speedwell, very few patients have jobs, many having been unemployed for a number of years and living on unemployment benefits (£42 a week). Many patients with chronic mental illness exist on invalidity benefits (£44 a week). (A pint of milk and a loaf of bread cost approximately £1.)

Over the past 5 years, the number of homeless people in Britain has increased markedly. It has been argued that the closure of the large mental hospitals is partly responsible for this increase, as are other factors such as lack of cheap rental accommodations, a decrease in the numbers of dwelling units available, an increase in unemployment, and changes in social security benefits. In general, mental illness in the homeless ranges from 41% to 93%, with alcohol dependence occurring in more than 60% (Morrisey and Levine 1987). About 5% of our clinic population are literally homeless. This group creates therapeutic problems, since they are frequently on the move, living in temporary hostels for a short period of time and then moving on. Building up a therapeutic relationship is difficult under these circumstances.

The relentless poverty endured by these patients transcends the traditional English notions of social class with subtle gradations based on income, education, accent, vocabulary, dress, table manners, and so forth. The material gulf between the patients and the staff is immediately obvious to any visitor. Almost none of the patients has a car, they cannot afford vacations, their clothes are shabby, and a high proportion are the victims of burglaries as soon as they are admitted to a hospital. The material poverty of the patients and their generally trusting attitude evokes in staff a far more obviously paternalistic caring attitude than would be seen in a middle-class suburb. There is more physical contact between staff and patients and more embracing and hugging than would normally be deemed proper in the English context. In this setting, medicalizing deprivation is a great risk. Although we do not see anything as extreme as Nancy Sheper Hughes's description of the distribution in northeast Brazil of minor tranquilizers to deal with chronic hunger pangs (construed as "nervos"), one of our patients actually reported that she was suffering from "depression" every Sunday. Close questioning revealed that this single mother with five children had regularly run out of money by the end of the weekend and could not afford food, so the children's demands became intolerable, and she would begin to feel desperate but labeled her anguish as "depression." The social class division in our service is then crudely economic. The staff have financial security and long-term jobs, whereas the patients' life chances are curtailed by the dual barrier of the stigma of major mental illness and residence in an area of endemic high unemployment.

Many of our patients are also subject to racism. In fact, Deptford is close to Bermondsey, the major bastion of the British National Party, an extreme right-wing organization whose policies are virulently racist. A number of studies have demonstrated that ethnic minorities are more disadvantaged than other residents in deprived areas and have inferior jobs, are paid less, and have poorer housing than the general population (Smith 1977). According to the Community Relations Commission (1977, p. 2), "The urban deprivation and social disadvantage experienced by ethnic minorities differ from those of other residents in urban deprived areas, in degree, in kind, in their causes, and consequences. Ethnic minorities are more likely to be socially disadvantaged and multiply deprived than the rest of the population, they experience distinctive clusters of multiple deprivation, and a major cause of their deprivation is the racial discrimination which they face." The same situation exists today.

It is certainly our experience that the African-Caribbean and African community experiences overcrowding, lack of amenities, high unemployment, and low family incomes. With large-scale unemployment and the resurgence of crude nationalism across Europe, one might anticipate a recrudescence of anti-Semitic xenophobia, but so far the targets of explicitly racist political extremists (the British National Party and the National Front) have been people of South Asian and African-Caribbean origin. A series of racially motivated murders of young black men has taken place in south and east London.

As psychiatrists, our first priority must be to combat racism within the mental health care system. Hospital records indicate that a disproportionate number of black patients, both those born in Britain and those born in the Caribbean and West Africa, are compulsorily detained under the Mental Health Act. The degree of overrepresentation is between two and four times the rate for the indigenous white population. African-Caribbeans are more likely to be admitted following arrest under Section 136 of the Mental Health Act. (Under this legal provision, the police have powers to detain people for up to 72 hours in a police station if the officer considers detention to be in the individual's own interest or for the protection of others [Lipsedge 1993].) The disproportionate number of compulsory admissions, the higher doses of neuroleptics prescribed, and the selective transfer of African-Caribbeans to locked wards indicate that the professional assessment of dangerousness is influenced by skin color.

The microcosm of the English maximum security hospital exposes the extent of racist stereotyping. Over the past 7 years, three young Afro-Caribbean men from south London have died at Broadmoor Secure Hospital following violent confrontations with staff and the forced injection of major tranquilizers. In the most recent case, Orville Blackwell's death in a seclusion room followed a forced injection that the staff argued was justified because Blackwell had refused to go to occupational therapy (Lipsedge 1994).

Over the past 40 years, there has been a process of deinstitutionalization with an emphasis on community care in Britain, and the decline in the number of inpatients has continued at an even rate since 1954 (Thornicroft 1988). Establishing outpatient clinics in general hospitals has been the trend, although recently outpatient clinics have been transferred from hospital sites and consultation clinics have been established in primary care settings. In Britain, 19% of all psychiatrists work at least partly in primary care settings (Strathdee and Williams 1984). Family practitioners (called GPs) play an important role in the care of those with acute chronic mental disorders, and the GP is the only source of continuing care for many patients with severe long-term disorders. Much psychological distress is first presented to the GP, who may then refer the patient to the psychiatric services. In Britain, psychiatric care is sectored, split into small, geographically defined areas as the unit of service provision. Each consultant psychiatrist is responsible for a given sector and has a defined responsibility for each patient requiring care.

Over the past few years, a growing number of community mental health centers have been established in Britain. They function as resources for crisis intervention, coordinating multidisciplinary teams, and as a consultation service. Speedwell is the community mental health center for Deptford. It was established in 1981 and functioned as a day hospital until 1990. The staff includes one consultant, one senior resident, one senior house officer, four community psychiatric nurses, one psychologist, one occupational therapist, one social worker, one administrator, and one secretary. Patients are referred by their GPs, social workers, other psychiatrists, the courts, and occasionally the church. Patients are assessed on an outpatient basis and sometimes on domiciliary visits. A "depot clinic," which patients with schizophrenia attend regularly for depot injections, has been established. A number of groups including the link group (patients close to discharge from the inpatient unit attend to learn coping skills in the community), a women's group, a social group, and an anxiety management group are available. Also, there is regular liaison with various ethnic minority support groups such as the Afro-Caribbean Mental Health Project, Isis, Fanon, and the Vietnamese Group.

Apart from their responsibilities at the mental health center, the doctors are involved in the care of inpatients accommodated on Cornelius Ward, a 12-bed ward at Guy's Hospital, a large teaching hospital in south London. The ward is full most of the time, and only the sickest patients are admitted there, more often than not compulsorily under a section of the 1983 Mental Health Act. The average duration of stay is about 3 weeks. The inpatients are reviewed regularly during two ward rounds each week. The vast majority of patients are managed on an outpatient basis at Speedwell, where they most commonly are allocated to the following diagnostic categories: acute situational crises, brief reactive psychoses, acute and chronic schizophrenia, affective disorders, personality disorders and repetitive self-harm, alcoholism, and comorbidity (i.e., psychosis plus drug abuse, especially of crack cocaine). Schizophrenia and affective disorders figure predominantly among the inpatients. Every week the doctors at Speedwell see about 60 patients. The majority are recurrent attendees, who are regularly reviewed in the outpatient service. New patients are discussed at the weekly referral meeting and are seen shortly afterward by a member of the multidisciplinary team.

With this background established, we now consider, through a few patient cases from our practice, what problems two middle-class, white, Jewish psychiatrists encounter in communicating with clients of different classes, cultures, and religions from their own.

At our Friday morning intake meetings, referrals are read aloud. The following is a typical referral:

Dear Dr. Lipsedge:

Please could you assess Miss A, a thirty-year-old lady, fairly urgently. She has recently been admitted to hospital having taken an overdose of 30 paracetamol. The overdose was impulsive and was precipitated by an argument with an ex-boyfriend who she claims has been abusing her. This is her third overdose, the first two occurring in 1987 and 1988 in what sounds like similar circumstances. She has also cut herself on a number of occasions although I do not have the exact details of these.

Miss A was born in Deptford but her parents split up shortly after her birth. Her mother was a heroin addict, and she was taken into care from the age of three to six. While she was there, she claims she was sexually abused and this continued when she was returned to her father's care. She spent a lot of time playing truant from school, and herself became addicted to heroin for a short period in 1988. A major problem as she stated to me is her extreme difficulty in establishing relationships. She has had two long-standing relationships in which she was beaten up and abused. Her first boyfriend went to prison shortly after the birth of her child Edward who is now eight. She has recently split up with her current boyfriend who was drinking heavily. She lives with her son in a council flat which she finds very noisy. She has a number of financial problems and is in some debt. She is relatively isolated and has few friends. When I saw her, Miss A seemed very low in mood, hopeless, and expressing suicidal ideas although no intent. I have started her on fluoxetine 20 mg a day. Thanks for your help.

Signed Dr. J.

As this letter is read aloud, I glance around the room and can see the look of dismay and despair on the team members' faces. Since no one else has volunteered to see Miss A, I offer myself, although my initial feeling is one of irritation. What can I do for her? She is multiply deprived. Where do I begin? Do I look at her mood, her sexual abuse, or her social problems? She needs mothering, money, and love, none of which I can provide. I realize that the reason that I am irritable is because I feel impotent in these circumstances.

I arrange to see her as an outpatient a couple of days later, and she turns up with her 8-year-old son. Initially, she is reluctant to talk and sits with her head down, looking very distrusting of me. She then recounts at length how she has had a life of constant physical and emotional abuse. She describes her life as being one of total failure "from the minute go." She has had to survive on very little for most of her life and can no longer bear to live in her overcrowded, noisy flat in Deptford. She sees little hope for the future and frequently has suicidal thoughts. She appears angry more than depressed, and her narrative is frequently interspersed with bitter questioning: "How can you understand what has happened to me, what it is like to be abused and to worry every day where money is coming from?" I sit back in my chair and think to myself that she is right. I earn a regular salary, live in reasonable accommodation, and do not have to worry about the basic necessities of life. I have never been abused. How many of her experiences can I share or even begin to understand?

Religion and Mental Health

Many of our patients are intensely religious, the majority being Christian or Muslim. Among the African and African-Caribbean patients, a large number belong to various Pentecostal churches such as the Celestial Church of Christ. For them, religion is not just an important part of their lives but rather the central focus around which everything else revolves. Religion provides an overarching framework in which they conceptualize their world. It structures their everyday experiences and plays an important role in articulating their distress, providing an explanation of suffering and misfortune, and acting as a focus of identity.

As Wilson (1992, p. 31) states, "All religions provide a vocabulary of sufferings, whether these are personal, communal, societal, or even universal in kind and they provide no less a repertoire of methods for their relief." At one level, the explicit and manifest function of religion is to offer its practitioners the prospect of salvation and to provide them with appropriate guidance for its attainment. Kiev (1964, p. 129) aptly summarizes how Pentecostalism provides a justification of present misfortune and sin and the guarantee of redemption by divine grace, both immediately and in the future: "These churches would seem to provide a form of social integration for some West Indian immigrants in a situation of relative social and cultural anomie. They would seem to have a special appeal for an emotionally isolated group in an urban society, because they provide a universal theme, a structured world view. The gifts of the spirit compensate for the lack of material gifts, and the gift of 'Tongues' provides the inarticulate with an opportunity to speak. Religious status is substituted for social and racial status."

Apart from one study (Rogow 1970), which concluded that psychiatrists were less likely than other doctors to be members of churches, little data relating to the religiosity of psychiatrists is available. It is our personal experience that psychiatrists with a scientific rationalistic background are generally hostile to religion, seeing it as atavistic, irrational, meaningless, arbitrary, and undertaken in the service of myths and ideas that could, empirically, be shown to be either unprovable or patently false. They agree with Freud (1930, p. 74) that belief in God is "so patently infantile, so incongruous with reality, that to one whose attitude to humanity is friendly it is painful to think that the great majority of mortals will never rise above this view of life."

It is also our experience that many psychiatrists lack knowledge about the belief systems, values, and sanctioned behaviors of the various religious groups with whom they work. For many, religion is important only insofar as it is a cultural value that structures the content of delusions; some believe that religious interest in a patient obscures the appropriate diagnosis: In West Indians, mania "is complicated with delusions of a religious character" (Donald 1876, p. 77). Cultural naïveté may result in misdiagnosis, whereby culturally sanctioned phenomena may be misdiagnosed as mental illness. For example, glossolalia may be misdiagnosed as schizophrenic speech disorder and possession as schizophrenic passivity. However, there is always the risk that the opposite may occur; the psychiatrist may miss serious mental illness, seeing it instead as culturally acceptable behavior, with disastrous consequences for the patient. It is not simply that psychiatrists and their patients sometimes do not share the same belief systems but that they often have different worldviews, modes of experiencing reality (Tambiah 1992), and ways of conceptualizing the universe.

Psychiatrists adopt a scientific, logical, causal viewpoint, whereas their patients adopt a religious perspective in which humans are intimately connected to their kinship group, nature, and the cosmos as a whole; in which the sacred continuously influences the profane world of human experience; and in which the construct of self is closely tied to that of others. In line with this perspective, the patients' constructions of mental illness are profoundly different from those of the psychiatrist, and experiences such as mind-to-mind communication may be accepted as the norm (see example in Marsella and White 1986). Because mental illness may be conceptualized as resulting from disharmony between the patient and the spirit world or the rest of the cosmos, the appropriate solution is not via medication but by reestablishing a harmonious relationship through prayer, ritual, sacrifice, or diet. This view may result in problems of negotiating treatment.

Ahmed is a 14-year-old boy who was born in Deptford but whose parents come from Pakistan. When Ahmed was 11 years old, he spent 2 years living with an uncle in a Pakistani village. His uncle was known to practice magic and had a large clientele. Having been educated in England, Ahmed was at first rather skeptical about his uncle's occult powers. His uncle explained that he sold talismans and was able to curse his clients' enemies in return for a fee. Ahmed wondered why, if his uncle was such a powerful magician, he was not able to use magic in his own interest to become fabulously rich. However, eventually Ahmed became convinced that his uncle really did have the ability to commune with spirits. When Ahmed returned to England, about a year before we saw him, he began to receive visits at night from a female figure, who told him that her name was Sophie. She was a large, hairy woman wearing a cloak. Her breasts were pendulous and were slung back over her shoulders. Her legs and feet pointed backward. She would appear out of the blue, and Ahmed would then feel a "rush" in his bottom and Sophie would get inside of him. In addition to Sophie, he had visits from a number of other spirits, including angry tree spirits who wished to punish him because he had urinated against a sacred tree while in Pakistan.

More recently the spirits had changed and become more benign. A kind, middle-aged man with a long beard would visit him at night and ask him to travel with him. Ahmed would then accompany him to an unfamiliar place, where he saw gigantic bananas. This was a happy land, far away. After traveling there during the night, he would come back and on occasions find himself outside his sister's bedroom. He would knock on the window and she would let him in, and then he would go back to his own room. Ahmed's parents noticed him apparently talking to himself in a strange voice and making bizarre, convulsive movements. They took him to consult a mullah, because they thought that he might be possessed. The mullah interviewed Ahmed and informed his parents that there were no spirits inside him and that he was suffering from a mental illness. His parents took him to see the family doctor, who in turn sought our opinion. Ahmed was rather ambivalent about the visits from these spirits. He had been frightened by the hag, Sophie, but he had learned to utter a sura from the Koran that helped to keep her at bay. He was very positive about the kind, bearded man who took him away to the enchanted land. He also described how he could invoke a magical power that gave him superhuman strength, which had served him well when fighting bullies at school.

We felt that these experiences were not pathological when considered in terms of rural Pakistani culture. The fact that the mullah had diagnosed mental illness as opposed to possession indicates the fallibility of relying on indigenous priests and healers to assist in disentangling the perennial transcultural problem of psychopathology versus culturally acceptable belief. We speculated that the mullah wished to dissociate himself from Ahmed's possessing spirits because of the potential threat they represent to orthodox Islam. (Lewis [1989] has made a helpful distinction between peripheral spirits and the mainstream of Islamic theology.) From the Western psychiatric point of view, some of these experiences could be labeled as hysterical dissociative states or DSM-IV possession states (American Psychiatric Association 1994). We were attracted by a psychodynamic interpretation of these unusual experiences: we speculated that the hag, Sophie, was a repository of guilt for emerging sexuality, whereas the magical visits to a never-never land where people never grow up, where kindness reigns, and where food is plentiful represents a retreat from adult responsibility. When talking to Ahmed, we found that he was certainly familiar with the Superman theme, which resonated with his invocation of a powerful spirit to help him fight his enemies, and also, of course, the story of Peter Pan.

Psychiatrists with an interest in cultural issues might be diverted by religious or cultural flavor and miss a diagnosis of major mental illness, with damaging consequences for patients and their families. A Nigerian woman presented with a brief reactive psychosis during which she declared that she had prophetic powers. After 2 days on the ward she seemed to have recovered, and we were falsely reassured by her statement that she was regarded as somebody who is *like* a prophet rather than a *true* prophet herself. That night she jumped through a ward window with no warning and died.

In Deptford there is a Vietnamese community, whose members came to the United Kingdom about 15 years ago. Few can speak English, and we encounter many problems in our work among them apart from linguistic ones. Mrs. V is a 30-year-old Vietnamese woman who lives in Deptford with her mother and 3-year-old son. She came to the United Kingdom from Saigon. Her family members are practicing Buddhists. She has been diagnosed as having schizophrenia and is regularly reviewed by one of our community psychiatric nurses, who gives her a depot injection. Over the past 10 years, she has had a number of relapses, mainly due to her stopping medication. On each discharge summary is written the following: "Throughout her admission she has been guarded and suspicious and has been very reluctant to discuss her feelings. Her compliance with medication is poor, and, thus, she does not have a good prognosis. She has no insight, and her family refuses to admit that she is mentally ill."

I was asked by the community psychiatric nurse to visit the patient at home, since she had been behaving strangely, talking to herself, and taking her clothes off in public. She had refused her depot medication. I arranged to visit with the nurse and a member of the Vietnamese health project, Dr. K, who is medically qualified but does not practice medicine in Britain. Dr. K advises on the mental health needs of Vietnamese clients and functions as an advocate, putting forward the patient's case and advising us about whether the patient is ill. As we were driving to Mrs. V's house, I described how difficult it had been for the family to accept that she was mentally ill. Dr. K explained to me the possible origin of this problem, noting that there is no term for mental illness in the Vietnamese language. Disturbed behavior is perceived as a manifestation of "nerve weakness" and is described as "flame burst out of the brain," which is relieved by medication, food, and herbs that help to "neutralize" the "flame." Vietnamese philosophy emphasizes the harmonious relationship between two opposing forces, those of yin and yang. When there is an excess of either the cold or the hot element, illness ensues.

Mental illness is seen as resulting from an excess of yang, a hot element. Drugs such as neuroleptics are considered hot and are countertherapeutic. Sometimes the family deliberately reduces the dosage or stops medication altogether to attenuate the deleterious effects of Western medicine. Herbs may also be taken for this purpose. Western medicine is seen by many as a form of magic that should therefore be effective within a few days. Long-term medication, with its side effects, is unacceptable. Much stigma is attached to being mentally ill. It is seen as disgraceful and difficult to treat and affects the whole family's economic status and future. The patient and his or her siblings may not be able to marry or be employed because of the misfortune it may bring. Consequently, families are very reluctant to accept that one of their members is mentally ill. The culture prohibits expressing feelings or interpersonal conflicts.

Questions asked by professionals can be interpreted as intrusive. This reluctance to speak may be misdiagnosed as suspiciousness or being guarded and may result in the prescription of more medication. Patients and their families are not familiar with psychological forms of treatment and in any case are reluctant to talk about their personal feelings to strangers. Negotiations about treatment can be very difficult in this group because of different explanatory models (Kleinman 1988a).

When we interviewed Mrs. V she appeared thought disordered to Dr. K and seemed to be hallucinating. She was admitted compulsorily to our psychiatric unit under a section of the 1983 Mental Health Act. She was treated against her will, and after a couple of weeks, when her mental state had improved considerably, she was discharged into the community. A week after discharge, the visiting community nurse was told by her family that they did not want her to take medication anymore and wanted to try Chinese herbal medicine. She has been on this regimen for some weeks now, and so far her mental state has remained stable.

Religion, Suffering, and Meaning

Mr. G is a 48-year-old married man who attends my outpatient clinic. He has suffered from manic depression for a number of years, and his symptoms are currently well controlled by lithium. He has been unemployed for a number of years and spends much of his time repairing his beaten-up car. He frequently expresses to me that he has underachieved and would like to take a course in something stimulating.

He was born in east London and is the son of Jewish parents. His childhood and schooling were uneventful, and he left school at the age of 17 to train as a tailor. He worked for most of his life in various shops but for the past 4 years has been receiving invalidity benefits because of recurrent hypomania. Currently he lives with his 30-year-old wife and two children, 3 and 6 years of age. The marital relationship is somewhat strained because of the overcrowding in their small, two-bedroom council flat. Mr. G, who is one of my few Jewish patients, sees me regularly for psychiatric review. Whenever he sees me we talk about Jewish matters, although he is not a practicing Jew and knows little about the religion.

On one appointment, he took out a list of questions, which he then read to me: "Why do we get old? Why are some people wealthy and some poor? Why have I suffered so much from my mental illness? I'm concerned about what happens when I die, where will I go? How can I be sure there is a God?" I sat back in my chair quite astounded. How could I answer these questions? Is it my job to do so? Who can answer them? Are they in fact answerable? Throughout our careers as doctors we witness suffering. Our medical education allows us to answer questions about how the disease comes about and what treatment to prescribe in certain conditions. In a well-written and somewhat moving book, *The Illness Narrative: Suffering, Healing, and the Human Condition,* Kleinman (1988b, p. 29) makes the cogent point that biomedicine cannot deal with issues of human suffering, and problems of bafflement (why me?), the moral order, and evil are not resolved. "Clinical and behavioral science also possess no category to describe suffering, no way of recording this most thickly human dimension of patients and families' stories of experiencing mental illness. Symptom scales and survey questionnaires and behavioral checklists quantify functional impairment and disability, rendering quality of life fungible. Yet about the suffering they are silent." A little later he asks, "what is the metric in biomedical and behavioral research for these existential qualities?" and lacking such understanding, can the professional knowledge that medical science creates be all-adequate for the needs of patients, their families, and the practitioner?

Although many systems of healing cross-culturally, like religious and moral systems, address the problem of bafflement, it is largely ignored by biomedicine. Our biomedical training does not provide a coherent framework for understanding suffering and the "why" questions such as "Why me?" or "Why now?" (as opposed to the "how" questions). Many people believe that we live in a secular society. By secularization, they mean the decline in the social significance of religious beliefs and institutions. Although many see this change in a positive light, others have decried the loss of religious belief, emphasizing that religion provides a framework for understanding suffering and evil in the world. It addresses the theological problem of the existence of suffering and evil in the world and the religious or theological solutions or resolutions that are proposed to reconcile this problem.

What, then, replaces religion in secular society as a way of understanding suffering and evil? Who sits in God's chair? What role does psychiatry play in this process? In the West, there are a number of explanations for misfortune and suffering: "the nature of the physical world," "just bad luck," "we cannot control what happens," "a random event," "because of bad genetic effects," and a "natural part of life." Although we may accept that illness is part of nature and that it happens to people through chance or bad luck, this is not saying very much. The search for meaning by the sufferer is strong, however. As Kushner (1981) cogently argues in *When Bad Things Happen to Good People,* although it may be argued and intellectually acknowledged, suffering is not the will of God; it is still difficult for many to emotionally accept that "nothing makes bad luck happen—it just happens."

As Atkinson (1993) states, "The randomness of the universe may be an appropriate explanation for much human suffering, but the second law of thermodynamics does not offer much in the way of consolation." In modern-day Western society, although religious frameworks may no longer be fashionable as explanations of misfortune and suffering, they remain, albeit in modified form. Perhaps the commonest idea deriving from Judeo-Christianity is that of suffering as punishment. The view of punishment as retribution for sin is the simplest and probably the commonest view associated with suffering (Isaiah 3:10, Proverbs 12:21). Illness is something brought upon people by their own behavior or that of their family (Deuteronomy 5:9). Illness has a disciplinary or purifying function. The individual is responsible for his or her illness, which is blamed on his or her "lifestyle." For instance, "A" got lung cancer because he smoked; "B" suffered a heart attack because of her unhealthy diet high in saturated fats. Perhaps the best example is that of human immunodeficiency virus (HIV) contracted through aberrant sexual behavior. We talk of innocent victims to denote those who have been exposed to acquired immunodeficiency syndrome (AIDS) through blood transfusions or babies born to infected mothers. Some even imply that a higher power decides to inflict the suffering.

Another Judeo-Christian idea is that suffering becomes a liberation from this world's pain and a gateway to a better place. Laing's (1967) view that schizophrenia is a transcendental experience and not a breakdown but a breakthrough to inner worlds fits this liberation model. Treatment is no more than repression.

Without religion, there is no coherent framework for understanding suffering; we may identify the proximal causes, but the distal causes are largely neglected. The psychiatrist faced with these issues can appeal only to his or her common sense or moral or religious background to answer them. Science and economics can never answer these questions, although attempts are being made (for instance, the increased interest in the West in parapsychology and the occult may address some of these issues). For many, modernity is a time of existential crisis in which each person must find his or her own individual solutions.

As our experience indicates, psychiatrists are often in the position of treating patients different from themselves. What is imperative is that the sensitive therapist be aware of what cultural distinctions exist, whether they be ethnicity, religion, lifestyle, or socioeconomic level. Psychiatrists must be resourceful in learning about other cultures. Understanding the complete cultural identity of patients not only allows psychiatrists to best diagnose and treat their patients but also helps them to prevent misdiagnosis and mistreatment.

References

Allen VL: Psychology of poverty: problems and prospects, in Psychological Factors in Poverty. Edited by Allen VL. Chicago, IL, Markham, 1970, pp 367–383

American Psychiatric Association: Diagnostic and Statistical Manual of Mental Disorders, 4th Edition. Washington, DC, American Psychiatric Association, 1994

Atkinson JM: The patient as sufferer. Br J Med Psychol 66:113–120, 1993

Bernstein B, Henderson S: Social class differences in the relevance of language to socialisation. Sociology 3:1–20, 1969

Brenner SO, Bartell R: The psychological impact of unemployment: a structural analysis of cross-sectional data. Journal of Occupational Psychology 56:132–136, 1983

Community Relations Commission: Ethnic Minorities and Employment. London, Community Relations Commission, 1977

Donald JS: Notes on lunacy in British Guiana. J Ment Sci 22:76–81, 1876

Fagin L: Unemployment and Health in Families. London, Department of Health and Social Security, 1981

Frese M, Mohr G: Prolonged unemployment and depression in older workers: a longitudinal study of intervening variables. Soc Sci Med 25:173–178, 1987

Freud S: Civilization and its discontents (1930[1929]), in Standard Edition of the Complete Psychological Works of Sigmund Freud, Vol. 21. Translated and edited by Strachey J. London, Hogarth Press, 1961, pp 59–145

Jahoda M, Lazarsfeld PF, Zeisel H: Marienthal: The Sociography of an Unemployed Community. New York, Aldine-Athenton, 1972

Kiev A: Magic, Faith, and Healing. New York, Free Press, 1964

Kleinman A: Rethinking Psychiatry. New York, Free Press, 1988a

Kleinman A: The Illness Narrative: Suffering, Healing, and the Human Condition. New York, Basic Books, 1988b

Kushner HS: When Bad Things Happen to Good People. New York, Schocken, 1981

Laing RD: The Politics of Experience. Harmondsworth, Penguin, 1967

Lewis IM: Ecstatic Religion: An Anthropological Study of Spirit Possession and Shamanism, 2nd Edition. London, Penguin, 1989

Lipsedge M: Mental Health: Access to care for black and ethnic minority people, in Access to Health Care for People From Black and Ethnic Minorities. Edited by Hopkins A, Bahl V. London, Royal College of Physicians of London, 1993

Lipsedge M: Dangerous stereotypes. Journal of Forensic Psychiatry 5:1565–1573, 1994

Marsella A, White G: Cultural Conceptions of Mental Health and Therapy. Dokdrecht, Holland, D Reidel, 1986

Morrisey J, Levine I: Researchers discuss late findings and examine needs of homeless mentally ill persons. Hosp Community Psychiatry 38:811–812, 1987

National Census, London, Her Majesty's Stationery Office (HMSO), 1991

Rogow AA: The Psychiatrists. New York, Delta, 1970

Rueth T, Heller A: Unemployment: a factor in mental health crisis. American Journal of Social Psychiatry 3:49–51, 1981

Smith D: Racial Disadvantage in Britain. Harmondsworth, Penguin, 1977

Strathdee G, Williams P: The silent growth of a new service. Journal of Royal College of General Practitioners 34:615–618, 1984

Tambiah S: Magic, Science, and the Scope of Rationality. Cambridge, Cambridge University Press, 1992

Thornicroft G: Progress towards DHSS targets for community care. Br J Psychiatry 153:257–258, 1988

Townsend P: Poverty in the United Kingdom. London, Allen Lane, 1979

Wilson B: Religion in Sociological Perspective. Oxford, Oxford University Press, 1992

CHAPTER 8

Clinical Applications of Cultural Psychiatry in Arabian Gulf Communities

M. Fakhr El-Islam, F.R.C.P., F.R.C.Psych.

In this chapter, I use the term *culture* to mean the social heritage of beliefs, attitudes, and practices. Culture is an important determinant of the behavior of various individuals and plays pathogenic, pathoplastic, prognostic, and therapeutic roles in relation to psychiatric disorders. The Arabian cultural perspective is important for scholars and practitioners in psychiatry, psychology, sociology, and anthropology. The two major reviews (El-Islam 1982a; Racy 1970) dealing with the subject need to be supplemented by recent research findings pertinent to clinical methods in transcultural psychiatry. In this chapter, I describe the picture of Arabian culture, how it differs from other cultures, and the effects of recent cultural changes on clinical practice. After a description of cultural (including religious and socioeconomic) background, I provide an account of common native healing rituals and describe culture as a pathogenic factor, a pathoplastic factor, and a resource.

Cultural Background

Pre-Islamic Arabs were pagans and lived in nomadic tribes. They were not unified under one ruler in the Arabian peninsula, though their neighbors across the gulf were united into one country, Persia, ruled by one ruler, or *Kysra*. They accorded women an inferior status and practiced female infanticide for fear of the disgrace females could bring on the family later by premarital pregnancy. They were proud of the number of male children and number of wives they had; females were regarded as objects of sexual gratification and procreation only.

With the onset of the Islamic religion 14 centuries ago, infanticide was prohibited and considered a premeditated murder, and the number of wives was limited to four, all of whom were to be treated fairly as equals by their husband (Hammudah 1977). It was the woman's role, however, to remain indoors and be devoted to nurturing family members inside of the house. Filial piety, respect of elders, and nepotism continued as cherished characteristics of Arab families from pre-Islamic into Islamic eras, although nepotism is not part of the Islamic doctrine. Western writers and orientalists often fail to make the distinction between the behavior of present-day Muslims and the teachings of the Islamic religion from which Muslims have recently chosen to depart. The Islamic prohibition of alcohol is based on its interference with the mind. Allocation to daughters of half of the wealth inherited by sons is rationalized in Islam by the moral obligation of family males to protect and provide for females.

Arab beliefs in spiritual (jinni) possession, envy by others' evil eyes, and sorcery or witchcraft continued from pre-Islamic into Islamic epochs. These beliefs have been invoked to explain changes of human behavior. The main belief introduced by Islam as its first pillar is the unitary concept of God and the prophethood of Muhammad as God's last messenger or apostle to humanity. The main observances introduced by Islam are the five daily prayers, the fast of 1 month every year (Ramadan), the obligatory giving away of money or equivalents (*zakat*) to the poor, and the performance of pilgrimage (hajj) by those who are healthy and wealthy. Muslim pilgrimage rituals include ritual sacrifices of sheep and lambs, symbolic stoning of the devil, and prayers and meditation around and near the holy shrine (Kaaba) in Mecca, Arabia (Al-Subaie 1989). The performance of hajj is believed to clear humans of sins of all kinds and to compensate for material loss or sacrifice by heavenly rewards in later life, leading to the sense of internal tranquillity and harmony that many people seek.

Recent social changes have encroached on the time-honored patterns of family relationships and encouraged variable degrees of individuation in various family members (Kinzie et al. 1972). Family decisions (e.g., arranging marriages) are challenged by youth, who like to make individual decisions independently. The family-nurturing monorole of women is challenged by their discovery of their potential for multiple roles after their recent access to education and social intercourse. Interdependence and group ego development are giving way to competitive individualism and even egoism.

The acquisition of wealth through oil discoveries by Arabian Gulf communities in the 1960s reduced achievement motivation and the value placed on work for livelihood. Current civilian laws in Arabian Gulf countries try to maintain the superiority of indigenous members of the community as wealth owners in the face of imported expatriate professionals and technical experts who run the community's modern services. Ownership of property and businesses, sponsorship of expatriates, and higher education are formally limited to the indigenous members of the population. However, because the proportion of the indigenous to the expatriate is 1:2 in most Arabian Gulf countries, indigenous members experience themselves as minorities in their own countries. This circumstance has led to covert conflicts between the indigenous and expatriate communities concerning their independence versus interdependence, their authority versus responsibility, and their traditional values versus imported ones.

Common Native Healing Rituals

The most commonly practiced rituals make use of verses from the holy book, the Koran, for reciting verses, tying written verses to the body in the form of amulets, and drinking the washings of Koranic verses written on a plate. Individuals approach religious healers with appeals for God's mercy, compassion, and forgiveness in order to employ Koranic verses in favor of their clients, although the Islamic religion prides itself on being uniquely devoid of the religious figures (i.e., the clergy) who mediate between God and humans in other religions.

Rituals exorcising bad spirits (jinni) include the elaborate trance-based rituals imported from Africa (Prince 1980), as well as caning or tying rituals, employed to compel the spirits to leave the body of the victim. They are used mainly as vehicles of suggestion in treating dissociation disorders. Anti-envy rituals are held to prevent or remove the damage to health or wealth resulting from other people's evil wishes and envious eyes. Anti-envy rituals, charms, and symbols usually include the number 5, which is represented in Arabic by a circle that can also symbolize an eye. Some charms contain the figure of a human eye and may be used as pendants.

Elaborate antisorcery practices by native healers involve the use of "traces" of material that belong to the victim (e.g., hair or clothes) to negotiate a disengagement with the responsible adverse spirits or counter the influence of those who employed these spirits to harm the victim (e.g., to make him impotent) or to spoil his or her harmony with others. Similar principles were described by Jilek and Jilek-Aall (1990) in Thailand. Cautery is used primarily to counter painful conditions, but head cauterizations may be practiced to drive away the jinni, presumed to have overwhelmed the minds of psychotic individuals.

Patients may relieve their guilt by visiting the graves of dead *sheikhs* (saint equivalents), which they regard as shrines and where appeals for forgiveness, success, and problem solving can be petitioned in an atmosphere of submissive humility. Apart from visits to the grave of the prophet Muhammad in Madina, Arabia, this ritual is not practiced in Arabian Gulf communities, although Mediterranean and African Arabs may indulge in its practice.

Culture as a Pathogenic Factor

In most Arabian Gulf communities, the monorole of marriage and mothering is all that is traditionally expected of women. No other role is a sufficient alternative. Under the term *culture-bound neurosis,* a syndrome has been described in women who fail to marry or fail to have children (El-Islam 1975). The syndrome is also described in women who live the threat of breakup of their marriage or the threat of losing their fertility through gynecological problems. It consists of feelings of dizziness, fatigue, palpitation, tightness in the chest, and nausea. Women affected by this syndrome portray themselves as "physical wrecks." The culture-conditioned stress of failure to fulfill the prescribed role of women leads to hypochondriacal developments (Dubovsky 1983; Racy 1980) that arouse attention and sympathy in others toward women who would otherwise be regarded as social failures. The psychosocial origin of the symptoms is forsaken, and the sequence of reasoning is reversed, since these women are considered to be too physically ill to marry or reproduce. Most patients undergo elaborate physical investigation in search of a presumed organic etiology. The more the patient's investigations yield negative results, the more she becomes a hypochondriacal invalid. Many of these women state that their doctors are looking for something they cannot find and wonder whether cases like theirs have ever been encountered by doctors.

The syndrome is distinctly more common in illiterate than literate women, presumably because the latter might be able to feel their worth through pursuits other than marriage and procreation. Secondary gain, in the form of attention by medical personnel and family members and trips for treatment abroad in more developed countries, tends to fix and prolong the symptoms of this syndrome. Only psychiatrists who have cultural insight recognize the roots of the problem. Rather than indulgence into injudicious investigation and use of psychotropic medication, psychotherapeutic support of these patients helps to reinforce a sense of identity by guidance to other roles that could actualize the patients' potentials. When these patients are entrusted with care of others' children, they may show envy and anger unless they manage to identify with the children whom they care for. Voluntary work and other unorthodox modern roles can be entertained by the educated minority. Looking after the sick and elderly in the extended family is the most acceptable alternative role in this community.

According to Wittkower's classification (1968) of value-oriented cultural stresses, this syndrome seems to be initiated and sustained not only by existing native value orientations about the monorole of women but also by coexisting value orientations about women's multiple roles among expatriates living in the Gulf region. A change of native value orientation is possible only in the minority of educated women. Similar somatization syndromes among Australian aborigines (Bianchi 1970) and in Muslim women in India (Jankiramaiah and

Subbakrishna 1980) were attributed to the breakdown of traditional cultural mechanisms.

Intergenerational conflict between youth and their parents has been implicated in patients presenting for psychiatric help. It is prominent in 57% of cases of parasuicide (deliberate self-harm), 20% of minor psychiatric disorders, and 17% of schizophrenic illnesses (El-Islam 1974, 1976, 1979). Conflict between traditional parental attitudes and modern attitudes of young people involves primarily family relationship patterns, types of marriage, and roles of women. Over the past 25 years, schools, the mass media, mixing with expatriates employed in Arabian Gulf countries, and tourism abroad have introduced the younger generation to nontraditional values that make them seek equality rather than hierarchy in family relationships, love rather than arranged marriages, and a multirole rather than a monorole for women in society. Also, occupational achievements of the young may be secretly envied though overtly criticized by parents who have not had a range of occupational opportunities comparable with that of their "petrol-generation" children. However, many young persons lack achievement motivation, since they "have only to stretch out their hands to have ripe fruits of prosperity fall into them" (Graz 1976, p. 7). Before the discovery of oil, members of the parental generation had to work very hard in the dangerous occupation of diving for pearls for the sake of relatively little profit. They are therefore disappointed with and critical of the meager achievement drive of their children, who adopt new culture-alien attitudes. Sometimes "it is not clear who [is] doing the more protesting: the young against their elders or the elders against their children" (McNamara 1968, p. 11).

Recognition of intergenerational conflict is important for therapy and prevention. Family counseling supports a broad concept of normality that encompasses both the old cultural traditions and the new modern methods. Diversity in the family is accepted for resolving intergenerational conflict. This understanding helps to improve relationships within the family as a whole, and many parents expressed their intention to use insights gained through family therapy to avoid conflict with their younger children as they come of age. Young patients struggle not only interpersonally with their parents but also intrapersonally with their internalized object relationships representing parental values. Relief of their guilt through conflict resolution helps them to find their way between two worlds, one dying and the other not yet living.

In a community survey, however, intergenerational conflict was not significantly associated with psychiatric symptoms in high school students, though interparental conflict in nontraditional attitudes had a significant association with symptoms in either parent (El-Islam et al. 1986, 1988a). Similar findings were made by Furnham and Shiekh (1993) in second-generation Pakistani immigrants who proved to have no excess of psychological symptoms. It has been concluded that pronounced intergenerational conflict, by diminishing family support, may be instrumental in instigating professional help seeking in clinical matters, whereas milder intergenerational conflicts in community samples can be managed by the normal supportive family atmosphere without generating symptoms.

In a survey of psychiatric symptoms associated with oral contraceptives, some cultural roots have been implicated (El-Islam et al. 1988b). Pronatalist attitudes in Arabian communities have pre-Islamic and Islamic cultural roots (Good 1980). Arabs have always regarded a large number of children, especially male children, as a source of power for the family. Women who produce many children enjoy high status in the family, and their husbands are less likely to acquire additional wives. Moreover, the Islamic prophet stated that multiplication of Muslims into a large nation will be a source of his pride on the day of judgment. A woman who resorts to contraception voluntarily abrogates her culturally defined monorole of reproduction. She may feel that she is interfering with God's will, a belief shared by Catholic Christians. In the early days of Islam, however, three methods of birth control were allowed in order to dissuade pagan Arabs from infanticide. These methods included periods of abstention from sexual intercourse, marriage to one wife only, and the practice of coitus interruptus if both parties agreed to it (El-Nassery 1971).

At present, socioeconomic and health factors make it mandatory for many families to resort to contraception for family planning and for control of the number of births. If women who believe contraception is wrong from a religious or sociocultural point of view have to resort to contraception, a state of cognitive dissonance, associated with a significant excess of psychiatric symptoms, results. Development of psychiatric symptoms is much less likely in women who believe that their contraceptive practice is permitted by their value systems. Symptomatic women often feel guilt ridden and regard their symptoms as retributions for transgression of religious or cultural values about procreation. Also, psychiatric symptoms are more likely and more marked in women taking oral contraceptives than in women who use intrauterine contraceptive devices. This higher prevalence may be attributed to the daily intake of pills acting as a repetitive guilt inducer, whereas the continuous presence of intrauterine contraceptives tends to be forgotten.

A lack of cultural stress on the value of work in the indigenous population in Arabian Gulf countries has led to very low levels of work-centered achievement motivation. In a study of the role of recent stressful life events in precipitating depression (El-Islam et al. 1983), work-related stress was much less likely among indigenous Qataris and Kuwaitis than among expatriate Arabs in Qatar and Kuwait, respectively. In a study of Arab patients with myocardial infarction (Emara et al. 1986), indigenous Kuwaitis had a lower incidence of type A behavior and work-related precipitating factors than non-Kuwaiti Arabs in Kuwait. Drive, including achievement motivation, and job involvement were the components of type A behavior that differentiated most between the indigenous and expatriate groups.

Culture as a Pathoplastic Factor

Culture plays an important part in determining the pattern of psychiatric symptoms. In various cultures, some symptoms are more common than others, since expressions of mental ill health vary according to the traditional schemata of illness imprinted during the formative years of individual development.

Somatization is the expression of emotional problems in bodily symptoms. The predominance of somatic over behavioral and emotional presentations of psychiatric disorder to medical and psychiatric services in Arabian Gulf communities is well documented (El-Islam 1975, 1978; El-Islam et al. 1988c). It is traditionally believed that doctors deal only with the human body and that health problems can be communicated to them solely through bodily symptoms. Emotional distress (e.g., fear or low-spiritedness) is traditionally attributed to weakness of self or weakness of faith and is therefore not brought to the attention of doctors (Furnham and Malik 1994). Overtly disturbed behavior is also traditionally believed to lie outside of the domain of doctors, because it is attributed to supernatural agents (e.g., the evil eye, the devil, or the spirits known as jinni). Therefore, patients whose main symptoms are behavioral are culturally held to need native healing by traditional or religious healers endowed with supernatural powers that can undo the envy by evil eyes or deal with the evil spirits responsible for sorcery.

Somatic symptoms are culturally approved excuses for role failure. Unlike emotional symptoms, no individual weakness is held responsible for bodily symptoms. Disturbance or loss of significant interpersonal relationships is traditionally expressed by chest symptoms attributed to the heart. A sense of tightness in the chest is the commonest somatic symptom in all psychiatric disorders presenting to doctors. It is experienced as a reduction in chest capacity, and patients often sigh repeatedly in order to test whether their chests can physically contain the amount of air they should accommodate. Losses of appetite and libido are traditionally signs of ill health in general and do not have the same significance for the diagnosis of major depression in Arab patients as they have in Western patients. Left-sided bodily pains are traditionally held to be connected in one way or another to the heart. Nausea is a traditional symbol of rejection. Low back pain is the most frequent expression of sexual difficulties, especially in men, in whom the back is the traditional symbol of strength, masculinity, and virility. Genital worries are believed to indicate urinary problems.

A delusion is clinically defined as a false belief, firmly held against reasoning and out of keeping with the cultural background of the individual holding it. A delusory cultural belief, on the other hand, "receives general acceptance within a cultural unit but appears to outsiders to lack objective verification or even to be objectively disprovable" (Murphy 1967, p. 684). Though a delusion is a sign of psychotic disorder, delusory cultural beliefs are not indicative of pathology.

Psychotic patients' delusions may be formed by misconstruing delusory cultural beliefs, which become culturally alien experiences that their peers do not hold in the socioculturally shared belief systems. The strange experiences associated with the onset of a psychotic disorder may also be attributed to current secular environmental events, especially those that are topical, relatively new, or ambiguous (e.g., satellites, spying devices, or ethnic prejudice).

Culture-centered delusions are therefore false beliefs that transgress culturally approved boundaries (El-Islam 1980). For example, sorcery is traditionally held responsible for marital disharmony and impotence, but it is a delusion to attribute to sorcery the loss of a job or the conviction of being poisoned. Only an Arab psychiatrist from within the community can appreciate and define the boundary between delusions and normal culturally shared beliefs. The profound influence of culture on sustaining supernatural beliefs in the face of modern education has been borne out by one study (El-Islam and Malasi 1985), which revealed that culture-centered explanations of delusional content are as likely to be found in the most educated as in the illiterate schizophrenic patient in Kuwait. Patients who spent several years of graduate education in Western institutions still explained their delusional experiences in terms of their beliefs about the influences of sorcery, jinni, and envy by the evil eyes of others. Traditional beliefs, part of their social heritage since their formative years, were not erased by later secular education about objective facts and thinking.

In recent international psychiatric classifications, Schneider's first-rank symptoms have been accorded an important place in the diagnostic criteria for schizophrenia. A cautious emic rather than etic approach is essential to differentiate Schneider's delusions of influence, delusions of passivity, audible thoughts, and running commentary hallucinations from culturally shared beliefs about the influences of God's will and of the devil (shaitan), inspiring and intimating human beings to do wrong (Al-Ansari et al. 1989).

Morbid fears have patterns that reflect the cultural background of the community (El-Islam 1994). Fear of death, in the form of panic attacks, usually involves not only fear of the end of life but also fear of torture in one's grave after burial and fear of punishment by hellfire in the later eternal life that follows doomsday. Agoraphobia is rarely found in women, since women are not expected to go outdoors on their own; they are always escorted outdoors by men. Moreover, being home-bound, which indicates severe agoraphobia in Western women, is a virtue in women in Arabian Gulf communities, where home is considered the natural place for women and going outdoors is a transgression of cultural mores. Because of an ultraconservative sex rearing, many young girls grow up associating sex with physical harm and disgrace; instances of coitophobia in newlywed girls have led to divorce or professional help seeking.

Obsessional ruminations are invariably attributed to the devil, who has the same name, *Wisswaas,* as ruminations in the Arabic language. By attributing unacceptable thoughts and religious doubts to the devil, individuals greatly mitigate the harboring of guilt feelings (El-Islam 1982a). Compulsive symptoms usually involve blasphemous ruminations, checking and cleanliness rituals related to religious observances *(taharah),* and fear of loss of control over one's own aggressive impulses to harm family members in breach of culture-honored filial piety.

Because alcohol consumption is forbidden by the Islamic religion (Baasher 1981; Suliman 1983), adolescents may resort to alcohol as an anticultural, antiparental act of rebellion (Bilal and El-Islam 1985). Many individuals who consume alcohol are brought by their relatives for psychiatric treatment, although they fulfill none of the criteria for dependence or loss of control over their drinking behavior. Their relatives equate breach of cultural sanctions against alcohol with the need for psychiatric attention. A study of guilt feelings in Kuwaiti depressive patients (El-Islam et al. 1988b) revealed that guilt feelings could be elicited in two-thirds of patients, although they are rarely volunteered by patients on presentation for psychiatric services. Though well-known as a "shame society," Arabian communities exhibit guilt as well. The guilt is usually linked to religious wrongdoing.

Suicide is rare in Arab nations, even in individuals with major depression, perhaps because the Islamic religion strongly disapproves of suicide (Okasha and Lotaif 1979). Those who take their own lives are condemned to eternal hellfire in later life, and it is blasphemous to give up hope that God's help is forthcoming (El-Islam et al. 1988b). However, deliberate self-harm (parasuicide) is not uncommon among young, culturally subdued females as a method of pathological care eliciting and sometimes ends in self-inflicted death (Suleiman et al. 1989). Like obsessional ruminations, suicidal thoughts are normally resisted as intimations from the devil; Muslims believe disorders occur only if a patient's religious faith is not strong enough to neutralize the devilish activities (Horikoshi 1980).

Culture as a Resource

Multicenter studies of schizophrenia point to the better outcome of schizophrenia in developing countries compared with developed industrial societies (Jablensky et al. 1980). The different prognosis may be due to overrepresentation of transient, psychogenic, or schizophreniform psychoses in samples from developing countries. However, the outcome was found to be better for patients living in extended (traditional) families than in nuclear (modern) families in the Arabian Gulf community in Qatar for both schizophrenia and schizophreniform psychoses independently studied (El-Islam 1979). The role of extended families (El-Islam 1982b) was distinguished by warm concern about their patient members in accordance with cultural nurturing traditions; this attitude was manifest in their patients' earlier presentation for treatment, better leisure time occupation, and frequent participation in social visits to relatives. Flexible role expectations led to extended family tolerance of patients' minor oddities in behavior and brief withdrawals. Moreover, extended families contained more patients whose delusions involved culturally recognized supernatural agents. When compared with delusions centered on secular matters, culture-centered delusions were found to be more likely to remit with treatment (El-Islam 1980). As these delusions lose the extracultural details that rendered them abnormal, their experience is readily contained in the repertoire matrix of traditional socially shared beliefs, and the experience becomes understandable to both patients and their families. On the other hand, a sense of alienation from the family and from the cultural background will always exist in relation to material-centered delusions, which remain nonunderstandable, since neither the patient nor his or her family can fit them into any belief system or schema.

Psychiatric disorders with marked intergenerational conflict were more likely than other psychiatric disorders to remit (El-Islam 1983). In family therapy, traditional family elders contribute to the resolution of intergenerational conflict by sacrificing low-order traditions (e.g., arranging marriages) to preserve high-order traditions (e.g., filial piety).

Traditional and religious methods of treatment that derive from cultural beliefs help many patients through suggestion, catharsis, identification with models, and guilt reduction (El-Islam 1967). Various forms of healing practices, such as zaar ceremonies, are carried out in groups, heightening suggestibility and enhancing identification with others. They relieve the patient's guilt through sacrifices. They exorcise the possessing evil spirits and clear the envy of others' evil eyes by use of verses from the holy Koran. In contrast to Western psychiatric treatment, which encourages and depends on undoing the projections responsible for patients' delusions and hallucinations, traditional healers reinforce patients' projection onto supernatural agents, and patients are impressed by their healers' ability to share their understanding (El-Islam 1992). Attempts to combine or integrate Western and traditional treatment have met with varying degrees of success (Asuni 1979; Baasher 1983).

Pilgrimage (hajj) performance in the holy city of Mecca helps to ameliorate the suffering of some patients. Some depressed patients, who regard their sufferings as God's retributions for wrongdoing, are likely to feel forgiven after their pilgrimage and hence relieved of their guilt.

The role of the traditional family as the main social service agency is established in Arabian Gulf communities. Families run the affairs of their members, healthy and sick alike, by group decisions. Family members informally help psychiatrists to secure hospitalization for psychotic patients who are too ill to recognize their need for hospital treatment. In most Arabian Gulf communities, this care obviates the need for mental health legislation and for formal certification of patients for compulsory admission. The family is also traditionally involved in the patient's discharge from the hospital and in assuring the individual's continued welfare in the community. Professional help seeking is always a family decision (El-Islam and Abu-Dagga 1990a). The family continues to arrange marriages for its members, especially for schizophrenic patients, whose emotional and social skills are not sufficient to secure a love marriage (El-Islam and Abu-Dagga 1990b). Many of these family members choose to continue their married lives within the household of the extended family.

Western types of psychotherapy are not likely to be appreciated in traditional Arabian Gulf communities, since talking is not considered a replacement for situation manipulation or medication (Racy 1970). Group therapies are likely to boost feelings of stigmatization—because psychiatric symptoms are "publicized" to others—rather than foster mutual support by group members. Shame is still an important feeling closely associated with psychiatric symptoms in Arab patients, who would deny all problems readily in situations where their "weakness" could be exposed to others.

The relative underrepresentation of female patients in psychiatric services in Arabian Gulf communities has been attributed to the protective effects of culture, such as not exposing women to life stresses and not expecting them to have a primary role in making decisions (El-Sendiony 1981). In the extended family, sick women receive support from other women in the household, who take over their roles in domestic chores until they recover (El-Islam 1982b). The presentation of young, unmarried females to psychiatric services is avoided at all costs in Arabian Gulf communities, because the stigma involved may jeopardize their chances of being sought in arranged marriages (El-Islam and Abu-Dagga 1990b).

References

Al-Ansari EA, Emara MM, Mirza IA, et al: Schizophrenia in ICD-10: a field trial of suggested diagnostic guidelines. Compr Psychiatry 30:416–419, 1989

Al-Subaie A: Psychiatry in Saudi Arabia: cultural perspectives. Transcultural Psychiatric Research Review 26:245–262, 1989

Asuni T: Modern medicine and traditional medicine, in African Therapeutic Systems. Edited by Ademywagun ZA. Waltham, MA, Brandeis University Crossroads Press, 1979, pp 176–181

Baasher T: The use of drugs in the Islamic world. British Journal of Addiction 76:233–243, 1981

Baasher T: Relationship between traditional and modern medicine. Bulletin de l'Association Francaise de Psychiatrie et Psychopathologie Sociable 15:101–103, 1983

Bianchi GN, McElwain DW, Cawte JE: The dispensary syndrome in Australian aborigines: origins of their bodily preoccupation and sick role behaviour. Br J Med Psychol 43:375–382, 1970

Bilal AM, El-Islam MF: Some clinical and behavioural aspects of patients with alcohol dependence problems in Kuwait psychiatric hospital. Alcohol Alcohol 20:57–62, 1985

Dubovsky S: Psychiatry in Saudi Arabia. Am J Psychiatry 140:1455–1459, 1983

El-Islam MF: The psychotherapeutic basis of some Arab rituals. Int J Soc Psychiatry 13:265–268, 1967

El-Islam MF: Hospital-referred parasuicide in Qatar. Egyptian Journal of Mental Health 15:101–112, 1974

El-Islam MF: Culture bound neurosis in Qatari women. Soc Psychiatry 10:25–29, 1975

El-Islam MF: Intergenerational conflict and the young Qatari neurotic. Ethos 4:45–56, 1976

El-Islam MF: Transcultural aspects of psychiatric patients in Qatar. Comparative Psychiatry East and West 6:33–36, 1978

El-Islam MF: A better outlook for schizophrenics living in extended families. Br J Psychiatry 135:343–347, 1979

El-Islam MF: Symptom onset and involution of delusions. Soc Psychiatry 15:157–160, 1980

El-Islam MF: Arabic cultural psychiatry. Transcultural Psychiatric Research Review 19:5–24, 1982a

El-Islam MF: Rehabilitation of schizophrenics by the extended family. Acta Psychiatr Scand 65:112–119, 1982b

El-Islam MF: Cultural change and intergenerational relationships in Arabian families. International Journal of Family Psychiatry 4:321–329, 1983

El-Islam MF: Transcultural aspects of schizophrenia and ICD-10. Curare 15:227–230, 1992

El-Islam MF: Cultural aspects of morbid fears in Qatari women. Soc Psychiatry Psychiatr Epidemiol 29:137–140, 1994

El-Islam MF, Abu-Dagga SI: Illness behaviour in mental ill-health in Kuwait. Scandinavian Journal of Social Medicine 18:195–201, 1990a

El-Islam MF, Abu-Dagga SI: Marriage and fertility rates of schizophrenic patients in Kuwait. Med Principles Pract 2:18–26, 1990b

El-Islam MF, Malasi TH: Delusions and education. Journal of Operational Psychiatry 16:29–31, 1985

El-Islam MF, Mohsen MYA, Demerdash AM, et al: Life events and depression in transit populations. Int J Soc Psychiatry 29:13–20, 1983

El-Islam MF, Abu-Dagga SI, Malasi TH, et al: Inter-generational conflict and psychiatric symptoms. Br J Psychiatry 149:300–306, 1986

El-Islam MF, Malasi TH, Abu-Dagga SI: Interparental differences in attitudes to cultural changes in Kuwait. Soc Psychiatry Psychiatr Epidemiol 23:109–113, 1988a

El-Islam MF, Malasi TH, Abu-Dagga SI: Oral contraceptives, sociocultural beliefs, and psychiatric symptoms. Soc Sci Med 27:941–945, 1988b

El-Islam MF, Moussa MAA, Malasi TH, et al: Assessment of depression in Kuwait by principal component analysis. J Affective Disord 14:109–114, 1988c

El-Nassery MM: Family planning viewed in the light of the Islamic code, in Family Planning. Edited by Nazer ER, Zayed MY, Najjar YJ. Beirut, International Planned Parenthood Federation (IPPF) United Publishing House, 1971, pp 39–67

El-Sendiony MFM: The effects of Islamic sharia on behavioural disturbances. Makka, Ummal Qura University, 1981, pp 24–30

Emara Mk, El-Islam MF, Abu-Dagga SI, et al: Type A behaviour in Arab patients with myocardial infarction. J Psychosom Res 30:553–558, 1986

Furnham A, Malik R: Cross-cultural beliefs about depression. Int J Soc Psychiatry 40:106–123, 1994

Furnham A, Shiekh S: Gender, generational, and social support correlates of mental health in Asian immigrants. Int J Soc Psychiatry 39:22–33, 1993

Good MD: Of blood and babies: the relationship of popular Islamic physiology to fertility. Soc Sci Med 14B:147–156, 1980

Graz L: Qatar. ICAA News 4:7, 1976

Hammudah A: The family structure in Islam. Washington, DC, American Trust Publication, 1977

Horikoshi H: Asrama: an Islamic psychiatric institution in West Java. Soc Sci Med 14B:157–165, 1980

Jablensky A, Schwarz R, Tomor T: WHO collaborative study on impairments and disabilities associated with schizophrenic disorders. Acta Psychiatr Scand 62(suppl 285):152–163, 1980

Jankiramaiah N, Subbakrishna DK: Somatic neurosis in Muslim women in India. Soc Psychiatry 15:203–206, 1980

Jilek WG, Jilek-Aall L: The mental health relevance of traditional medicine and shamanism in refugee camps of northern Thailand. Curare 13:217–224, 1990

Kinzie JD, Sushama PC, Lee M: Cross-cultural family therapy: a Malaysian experience. Fam Process 11:59–67, 1972

McNamara RS: The essence of security. The Times (London), August 31, 1968, p. 684

Murphy HBM: Cultural aspects of the delusion. Stadium Generale 20:684–692, 1967

Okasha A, Lotaif F: Attempted suicide: an Egyptian investigation. Acta Psychiatr Scand 60:69–75, 1979

Prince R: Variations in psychotherapeutic procedures, in Handbook of Cross-Cultural Psychology, Vol 6. Edited by Triandis HC, Draguns JG. Boston, MA, Allyn & Bacon, 1980, pp 291–349

Racy J: Psychiatry in the Arab East. Acta Psychiatr Scand Suppl 211, 1970

Racy J: Somatization in Saudi women: a therapeutic challenge. Br J Psychiatry 137:212–216, 1980

Suleiman MA, Moussa MAA, El-Islam MF: The profile of parasuicide repeaters in Kuwait. Int J Soc Psychiatry 35:146–155, 1989

Suliman H: Alcohol and Islamic faith. Drug Alcohol Depend 11:63–65, 1983

Wittkower ED: Transcultural psychiatry, in Modern Perspectives in World Psychiatry. Edited by Howells JG. Edinburgh, Oliver & Boyd, 1968, pp 697–712

CHAPTER 9

Ethnicity and Psychopharmacology
The Experience of Southeast Asians

J. DAVID KINZIE, M.D.
TIMI EDEKI, M.D., PH.D.

The era of cross-cultural psychopharmacology can be said to have begun in 1969 when Murphy described ethnic differences in drug use throughout the world. Overall et al. (1969) later reported that blacks improved more than whites from a variety of short-term psychotherapeutic agents. Raskin and Crook (1975) found that depressed black patients taking tricyclic (imipramine) antidepressants (TCAs) evidenced a higher rate of improvement than did whites after 1 week of treatment. Of special interest was the finding that chlorpromazine was the most efficacious for black women, whereas imipramine was more efficacious for black men. In 1979 Yamamoto and co-workers found that Asian Americans needed lower doses of antidepressant and neuroleptic medicines for effectiveness compared with Caucasians. This finding was confirmed, at least partially, by Lin et al. (1986), who found that Asian patients required lower neuroleptic and tricyclic doses.

These studies provided evidence for racial and ethnic differences in psychopharmacologic effects. They also opened up a variety of biological studies that determined the magnitude of these effects, the underlying biological mechanisms, and the practical clinical significance. The field clearly came of age with the awarding of a National Institute of Mental Health (NIMH) grant for a research center on the psychobiology of ethnicity in 1990, headed by Dr. Keh-Ming Lin. The center sponsored a book by Lin et al. (1993b) entitled *Psychopharmacology and the Psychobiology of Ethnicity*.

In this chapter we 1) present studies of the psychobiology of psychotropic drug use, 2) describe the current data on treatment of major psychiatric disorders during Kinzie's 15 years of experience with Indochinese refugees, and 3) offer practical guidelines for the treatment of psychiatric disorders of patients from other cultures. Throughout this chapter, references are made to Kinzie's experience in the Indochinese Psychiatric Clinic in Portland, Oregon. For more than 15 years, Vietnamese, Cambodian, Laotian, and Mien patients have been treated there. Currently, the Portland clinic employs six faculty psychiatrists, treating a total of 550 patients. A wide variety of treatment modalities have been used, including psychotherapy, social therapy, and a series of rehabilitation services. However, in this chapter we concentrate on the use of psychotropic medication.

Ethnic Differences in Drug Response

Ethnic differences in drug response have led to a better understanding of the complexity of transcultural pharmacology (Blackwell 1971) and a warning not to extrapolate clinical findings from one culture to another (Lewis et al. 1980). Ethnic differences in drug response may consist of different mean capacities in drug metabolizing or different frequencies of this capacity by the occurrence of genetic enzyme variants (Kalow 1982). An example of the former is presented in a study of racial differences in propranolol pharmacokinetics between blacks and whites, showing lower serum concentrations in black men (Johnson and Burlew 1992). An example of the latter is the finding that approximately 50% of Chinese and Japanese subjects lack the active form of aldehyde dehydrogenase (Kalow 1982; Lin et al. 1992). These Asians would be poor eliminators of the alcohol metabolite acetaldehyde, which is responsible for the flushing response seen after ingestion of alcohol.

Ethnic Differences in Drug Metabolism

The cytochrome P450 enzymes (CYP) that are important in the metabolism of psychotropic drugs include CYP2D6 and CYP2C19. These enzymes are polymorphically distributed in different populations. The presence of these enzymes is genetically determined, and certain individuals with reduced amounts are referred to as poor metabolizers (PMs), in contrast to extensive metabolizers (EMs), who have normal amounts of the enzyme (Eichelbaum and Gross 1990). PMs have a reduced ability to metabolize drugs that are substrates of these enzymes.

CYP2D6 is responsible for the metabolism of dextromethorphan and more than 30 drugs that are commonly used clinically (Daly et al. 1993). This enzyme also metabolizes several psychotropic drugs such as tricyclic antidepressants, selective serotonin-reuptake inhibitors (SSRIs), and neuroleptic agents such as thioridazine (Shen and Lin 1991). Dextromethorphan, an over-the-counter cough preparation, and debrisoquin are probe drugs often used to screen for deficiency of this enzyme in populations. Using this drug, it was found that 7.7% of white children were PMs compared with only 1.9% of black children (Relling et al. 1991).

Another drug that exhibits genetic polymorphism is the anticonvulsant mephenytoin (Wilkinson et al. 1989). This drug is given as a racemic mixture of R and S enantiomers, and PMs have a relative deficiency in their ability to hydroxylate the S enantiomer (Kupfer et al. 1981; Wilkinson et al. 1989). The 4-hydroxylation of mephenytoin is carried out by CYP2C19 (Goldstein et al. 1994).

CYP2C19 is also involved in the metabolism of several psychotropic agents such as N-demethylation of diazepam (Bertilsson et al. 1989), imipramine (Skjelbo et al. 1991), hexobarbital (Adedoyin et al. 1994), and mephobarbital (Jacqz et al. 1986).

The distribution of the deficiency of CYP2D6 enzyme is racially determined and varies in different populations. For example, about 3–11% of the United States and European Caucasian population are PMs for the substrates of this enzyme, whereas the frequency is <1% in the Japanese and Chinese populations. On the other hand, as can be seen from Table 9–1, the frequency of the PMs for CYP2C19 substrates is very high in Oriental populations compared to Caucasian or African populations.

This fact could have important clinical implications in the therapeutic use of many psychotropic drugs in different populations. It also emphasizes the need to carry out drug studies in different populations,

Table 9–1. Frequency of mephenytoin poor metabolizers (PMs) in different populations

Population	Number studied	Percentage of PMs	Reference
African Americans	173	1.7	Edeki et al. 1994
African American elderly	27	18.5	Pollock et al. 1991
Americans (Caucasians)	156	2.6	Wedlund et al. 1984
American elderly (Caucasians)	123	4.1	Pollock et al. 1991
Canadian Caucasians	113	4.2	Jurima et al. 1985
Chinese	137	14.6	Bertilsson et al. 1992
Estonians	156	3.9	Kiivet et al. 1993
Indonesians	104	15.4	Setiabudy et al. 1994
Indians	48	20.8	Doshi et al. 1990
Japanese	24	22.6	Jurima et al. 1985
Koreans	206	12.6	Sohn et al. 1992
Spanish	373	1.34	Reviriego et al. 1993
Swedish	488	3.3	Bertilsson et al. 1992
Swiss	221	5.4	Kupfer and Preisig 1984
Vietnamese	37	22.0	Brosen et al. 1993

without extrapolating findings in one population, usually the Caucasian male, to other populations without appropriate studies.

Nongenetic Factors in Cross-Cultural Psychopharmacology

A variety of biological and nonbiological factors can influence the ethnic difference in psychotropic drug response. The biological factors include body size, dietary factors, commonly used nonpsychotropic medicines, and the frequency of smoking, which has been shown to affect the pharmacokinetics of haloperidol (Perry et al. 1993). The nonbiological factors include problems related to cross-cultural diagnosis and treatment. The early surveys did not use operationalized criteria of the disorders being treated, were often unclear about the target symptoms, and sometimes did not use placebo controls. In addition, the treating psychiatrists often reported the findings. Such approaches made comparisons of drug effects across culture difficult to interpret because of the poor methodology used.

Biologically oriented psychiatry infrequently recognizes the nonpharmacological factors in drug therapy that operate in all cultures. The nonspecific factors include the rate of placebo response in the population, the effects of the therapist's personality and his or her belief in the efficacy of medicine, the patient's personality and belief in the medicine, and especially the patient's expectation of therapy (Group for the Advancement of Psychiatry 1975; Smith et al. 1993). The patient's beliefs and expectations may be part of a culturally shared value system. In the Indochinese clinic, we commonly hear that "American medicine is too strong for the Vietnamese" or "American medicine is too 'hot' and causes imbalance" (in the yin-yang sense). Truly, many pharmacological and nonpharmacological variables need to be controlled before accurate cross-cultural comparisons can be made. However, noncompliance issues are so significant that they must be considered separately from other nonpharmacological factors.

Compliance

When our clinic first studied TCA plasma levels in the mid-1980s, we found a surprisingly high noncompliant rate among Vietnamese, Cambodian, and Mien patients (Kinzie et al. 1987). Among this group of 41, who had been prescribed long-term treatment with therapeutic oral doses of TCAs, 61% had no detectable levels of medicine. Therapeutic levels were found in only 15%.

A similar finding was obtained by Kroll et al. (1990), who found only 5 of 32 Southeast Asian patients taking antidepressant medicine had therapeutic plasma levels and 17 (53%) had undetectable levels. Interestingly, patients with undetectable levels had more side effect complaints than those with therapeutic plasma levels. A report from Benin, West Africa (Bertschy and Vadel 1992), on clomipramine found that only 42 of 92 patients could follow a 4-week treatment plan, and, of those, 12 had none or only trace amounts of antidepressants in the plasma (a compliance rate of 69% after a dropout rate of 51%; an overall compliance rate of 31%).

In the recent analysis of plasma TCA levels of 43 Southeast Asian patients who were determined for clinical purposes (i.e., in a nonrandom sample), we found none to only trace amounts in 40%. Thus, even in a well-established clinic, noncompliance with carefully prescribed medicine remains a serious problem. The reasons may relate to general cultural beliefs about Western medicines, individual fear, and intolerance of side effects. A common problem is the lack of awareness of the need for long-term maintenance to achieve relief. Clearly, for practical clinical therapeutic effects, compliance must be addressed with all patients. For cross-cultural studies, no comparisons of drug effects and side effects can be made unless there is certainty that the drug prescribed is actually taken in the appropriate amount.

The Antidepressants

A body of literature continues to develop on the cross-cultural treatment of depression. Several studies used single doses of a TCA and compared the pharmacokinetics in Caucasians and Asians. Rudorfer et al. (1984) reported high peak levels of desipramine in Asians, and Pi et al. (1986) found that Asians had an earlier time of peak concentration. Allen et al. (1977) found that Asians (Indian and Pakistani) had a significantly lower plasma level than English subjects following a 50-mg clomipramine dose. It is unclear how single-dose studies, usually done on volunteers and not depressed patients, relate to real clinical treatment in which high doses are used for a long time to achieve clinical remission. Therefore, this review concentrates on clinically relevant studies of antidepressants.

An early study (Ziegler and Biggs 1977) found no differences in plasma TCA levels between black and white patients taking amitriptyline, but black patients had 50% higher nortriptyline levels than whites. This difference was considered clinically relevant, given the therapeutic window of nortriptyline. In our study of imipramine (Kinzie et al.

1987) with Southeast Asians (noncompliant patients were eliminated from the study), it was found that plasma levels were dose related, and an oral dose of 150 mg/day of imipramine was required to reach the therapeutic plasma levels (7 of 9 at 150 mg/day had appropriate levels, whereas only 3 of 7 at doses of 100 to 125 mg/day had therapeutic plasma levels). Kroll et al. (1990) found that among another group of Southeast Asians, plasma levels of TCA correlated with clinical improvement. A sophisticated study from Japan (Shimoda et al. 1993) using clomipramine in 92 psychiatric patients found large individual variations in concentrations of the parent drug and its metabolite in plasma. However, there was a significant relationship between the daily dose of clomipramine and plasma levels. Only one poor hydroxylator was found in this group. An African study (Bertschy and Vandel 1992) found no higher plasma levels in Beninese patients than in Caucasian patients.

We recently analyzed our clinic data for nortriptyline and imipramine prescribed to Indochinese patients. Two aspects stand out: 1) at any one dose there is a three- to fourfold variation in plasma levels and 2), even so, there is a linear relationship between dose and plasma level. The nortriptyline dose needed to achieve the therapeutic window should be 50 to 75 mg/day. Imipramine usually needs to be taken in an oral dose of 150 mg or more daily to achieve a therapeutic plasma level. These doses are administered in the usual range for American patients (American Psychiatric Association 1994).

Newer antidepressants.   Just as data are beginning to accumulate regarding cross-cultural effects of TCA, the information runs the risk of quickly becoming irrelevant. The newer antidepressants, especially the SSRI antidepressants (fluoxetine, sertraline, and paroxetine), have rapidly become first-line drugs for outpatients with mild to moderate depression. They have the advantage of relative safety in overdoses and absence of anticholinergic side effects, about which many Asian patients complain. They clearly have caught on in our Indochinese clinic. Of 242 patients treated primarily with an antidepressant for depression, 41% received TCAs, 42% received SSRIs, and 17% received trazodone. Among the five physicians, use of SSRIs varies widely, from 17% to 79%, in the treatment of depression. Administration of SSRIs was associated with polypharmacy. Of the 77 patients taking SSRIs, 57 (74%) were also taking another psychotropic medication, usually for insomnia. The secondary medicine involved a low dose of trazodone, sedative TCAs, benzodiazepines, and even phenothiazines. Clearly, one of the major concerns of many Indochinese patients has been disturbed sleep or anxiety, for which the SSRIs seem ineffective or even exacerbating. The psychiatrists agree that TCAs may be more effective in treating severe depression. They also believe that the sexual dysfunction problems found with SSRIs have not been adequately addressed with the Southeast Asian populations because of the difficulty Asians have in discussing sexual issues.

The rapid change in outpatient treatment from TCAs to SSRIs seems to have resulted in greater patient acceptance but at a cost, including greater expense, polypharmacy to treat sleep and anxiety symptoms, and perhaps unreported side effects such as sexual dysfunction. An overlooked issue is the lack of adequate therapeutic drug monitoring to determine compliance, without which ethnic differences cannot be examined. It is difficult to make any statement about the SSRIs' relative effectiveness across cultures with the current state of clinical information.

Summary. Some impressions about cross-cultural differences in TCA use have been suggested, and some pharmacokinetics show differences in Asians and Caucasians. The clinical meaning of these reports is not clear. The high rate of noncompliance of TCAs in Asian and African populations confounds the issue. The high degree of plasma-level variation within each ethnic group seems to cloud ethnic differences. With current data (with the possible exception of nortriptyline with blacks), it seems that most patients from all studied ethnic groups require the usual American doses of TCA. However, this information may become irrelevant as the SSRIs supplant the TCAs. New research strategies will have to be developed to test whether SSRIs are differentially effective across cultures.

The Antipsychotics

Although it has been suggested that Asians need lower amounts of antipsychotics than Caucasians, the first report to systematically document these differences was published in 1981, when Asian patients were found to have more acute extrapyramidal (EPS) reactions than black or white patients (Binder and Levy 1981). Lin and Finder (1983) reported that Asians needed a significantly lower-dose maximum and stabilized neuroleptic drug than whites to control psychopathology. Lin and Finder's original report could not be replicated in another study (Sramek et al. 1986). However, in a study using a fixed dose of haloperidol, Chinese schizophrenic patients had 52% higher plasma levels than American non-Asian patients (Potkin et al. 1984). In a very thoughtful prospective study, Lin et al. (1989) observed Caucasian and Asian schizophrenic patients. During a fixed-dose phase, Asians had a higher serum haloperidol concentration and higher rating of EPS. Asians required a mean lower dose during a variable-dose phase. A suggestion from South Africa indicates that blacks tolerate neuroleptic side effects better than do whites (Pearlman 1984). Taken together, considerable evidence suggests that, at least for haloperidol, Asian schizophrenic patients can improve with lower doses. The evidence for black-Caucasian differences, however, is less compelling.

These data imply that one could probably use lower doses of neuroleptic medicine when treating the Southeast Asian schizophrenic patient. Our Indochinese clinic currently treats 66 Vietnamese and Cambodian patients with chronic schizophrenia, many of whom have been treated with neuroleptics for more than 5 years. This group consists of 29 males and 37 females, with ages ranging from 22 to 64 years. Although a number of antipsychotics are used, the most widely prescribed and probably best accepted by patients is perphenazine (N = 20). The decanoate form of fluphenazine and haloperidol was used in 22 patients, where males are greatly overrepresented (17 to 5). Compliance is a major concern for our clinicians, a difficulty overcome by regular intramuscular (IM) injections.

The dose range of the chronic maintenance phase varied from 1 mg daily of fluphenazine to 30 mg trifluoperazine. However, the highest dose was with the IM medication. One patient required 100 mg haloperidol decanoate IM every 2 weeks. When all of the medication prescribed was converted to chlorpromazine equivalence (Schatzberg and Cole 1991), the average daily dose for schizophrenic patients was 359.3 mg/day. This dose is not greatly dissimilar to reports of inpatients in Japan who received 276.8 mg/day of chlorpromazine (CP2E)

(Koshino et al. 1992) or in China, where patients received 311.3 mg/day (Ko et al. 1989). The dose used in our clinic is much less than that reported for American patients in a variety of settings (Baldessarini et al. 1984), where the equivalent of 1,000 mg/day of chlorpromazine is standard.

In summary, data from controlled studies and clinical reports support the idea that Asians need smaller doses of neuroleptic medicines than do American patients. Our experience with Vietnamese and Cambodians tends to support that finding. However, about one-third of the patients require long-acting IM medication, and, in these cases, the doses are generally in the recommended range. At this time, we have had limited experience with clozapine and risperidone.

Tardive dyskinesia. The development of tardive dyskinesia (TD) as a late neurologic side effect of antipsychotic drugs has been of concern to psychiatrists for many years. As has been pointed out in an American Psychiatric Association (1992) publication, the problem is complicated by issues of definition, assessment, and natural history of the disorder in chronic schizophrenia. Although prevalence rates reveal a wide variation, a long-term prospective study of Americans showed progressive cumulative incidence of 26% at 6 years of exposure to antipsychotic medicine (Kane and Smith 1982). In this light, a report from China involving psychiatric inpatients found a prevalence rate of only 8.4% (Ko et al. 1989), which was felt to be related to the use of low dosages of neuroleptics. However, a more recent report from Japan, also using low doses of neuroleptics, found a prevalence rate of 22.3% (Koshino et al. 1992). Koshino and co-workers felt that the older age of patients could account for the high prevalence rate.

In our clinic, the same nurse practitioner has performed systematic Abnormal Involuntary Movement Scale (AIMS) tests for the last 3 years. We have found a fluctuating course of the patients' TD, a finding also reported by others (American Psychiatric Association 1992). That is, some patients will show evidence of TD one year and none the following year. We have 46 schizophrenic Vietnamese and Cambodians who have been taking neuroleptics for at least 1 year and have undergone at least one AIMS test. If a criteria of AIMS rating of 2 or more is used (as in Ko's study), 14 patients have TD, for a point prevalence rate of 30%. If a rating of 2 or more in at least two parts of the body is used as the criterion, then six have TD, for a prevalence rate of 13%. Both results are comparable with other studies in the United States and abroad as quoted previously. Of the 14 cases of TD, 5 were mild (AIMS = 2–3) and 8 were moderate (AIMS = 4–8); only 1 case was severe (AIMS = 15).

Although our numbers are small, we have some suggestions of the factors related to TD in Southeast Asians. In this population of 24 males and 22 females, 13 of 14 with TD were males (χ^2, $P < .0009$). The presence and severity of TD was not related to ethnicity or age but related strongly to time on antipsychotic medicine (χ^2, $P < .0075$). Specifically, of the 20 who had been taking medicine for more than 5 years, 12 had signs of TD, and of the 5 who had been taking medicine for 11 to 13 years, all had TD. Overall, even in this small sample, we can find TD among Vietnamese and Cambodian schizophrenic patients in comparable rates with the United States population, although the condition is mostly labeled mild or moderate. Unlike in other reports (American Psychiatric Association 1992; Kane and Smith 1982), the at-risk population seems to be males with at least 5 years' exposure.

Lithium

Okpaku and colleagues (1980) pointed out that blacks have less Li^+ to Na^+ red cell countertransport activity than whites. This difference could result in blacks having high Li^+ ratios measured in vitro. A recent study has confirmed that Afro-Americans have a higher red blood cell to plasma lithium ratio than Caucasians and have increased side effects (Strickland et al. 1995). Clinical experience with Chinese bipolar patients (Yang 1985) found a good prophylactic effect of lithium at a mean plasma concentration of 0.5 mM/L. This dose is somewhat lower than the recommended dose for American patients (Schatzberg and Cole 1991). Our own experience with lithium is limited because of the low numbers of patients with pure bipolar disorder. In the more than 1,000 patients we have evaluated in 15 years, perhaps as few as 5 patients have truly had bipolar disorder. In our current population of 550 patients, only 7 patients are taking lithium, and all of these are also taking a neuroleptic. They are all diagnosed as schizoaffective, and pure bipolar disorder seems to be very uncommon in this group of refugees. When lithium is used, we have maintained patients in the usual United States therapeutic range of 0.8–1.2 mM/L.

Posttraumatic Stress Disorder

Awareness that refugees and many minorities throughout the world have suffered from violence and persecution is increasing. Many of these people will have experienced the prolonged symptoms of post-traumatic stress disorder (PTSD). In our clinic of Indochinese refugees, we found 70% met DSM-III-R criteria (American Psychiatric Association 1987) for current PTSD. Among Cambodians and Mien, the prevalence rate was more than 90% (Kinzie et al. 1990). A variety of pharmacotherapeutic agents including tricyclic antidepressants (Falcon et al. 1985), phenelzine (Kosten et al. 1991), fluoxetine (Nagy et al. 1993), and sertraline (Kline et al. 1994) have been used to treat symptoms of PTSD.

Almost all of our patients with PTSD also suffer from comorbid major depression. Therefore, we have begun administering TCAs to most patients. When an adequate plasma level is reached but symptoms are still present, we add clonidine. Clonidine is effective at reducing central nervous system norepinephrine hyperactivity, which is thought to mediate the arousal symptoms. This combination is well tolerated by our patients, and, in a prospective study, we found this combination effective in reducing depressive, intrusive, and hyperarousal, but not avoidant, symptoms (Kinzie and Leung 1989). In one study using only clonidine, we found marked reduction in nightmares in PTSD patients, but the mechanism for this reduction is unclear (Kinzie et al. 1994). Clonidine is of course effective in treating hypertension, which affects 30% of our patients. Alone (not combined with TCAs), clonidine can be used to treat both PTSD and hypertension. Furthermore, it can be administered by a weekly transdermal patch to overcome problems with compliance. Currently, we are using clonidine extensively in our clinic. One physician with 61 PTSD patients has 55 taking clonidine, 9 of whom use clonidine alone. Clonidine can be used successfully in conjunction with both TCAs and SSRIs.

Benzodiazepines

Several studies have shown single-dose pharmacokinetic and pharmacodynamic differences with benzodiazepines between Asians and Caucasians (Lin et al. 1993a). A comparative study of the pharmacokinetics of diazepam, carried out on 16 Chinese and 18 Caucasian patients, revealed that the apparent volume of distribution of diazepam was higher in the Caucasians than in the Chinese (Kumana et al. 1987). Since diazepam is a highly lipid-soluble drug, this observed interethnic difference is a reflection of the variation in body fat content. The authors concluded that in the relatively lean Chinese, diazepam more quickly attains steady-state serum concentrations. Another study examined the metabolism of diazepam in native Chinese who are poor and extensive metabolizers of S-mephenytoin (Zhang et al. 1990). This study revealed important interethnic differences in diazepam metabolism. Both Chinese EMs and PMs had slow metabolism of diazepam, which was found to be comparable with that of white PMs. It was implied that, unlike in Caucasians, CYP2C19 may have a different substrate specificity in the Chinese.

However, studies are lacking about the differential effect of benzodiazepines in clinical settings. We have little experience with benzodiazepines, which are rarely prescribed to our patients. Although many patients with depression have anxiety, most anxiety is controlled with treatment for depression. We usually do not administer benzodiazepines to patients with PTSD, since they tend to disinhibit patients, resulting in more nightmares and hyperarousal symptoms.

Clinical Guidelines

There are several important issues in pharmacotherapy for Southeast Asian psychiatric patients that have applicability to other refugee and minority groups. As Lin and Shen (1991) point out, issues of diagnostic problems, communication styles, differences between clinicians and patients, and the special expectations of psychiatric medication need to be considered before beginning drug therapy with refugees. With this cultural background in mind, the following clinical guidelines are suggested to aid in the pharmacotherapy of Southeast Asian and other immigrant groups.

1. Have a clear concept of the medicine's use. Diagnostic clarity and clear target symptoms that the medicine is to relieve must be defined.

2. With the patient, develop a joint agreement about the goals of the medicine (i.e., symptoms to be relieved). A patient sometimes may complain of certain symptoms (such as headaches or poor sleep) that may be a minor part of the clinician's consideration (such as treating a depressive disorder). However, both physician and patient could agree on the need for improved sleep in patients with depression.

3. Elicit the patient's concerns, expectations, and hopes for the medicine. The patient may expect quick relief and not understand the need for long-term maintenance for many psychiatric disorders. Discussion with family members about their concerns is very useful, and their support can greatly improve compliance.

4. Be hopeful and positive about the use of medicine and treatment in general. Instilling hope is a very helpful therapeutic approach.

5. Use medicine as only part of the treatment that also includes psychotherapy, social therapies, and a long-term commitment to treat patients. Group therapy, in which patients discuss benefits of medicine and encourage each other, has been particularly helpful.

6. Be aware of particular cultural groups' general concerns about medicine. We often hear that "American medicine is too strong" and "American medicine is too hot," the latter in the yin-yang imbalance sense.

7. Use only one medicine and the fewest number of pills initially. Sometimes the idea of American medicine being too strong is related to the sheer number of pills. Other medicines or increased dosages can be initiated as compliance is established.

8. Ask about other medicines the patient may be taking. To relieve symptoms, many patients see other doctors and are prescribed medications that can cause drug interactions. Also, many patients may take over-the-counter medications or herbal medicine. Asking about their experience and their compliance with these medications can give

the clinician useful ideas about the patient's likely compliance with the current prescription.

9. Reevaluate a patient frequently after starting a medicine regimen. Because the questions about medicines among refugees are so common and noncompliance so frequent, we recommend seeing patients weekly to address these issues as treatment begins.

10. Always ask about compliance and problems with medicine in a nonjudgmental manner. Let patients know that there are other choices, and treatment is not dependent on taking a specific medicine. Many patients are afraid to tell their doctors about problems with medicines for fear of upsetting them or being dismissed as clinic patients.

11. When possible, use medicines that have established plasma levels to determine compliance.

12. Be aware of the large variation in the individual pharmacodynamics of drugs, which occurs in all ethnic groups. The general effects of medicine (the lower doses of neuroleptics needed in Asians) can provide guidelines, but treatment must be based on individual responses.

13. Consider the side effects profile (i.e., sedative effects of some TCAs, such as imipramine, in depressed patients with insomnia; H_2-blocking activity of some TCAs, such as doxepin, in patients with ulcers; clonidine use for both PTSD and hypertension; and the less lethal potential from overdose of SSRIs) in choosing medicine.

14. Do not fine-tune medicine or the dosages. Once an acceptable medical regimen has been found, make adjustments slowly. Manage successes and failures of treatment without overreaction. The refugee's life is often full of multiple stresses and adjustments, and medicine is of minimal value on many of these occasions. Keep a general plan and a long-term perspective in mind, and check with patients about their general comfort with the program.

References

Adedoyin A, Prakash C, O'Shea D, et al: Stereoselective disposition of hexobarbital and its metabolites: relationship to the S-mephenytoin polymorphism in Caucasian and Chinese subjects. Pharmacogenetics 4:27–38, 1994

Allen JJ, Rack PH, Vaddadi KS: Differences in the effects of clomipramine on English and Asian volunteers: preliminary report of a pilot study. Postgrad Med J 53(suppl 4):79–86, 1977

American Psychiatric Association: Diagnostic and Statistical Manual of Mental Disorders, 3rd Edition, Revised. Washington, DC, American Psychiatric Association, 1987

American Psychiatric Association: Tardive Dyskinesia: A Task Force Report of the American Psychiatric Association. Washington, DC, American Psychiatric Association, 1992

American Psychiatric Association: American Psychiatric Association practice guidelines: practice guideline for major depressive disorders in adults. Am J Psychiatry 150(suppl 4), 1994

Baldessarini RJ, Katz B, Cotton P: Dissimilar dosing with high-potency and low-potency neuroleptics. Am J Psychiatry 141:748–752, 1984

Bertilsson L, Henthorn TK, Sanz E, et al: Importance of genetic factors in the regulation of diazepam metabolism: relationship to S-mephenytoin, but not debrisoquine, hydroxylation phenotype. Clin Pharmacol Ther 45:348–355, 1989

Bertilsson L, Lou LQ, Du YL, et al: Pronounced differences between native Chinese and Swedish populations in the polymorphic hydroxylations of debrisoquin and S-mephenytoin. Clin Pharmacol Ther 51:388–397, 1992

Bertschy G, Vandel S: Clomipramine plasma levels among depressed outpatients in Benin, West Africa: drug compliance and comparison with Caucasian patients. J Clin Psychopharmacol 12:334–336, 1992

Binder RL, Levy R: Extrapyramidal reactions on Asians. Am J Psychiatry 138:1243–1244, 1981

Blackwell B: Culture, morbidity, and the effects of drugs. Clin Pharmacol Ther 19:668–674, 1971

Brosen K, Skjelbo E, Flachs H: Proguanil metabolism is determined by the mephenytoin oxidation polymorphism in Vietnamese living in Denmark. Br J Clin Pharmacol 36:105–108, 1993

Dahl ML, Bertilsson L: Genetically variable metabolism of antidepressant and neuroleptic drugs in man. Pharmacogenetics 3:61–70, 1993

Daly AK, Cholerton S, Gregory W, et al: Metabolic polymorphisms. Pharmacol Ther 57:129–160, 1993

Doshi BS, Kulkarni KD, Chauhan BL, et al: Frequency of impaired mephenytoin 4'-hydroxylation in an Indian population. Br J Clin Pharmacol 30:779–780, 1990

Edeki TI, Goldstein JA, de Morais SM, et al: Genetic polymorophism of S-mephenytoin 4'-hydroxylation in African Americans. Pharmacogenetics 6:357–360, 1996

Eichelbaum M, Gross AS: The genetic polymorphism of debrisoquin/sparteine metabolism: clinical aspects. Pharmacol Ther 46:377–394, 1990

Falcon S, Ryan C, Chamberlain K, et al: Tricyclics: possible treatment for posttraumatic stress disorder. J Clin Psychiatry 46:385–389, 1985

Goldstein JA, Faletto MB, Romkes-Sparks M, et al: Evidence that CYP2C19 is the major (S)-mephenytoin 4'-hydroxylase in humans. Biochemistry 33:1743–1752, 1994

Group for the Advancement of Psychiatry (GAP): Pharmacotherapy and psychotherapy: paradoxes, problems, and progress. New York, Mental Health Media Materials Center, 1975

Guy W (ed): ECDEU Assessment Manual for Psychopharmacology, Revised (DHEW Publ No ADM 76-388). Rockville, MD, U.S. Department of Health, Education and Welfare, 1976

Jacqz E, Hall SD, Branch RA, et al: Polymorphic metabolism of mephenytoin in man: pharmacokinetic interaction with a co-regulated substrate, mephobarbital. Clin Pharmacol Ther 39:646–653, 1986

Johnson JA, Burlew BS: Racial differences in propranolol pharmacokinetics. Clin Pharmacol Ther 51:495–500, 1992

Jurima M, Inaba T, Kadar D, et al: Genetic polymorphism to mephenytoin $p(4')$-hydroxylation: difference between Orientals and Caucasians. Br J Clin Pharmacol 19:483–487, 1985

Kalow W: Ethnic differences in drug metabolism. Clin Pharmacokinet 7:373–400, 1982

Kane JM, Smith JM: Tardive dyskinesia: prevalence and risk factors, 1959 to 1979. Arch Gen Psychiatry 39:473–481, 1982

Kiivet RA, Svensson JO, Bertilsson L, et al: Polymorphism of debrisoquine and mephenytoin hydroxylation among Estonians. Pharmacol Toxicol 72:113–115, 1993

Kinzie JD, Leung P: Clonidine in Cambodian patients with posttraumatic stress disorder. J Nerv Ment Dis 177:546–550, 1989

Kinzie JD, Leung P, Boehnlein JK, et al: Antidepressant blood levels in Southeast Asian clinical and cultural implications. J Nerv Ment Dis 175:480–485, 1987

Kinzie JD, Boehnlein JK, Leung PK, et al: The prevalence of posttraumatic stress disorder and its clinical significance among Southeast Asian refugees. Am J Psychiatry 147:913–917, 1990

Kinzie JD, Sack RL, Riley CM: The polysomnographic effects of clonidine on sleep disorders in posttraumatic stress disorder: a pilot study with Cambodian patients. J Nerv Ment Dis 182:585–587, 1994

Kline NA, Dow BM, Brown SA, et al: Sertraline efficacy on depressed combat veterans with posttraumatic stress disorder (letter). Am J Psychiatry 151:621, 1994

Ko GN, Thong LD, Yan WW, et al: The Shanghai 800: prevalence of tardive dyskinesia in a Chinese psychiatric hospital. Am J Psychiatry 146:387–389, 1989

Koshino Y, Madokoro S, Ito T, et al: A survey of tardive dyskinesia in psychiatric inpatients in Japan. Clin Neuropharmacol 15:34–43, 1992

Kosten TR, Frank JB, Dan E, et al: Pharmacotherapy for posttraumatic stress disorder using phenelzine or imipramine. J Nerv Ment Dis 179: 366–370, 1991

Kroll J, Linde P, Habenicht M, et al: Medication compliance, antidepressant blood levels, and side effects in Southeast Asian patients. J Clin Psychopharmacol 10:279–283, 1990

Kumana CR, Lauder IJ, Chan M, et al: Differences in diazepam pharmacokinetics in Chinese and white Caucasians: relation to body lipid stores. Eur J Clin Pharmacol 32:211–215, 1987

Kupfer A, Preisig R: Pharmacogenetics of mephenytoin: a new drug hydroxylation polymorphism in man. Eur J Clin Pharmacol 26:753–759, 1984

Kupfer A, Roberts RK, Schenker S, et al: Stereoselective metabolism of mephenytoin in man. J Pharmacol Exp Ther 218:193–199, 1981

Lewis P, Rack PH, Vaddadi KS, et al: Ethnic differences in drug response. Postgrad Med J 56(suppl 1):46–49, 1980

Lin K-M, Finder E: Neuroleptic dosage for Asians. Am J Psychiatry 140:490–491, 1983

Lin K-M, Shen WW: Pharmacotherapy for Southeast Asian psychiatric patients. J Nerv Ment Dis 179:346–350, 1991

Lin K-M, Okamoto T, Yamamoto J, et al: Psychotropic dosage in Asian Americans. P/AAHRC Research Review 15:1–2, 1986

Lin K-M, Poland RE, Nuccio I, et al: A longitudinal assessment of haloperidol doses and serum concentrations in Asians and Caucasian schizophrenic patients. Am J Psychiatry 146:1307–1311, 1989

Lin K-M, Chang W-H, Poland RE, et al: Ethnicity and psychopharmacology: the Chinese case. Chinese Psychiatry 6:235–250, 1992

Lin K-M, Poland RE, Fleeshaker JC, et al: Ethnicity and differential responses to benzodiazepines, in Psychopharmacology and Psychobiology of Ethnicity. Edited by Lin K-M, Poland RE, Nakaski G. Washington, DC, American Psychiatric Press, 1993a, pp 91–105

Lin K-M, Poland RE, Nakaski G: Psychopharmacology and psychobiology of ethnicity. Washington, DC, American Psychiatric Press, 1993b

Murphy HBM: Ethnic variations in drug responses. Transcultural Psychiatric Research Review 6:6–23, 1969

Nagy LM, Morgan CA III, Southweek SM, et al: Open prospective trial of fluoxetine for posttraumatic stress disorder. J Clin Psychopharmacol 13:107–113, 1993

Okpaku S, Frazer A, Mendels J: A pilot study of racial differences in erythrocyte lithium transport. Am J Psychiatry 137:120–121, 1980

Overall JE, Hollister LE, Kimbell I, et al: Extrinsic factors influencing responses to psychotherapeutic drugs. Arch Gen Psychiatry 21:89–94, 1969

Pearlman T: Letter to the editor. Am J Psychiatry 141:157, 1984

Perry PJ, Miller DD, Arndt SV, et al: Haloperidol dosing requirements: the contributions of smoking and non-linear pharmacokinetics. J Clin Psychopharmacol 13:46–51, 1993

Pi EH, Simpson GH, Cooper TB: Pharmacokinetics of desipramine in Caucasian and Asian volunteers. Am J Psychiatry 143:1174–1176, 1986

Pollock BG, Perel JM, Kirshner M, et al: S-mephenytoin 4-hydroxylation in older Americans. Eur J Clin Pharmacol 40:609–611, 1991

Potkin SG, Shen Y, Pardes H, et al: Haloperidol concentrations elevated in Chinese patients. Psychiatry Res 12:167–172, 1984

Raskin A, Crook TH: Antidepressants in black and white inpatients. Arch Gen Psychiatry 32:643–649, 1975

Relling MV, Chessie J, Schell MJ, et al: Lower prevalence of the debrisoquin oxidative poor metabolizer phenotype in American black versus white subjects. Clin Pharmacol Ther 50:308–313, 1991

Reviriego J, Bertilsson L, Carrillo JA, et al: Frequency of S-mephenytoin deficiency in 373 Spanish subjects compared to other Caucasian populations. Eur J Clin Pharmacol 44:593–595, 1993

Rudorfer MV, Lane EA, Chang WH, et al: Desipramine pharmacokinetics in Chinese and Caucasian volunteers. Br J Clin Pharmacol 17:433–440, 1984

Schatzberg AF, Cole JO: Manual of Clinical Psychopharmacology, 2nd Edition. Washington, DC, American Psychiatric Press, 1991

Setiabudy R, Kusaka M, Chiba K, et al: Dapsone N-acetylation, metoprolol l-hydroxylation, and S-mephenytoin 4-hydroxylation polymorphisms in an Indonesian population: a cocktail and extended phenotyping assessment trial. Clin Pharmacol Ther 56:142–153, 1994

Shen WW, Lin K-M: Cytochrome P450 monooxygenases and interactions with psychotropic drugs. Int J Psychiatry Med 21:47–56, 1991

Shimoda K, Minowada T, Noguchi T, et al: Interindividual variations of demethylation and hydroxylation of clomipramine in an Oriental psychiatric population. J Clin Psychopharmacol 13:181–188, 1993

Skjelbo E, Brosen K, Hallas J, et al: The mephenytoin oxidation polymorphism is partially responsible for the N-demethylation of imipramine. Clin Pharmacol Ther 49:18–23, 1991

Smith M, Lin K-M, Mendoza R: "Nonbiological" issues affecting psychopharmacotherapy: cultural considerations, in Psychopharmacology and Psychobiology of Ethnicity. Edited by Lin K-M, Poland RE, Nakaski G. Washington, DC, American Psychiatric Press, 1993, pp 37–58

Sohn DR, Kusaka M, Ishizaki T, et al: Incidence of S-mephenytoin hydroxylation deficiency in a Korean population and the interphenotypic differences in diazepam pharmacokinetics. Clin Pharmacol Ther 52:160–169, 1992

Sramek JJ, Sayles MS, Simpson GM: Neuroleptic dosage for Asians: a failure to replicate. Am J Psychiatry 143:535–536, 1986

Strickland TL, Lin K-M, Fu P, et al: Comparison of lithium ratios between African-American and Caucasian bipolar patients. Biol Psychiatry 37:325–330, 1995

Wedlund PJ, Aslanian SW, McAllister CB, et al: Mephenytoin hydroxylatin deficiency in Caucasians: frequency of a new oxidative drug metabolism polymorphism. Clin Pharmacol Ther 36:773–780, 1984

Wilkinson GR, Guengerich FP, Branch RA: Genetic polymorphism of S-mephenytoin hydroxylation. Pharmacol Ther 3:53–76, 1989

Yamamoto J, Fung D, Lo S, et al: Psychopharmacology for Asian American and Pacific Islanders. Psychopharmacol Bull 15:29–31, 1979

Yang YY: Prophylactic efficacy of lithium and its effective plasma levels in Chinese bipolar patients. Acta Psychiatr Scand 71:171–175, 1985

Zhang Y, Reviriego J, Lou Y, et al: Diazepam metabolism in native Chinese poor and extensive hydroxylators of S-mephenytoin: interethnic differences in comparison with white subjects. Clin Pharmacol Ther 48:496–502, 1990

Ziegler UE, Biggs JT: Tricyclic plasma levels: effects of age, race, sex, and smoking. JAMA 238:2167–2169, 1977

CHAPTER 10

Religion and Mental Health
The Need for Cultural Sensitivity and Synthesis

DAVID LARSON, M.D., M.S.P.H.
MARY GREENWOLD MILANO, B.A., MGM
FRANCIS LU, M.D.

Introduction

Background. Surveys of the United States population over the past decade have established religion as an important cultural aspect in the lives of many Americans. When questioned about their religious beliefs, 95% of the general public espouse a belief in God (Gallup Report 1985). In addition, this belief in God seems to hold a great deal of meaning for the majority of the population, with nearly three-quarters of the population claiming that their approach to life is grounded in their religious beliefs (Bergin and Jensen 1990).

Indeed, just as cultural issues of ethnicity, gender, and race have been identified as being clinically relevant to the therapeutic setting, recent research has suggested that the religious culture of a patient should be considered in the treatment process as well (Lukoff et al. 1992). Given Lukoff and colleagues' observation that "the religious and spiritual dimensions of culture are among the most important factors that structure human experience, beliefs, values, behavior, and illness patterns" (p. 673), what effect might religion have on the therapeutic process?

Kroll and Sheehan (1989) demonstrated that the religious beliefs of mental health patients are nearly identical to those held by the general population. Such beliefs have also been found to have much clinical relevance to care, with the religious cultures of patients influencing their personal attitudes about illness. A 1990 study found that one-third of those surveyed believed that sickness was a punishment from God, while nearly four-fifths felt that good health was a blessing from God (Bearon and Koenig 1990). Another study, conducted on hospitalized psychiatric patients, supported the idea that a patient's religious beliefs could influence his or her perceptions of illness, with nearly half of the patients surveyed believing that leading a moral life could protect against illness (Sheehan and Kroll 1990).

A patient's religious culture has not only been found to affect attributional style but also may be associated with either clinical improvement or enhanced mental health outcomes (Gartner et al. 1991; Larson et al. 1992). In a review more than 20 years ago, Nancy Andreasen (1972) heralded the beneficial impact that a religious perspective can have in dealing with depression—a finding corroborated by a study of patients with hip fractures, in which the elderly who had greater levels of religious commitment experienced lower levels of depression and better clinical status at discharge (Pressman et al. 1990). Other studies have supported the finding that religion is associated with improvement in overall psychological functioning. For example, patients with schizophrenia who attended church or were given supportive aftercare by religious caregivers were found to have lower overall rates of rehospitalization (Chu and Klein 1985; Katkin et al. 1975). In addition, following participation in religious worship, a significant reduction in a number of psychiatric symptoms has been noted on both patient self-report measures and more objective measures such as electromyogram biofeedback instrumentation (Elkins et al. 1979; Finney and Malony 1985; Griffith et al. 1986; Morris 1982).

Furthermore, a patient's religious culture may possibly help protect against stress, with the religiously committed reporting much lower stress levels than the less committed, as shown in two past community studies (Lindenthal et al. 1970; Stark 1971). In a more recent community study, Williams et al. (1991) found that as the level of religious attendance rose, the adverse psychological consequences of stress in turn lessened, thus suggesting that religious commitment may also have a prophylactic effect against the deleterious effects of stress on one's mental health status.

Just as religion has been found to have a beneficial effect on mental health, religious commitment has also been found to play a role in the lowering of self-destructive behaviors. For example, Comstock and Partridge (1972) found that persons who did not attend church were four times more likely to kill themselves than were frequent church attendees. This finding was later supported by a systematic review of the literature concerning the relationship between religious commitment and suicide rates. The reviewers found a beneficial, negative relationship between religious commitment and suicide in nearly every published study located (Gartner et al. 1991).

Religion also appears to reduce the appeal of other potentially self-destructive behaviors such as alcohol and drug abuse. When Gorsuch and Butler (1976) conducted an early review of the drug abuse literature, they noted that religious commitment seemed to have a protective effect against drug abuse: "Whenever religion is used in an analysis, it predicts those who have not used an illicit drug regardless of whether the religious variable is defined in terms of membership, active participation, religious upbringing, or the meaningfulness of religion as viewed by the person himself" (p. 127). Gartner et al. (1991) confirmed the results of this earlier review 15 years later in their review of the literature, finding that even when studies employed weaker measures of religion such as denomination, religion was still associated with lower rates of drug abuse. Paralleling the drug abuse studies, Larson and Wilson (1980) found that those who abused alcohol rarely had a strong religious commitment. Indeed, of the alcoholic persons surveyed, 89% had lost interest in religion during their teenage years, whereas among the controls, 48% had increased interest in religion and 32% had no change in their religious practices during adolescence. Furthermore, a relationship between religious commitment and the nonuse or moderate use of alcohol has been well documented (Amoateng and Bahr 1986; Cochran et al. 1988). Most interestingly, Amoateng and Bahr discovered that whether or not a religion specifically proscribed alcohol use, those who were active in a religious group consumed substantially less than those who were not active.

Given the potential impact of a patient's religious culture on clinical symptomatology and outcomes, it is not surprising that therapy with religious patients can be more effective when it incorporates elements of the patient's belief system (Propst 1980; Propst et al. 1992). Indeed, for the more than 70% of the population for whom religious commitment is a central life factor, "secular approaches to psychotherapy may provide an alien values framework" (Bergin and Jensen 1990, p. 6). They continue: "A majority of the population probably prefers an orientation to counseling and psychotherapy that is sympathetic, or at least sensitive, to a spiritual perspective. We need to better perceive and respond to this public need" (p. 6).

Incorporating aspects of the patient's belief system into medical treatment does not necessitate that the therapist share the patient's belief system (Worthington 1986). Rather, it simply implies that the therapist must be sensitive to and recognize the importance of the patient's religious culture in the clinical setting. Propst and colleagues (1992) highlighted this finding in a carefully controlled study designed to examine the use of religion in therapy with samples of religious patients suffering from depression. The patients were divided into two treatment groups, with one group receiving cognitive behavioral therapy with religious content and the other group receiving the same therapy without religious content. Religious and nonreligious therapists were then divided between both treatment groups. Not surprisingly, depressed patients receiving therapy with religious content had better scores on measures of both posttreatment depression and adjustment than did patients whose therapy did not include religious content. Most importantly, the nonreligious therapists using the religious approach had the highest level of treatment effect, suggesting that a therapist does not need to personally value religion to deal sensitively with religious issues in treatment.

Religion and mental health providers.   Although nonreligious therapists can begin to deal effectively with religious issues in a therapeutic setting given even minimal training and education, as demonstrated by Propst et al. (1992), clinicians seldom receive this needed instruction. A recent survey of members of the American Association of Directors of Psychiatric Residency Training found that while religion was viewed as an issue of significant importance to the mental health field, religious issues were infrequently addressed in training (Sansone et al. 1990). Likewise, a study of the Association of Psychology Internship Centers found that none of the training directors had received any training or instruction on religious issues during their formal internship (Lannert 1991). What is most surprising, and regrettable, about this lack of clinical education is that when asked how often they encountered religious issues with their patients, nearly three-quarters of the directors surveyed said that they had addressed religious issues at least occasionally in the therapeutic setting.

Religion in psychiatric research. If clinical training does not provide sufficient information concerning religion's role in the therapeutic setting, could clinical research help mental health professionals better understand the impact that religious beliefs can have in mental health care? A systematic review of studies published in the four leading psychiatry journals from 1978 to 1982 suggests that clinical research is of little help in increasing field understanding of, or sensitivity toward, religion. The systematic review found that religion was infrequently considered in psychiatric research, and, when it was considered, it was generally measured inadequately (Larson et al. 1986a). Of the 2,348 reviewed articles, less than 2.5% (59 studies) included any type of quantified religious variable.

Even when clinicians attempted to include religious variables in their research, they seemed to lack even the most basic knowledge about how to best assess religion. Of the nearly 2.5% of published studies containing a quantitative religious variable, less than 1% assessed religion with minimal standards of acceptability using at least a single item measure of religious commitment (i.e., religious practices, attitudes, and beliefs) (Larson et al. 1986b, 1992). In addition, only one study employed the state-of-the-art approach to measuring religion—an already developed array of items assessing various aspects of religious practices, attitudes, and beliefs (Larson et al. 1986a). The majority of the published literature including a religious variable measured religion with the single, more static measure of denomination—a much less useful measure of religious commitment (Craigie et al. 1990; Williams et al. 1991). In addition, despite the fact that more than 90% of the population is affiliated with traditional denominational groups (i.e., Protestantism, Catholicism, or Judaism), only three studies focused on traditional religion. In contrast, 17 studies focused on sects or cults, despite the fact that less than 0.5% of the United States population is involved in these religious belief systems (Larson et al. 1986b).

Another systematic review of the two leading psychiatry journals found that the scientific methodology assessing religious commitment is seriously flawed (Larson et al. 1992). When a study had a hypothesis regarding religion, a study result was reported only 40% of the time. More importantly, when a study result was reported concerning a religious factor's association with a psychiatric measure, only 22% of the studies, fewer than one in four, had previously clarified a hypothesis about religion (Larson et al. 1992). In short, results were frequently analyzed and published without prior hypotheses, and religious hypotheses were frequently stated without reporting the corresponding findings.

Mental health's view of religion. Although disparities in the clinical understanding of religious cultures, inadequate training, and a lack of quality empirical research offer sufficient challenges to the mental health field in treating religion with clinical sensitivity, perhaps the greatest challenge to the American Psychiatric Association's call for religious sensitivity comes from those within the field who regard religion as being virtually equivalent to psychopathology. The view that religion is detrimental to mental health is a long-standing one. For instance, Freud (1966) saw religion as a "universal obsessional neurosis" and labeled mystical experience as "infantile helplessness" and a "regression to primary narcissism" (Freud 1959). Other clinicians have continued to associate religion with psychopathology, describing spiritual experiences as borderline psychosis (Group for the Advancement of Psychiatry 1976), a psychotic episode (Horton 1974), or temporal lobe dysfunction (Mandel 1980). Even the 1976 report by the Group for the Advancement of Psychiatry entitled "Mysticism: Spiritual Quest or Psychological Disturbance?" supported the long-standing view of religion as psychopathology, calling mystical experiences "a regression, an escape, a projection upon the world of a primitive infantile state" (Deikman 1977, p. 214). More recently, a professor emeritus in psychiatry at a noted university published an entire book labeling religion as a detrimental, destructive, and pathological force in human life (Watters 1992). Judging from the content of the book, it is difficult to fathom why so many in the United States population choose to participate in religious experiences. Indeed, according to the author, the addictive and clinically harmful nature of religion is responsible for a "kitchen sink" array of problems ranging from dependency, severe self-effacement, denial, ignorance, intolerance, and alienation to anti-social behavior, inadequate psychological development, sexual dysfunction, anxiety, low self-image, and schizophrenia.

This view of religion as psychopathology is not simply a fringe issue to some clinicians. In fact, Albert Ellis, the founder of rational-emotive therapy, has devoted several published articles solely to this topic. Ellis began a 1988 article entitled "Is Religion Pathological?" with the proposition that "unbelief, skepticism, and even thoroughgoing atheism not only abet, but are practically synonymous with mental health; and that devout belief, dogmatism, and religiosity distinctly contribute to, and in some ways are equivalent to, mental or emotional disturbance" (p. 27). Ellis supports his view of religion as pathology by claiming that there are multiple clinical problems associated with religious commitment, including 1) masochistic behavior, 2) social incompetence, 3) the inability to think scientifically, and 4) the absence of unconditional self-acceptance.

What is perhaps most surprising about Ellis's article is the startling absence of empirical evidence in his paper. Ellis himself recognizes the importance of using empirical research to investigate religion's effect on mental health when he notes that his view of religion "is tentative and revisable in the light of later substantiating or nonsubstantiating evidence" (Ellis 1988, p. 27). One wonders how Ellis would have treated religion had he taken his own advice and relied on objective evidence in forming his opinion. For example, when studies containing religious variables in the two leading journals of psychiatry were systematically reviewed, 84% of the religious–mental health associations located were found to be clinically beneficial, while 13% of the mental health–religion associations were harmful and 3% neutral (Larson et al. 1992)—findings that run counter to Ellis's hypothesized expectations.

Although the majority of studies including religion have found that religious commitment is associated with mental health benefits, a small minority of studies have found that religious commitment can have clinically harmful relationships. For example, members of a specific religious group, Pentecostals, do not seem to derive as many benefits as those in conservative or mainline denominations. Indeed, Koenig et al. (1993) found that Pentecostals have a significantly higher risk of developing anxiety disorders than do members of other religious denominations. However, when compared to the nonreligious, Pentecostals still had lower rates of anxiety disorder, indicating that religious commitment still provides some protection from anxiety disorders. Similar studies have found that Pentecostals seem to run a higher risk of alcoholism, depression, and psychiatric disorder than members of mainline or conservative denominations as well (Koenig et al. 1994). The rates of these problems, however, have not been compared with the rates of the same problems among the nonreligious to determine whether, as was found in the anxiety study, Pentecostals have higher rates of mental health problems than other religious groups but lower rates overall than the nonreligious. Although a small minority of studies have found some potentially negative mental health consequences from involvement with a specific religious group, the vast majority of published research studies have shown religion as having a positive influence on mental health. Despite these findings, however, religious commitment generally remains either ignored or even still maligned by the mental health community.

An indicator of religious insensitivity: the handling of religion in DSM-III-R.   Given the negative view of religion held by some mental health professionals, coupled with the inadequate handling of religion in clinical training and research, we decided to empirically assess the mental health field's handling and interpretation of religious issues in the clinical setting by evaluating the consensus handling of religious issues within a clinically relevant body of knowledge more formally produced and generally accepted by the mental health field. The most recent edition (at that time) of the *Diagnostic and Statistical Manual of Mental Disorders* (DSM-III-R) (American Psychiatric Association 1987) would more than qualify as such a document, since it has been consensually developed and agreed upon through a process including multiple iterations of field reviews. Thus, the study of how a section of DSM-III-R approaches issues of religion can reasonably be proposed as an indicator of the consensus treatment of religion by the mental health field.

The handling of religion in DSM-III-R was reviewed by two of the current authors in a brief report published in the *American Journal of Psychiatry* (Larson et al. 1993). Though limited in scope due to the shorter nature of a brief report, the article generated a great deal of professional as well as media interest (American Psychiatric Association

1994b; Neuhaus 1994; Steinfels 1994). Thus, given the demonstrated interest in the subject matter, we have decided to more fully develop the article for this chapter, explaining in more detail the review methodology, important results, and implications of the review findings.

Following up on a letter to the editor by Post (1990) in the *American Journal of Psychiatry* that noted examples of insensitivity to religion found in the Glossary of Technical Terms in Appendix C of DSM-III-R, we systematically reviewed two specific components of the glossary in order to assess how religion is handled in DSM-III-R. First, all definitions in the glossary were reviewed to determine the frequency that religion was presented as a clinically relevant factor—a potentially important issue that might be forgotten or neglected in the diagnostic or treatment process. Secondly, all definitions were further reviewed to determine how sensitively religious examples were used to illustrate psychopathology in each term's brief, illustrative case examples. As a result, we evaluated how frequently within the glossary

1. Religion was presented as a clinically relevant issue.
2. Other cultural issues were presented as clinically relevant issues.
3. Religion was used to illustrate psychopathology.
4. Other cultural issues were used to illustrate psychopathology.

Method

The religious content found in clinical reminders and in illustrative case examples of Appendix C of the Glossary of Technical Terms (*glossary* in the remainder of this chapter) was selected for systematic research review.

Background. The glossary, as described in DSM-III-R, "is generally limited to those [technical terms] that are used in either the descriptions and definitions or the diagnostic criteria of DSM-III-R and [consists of those technical terms] that are associated with several mental disorders" (American Psychiatric Association 1987, p. 391).

In other words, of the many technical terms that could have been selected for placement and definition in the glossary, the 100 selected by the reviewers were the most frequently used terms in DSM-III-R. Thus, for the layperson, the definition of these most frequently used terms would provide additional assistance in understanding the language used in DSM.

Review assumptions. We assumed that the finalizing of the glossary's 100 technical terms along with 1) all illustrative case examples and 2) all caveats concerning clinically relevant issues paralleled the same arduous and consensual review process used for the rest of DSM-III-R. The process of review, feedback, and field consensus has been extremely thorough: first with DSM-III (American Psychiatric Association 1980, pp. 1–12) and with DSM-III-R (pp. xvii–xxvii). Thus we assumed that the high standards of field agreement that were employed in finalizing one section of the DSM, such as the glossary, or even material within a section in the glossary, such as the illustrative case examples, should have varied little from the high standards employed for the finalizing of each edition of the DSM.

Sensitivity to religion as a clinically relevant issue. All 100 technical terms listed in the glossary with either major boldface headings or minor boldface subheadings were systematically reviewed for clinical "reminders" or caveats about specific issues requiring clinician sensitivity in diagnosis—issues that might be overlooked or neglected but that could be of important clinical relevance. For example, three "reminders" were found in the definition of the term mental disorder; they encouraged clinician sensitivity to sexual, political, and religious issues.

Sensitivity to religion in illustrative case examples. All 100 technical terms listed in the glossary with either major boldface headings or minor boldface subheadings were again systematically reviewed for religious content that was used in illustrative case examples within a term definition. The illustrative case examples were found to be one of two different types: 1) a statement made by a patient or 2) a description of the patient's behavior, thinking, or language.

Examples presented as a series of multiple symptoms as in *mood-incongruent psychotic features* (p. 402) or in *psychomotor agitation* (p. 404) were not included as illustrative case examples. In addition, examples presented as an array of additional psychiatric terms as in the final lines of the terms *psychotic* (p. 404) and *residual* (p. 405) were excluded as illustrative case examples.

Other cultural issues used for comparisons. All 100 technical terms listed in the glossary with either major boldface headings or minor boldface subheadings were systematically reviewed for a final time for other cultural issues that were 1) included in clinical reminders as potentially clinically relevant issues and 2) included in illustrative case examples. Other cultural issues were reviewed to provide comparisons with the frequency and handling of the cultural issue of religion in the glossary. Cultural issues selected for comparison with religion included 1) ethnicity, 2) race, 3) gender, 4) sexuality, and 5) the use of the general term *culture.*

Given the infrequent attention paid by psychiatric research, training, and care to religion, we expected the glossary to 1) remind the reader of the relevance of religion less frequently than other cultural issues in clinical reminders and 2) include religion in illustrative case examples far less often than the other cultural issues that were systematically reviewed.

Results

Sensitivity to religion as a clinically relevant issue. Thirteen technical terms included a reminder about an issue of clinical relevance: seven terms included one reminder, four terms included two issues, two terms included three issues, and no terms included four or more issues. Thus we identified 21, or ([7 × 1] + [4 × 2] + [2 × 3]), reminders of clinical relevance.

Of the 21 clinically relevant reminders, 6 (28.5%) had religious content. These six reminders were found in the definitions of the technical terms 1) delusion; 2) delusion of being controlled; 3) delusion, grandiose; 4) hallucination; 5) illogical thinking, and 6) mental disorder. The relevant portion of these six definitions referring to religion is found in Appendix I.

In contrast, among the remaining 15 clinical reminders, only 1 term related to ethnicity (incoherence), 1 term to sexuality (mental disorder), and 7 terms to the most general type of context—issues of culture or subculture (affect; delusion; delusion, bizarre; illogical thinking; magical thinking; neologisms; and overvalued idea). Surprisingly, no terms contained clinical reminders regarding issues of race or gender.

Sensitivity to religion in illustrative case examples. Of the 100 technical terms located, 29 terms that had one or more illustrative case examples were found, whereas 71 of the terms did not have illustrative examples. Of the 29 technical terms with examples, 18 terms contained only a single example, 6 terms contained two examples, 5 terms contained three examples, and no terms contained more than three examples. Thus we identified 45, or $[(18 \times 1) + (6 \times 2) + (5 \times 3)]$, illustrative case examples, including 14 statements made by a patient and 31 descriptions of a patient's behavior, thinking, or language.

Of the 45 illustrative case examples, 10 (22.2%) had religious content. The 10 illustrative examples citing religious content are found in Appendix II, which includes the three verbatim patient statements and the seven descriptions of patient behavior, thinking, or language having religious content. In contrast to the 10 with religious content, only 2 (4.4%) of the 45 case examples contained sexual content, and no case examples included content pertaining to ethnicity, race, gender, sexuality, or culture.

Discussion

Those who developed the glossary seemed to be aware of the particular need for clinicians to be reminded about the clinical relevance of religious issues. Although this sensitivity to religious issues in diagnosis is encouraging, it is also quite surprising when so little research attention has focused on religion. As already noted, nearly 30% of all clinical reminders in the glossary recognized the need for clinicians to be sensitive to religious practices and beliefs. In contrast, it was noteworthy that issues of sexuality and ethnicity had so few reminders and issues of race and gender had none.

Yet, while the DSM encourages sensitivity to religious issues, the glossary seems to have difficulty heeding its own urgings. The present findings indicate that "Appendix C: Glossary of Technical Terms" in DSM-III-R contains an overrepresentation of illustrative case examples portraying religion as a pathological state and thus should be of major concern to psychiatry. Illustrative case examples with religious content were used in the DSM-III-R glossary at a surprisingly high rate (22.2%) given that quantified religious commitment variables are included in psychiatric research in less than 1% of published studies (Larson et al. 1986a,b). Even more surprising was the frequent association of religion with psychopathology and the frequent presentation of negative inferences about religion in DSM-III-R, considering the frequent beneficial relationship that religion has been found to have with mental health status in psychiatric research (Gartner et al. 1991; Larson et al. 1992).

In addition, the inclusion of religious references to illustrate psychopathology occurred at a rate five times higher than did sexual references, while issues of ethnicity, race, gender, and culture were conspicuously absent among case examples illustrating psychopathology. These findings seem to imply that other cultural issues play a fraction of the role religion plays in illustrating and defining technical terms of mental illness. Such results are quite perplexing, considering the substantial attention paid by the mental health field to issues of ethnicity, race, gender, sexuality, and culture and the less-than-substantial attention paid to religion.

Although none of the individual case examples found would seem clinically implausible or outlandish, the context in which they are given (i.e., the definitions section of a major document of psychiatric nosology describing psychopathology) casts religious commitment in a negative and pathological light. Though current psychiatric research supports the notion that religious commitment is frequently associated with mental health benefit, this systematic review found that the illustrative case examples used in the glossary of the DSM-III-R suggest quite the opposite. Indeed, the overutilization of religion as case examples of psychopathology supports the simplistic traditional mental health notion that religious commitment fosters psychopathology and, conversely, that religion is not associated with psychiatric well-being (Ellis 1980; Watters 1992). Although these findings cannot be used to imply that all other sections of the DSM-III-R will reveal similar findings, the field should be concerned if even one section shows such frequent, insensitive notions about religious commitment.

Given past research showing widespread neglect and misinterpretation of religious issues (Larson et al. 1986a), the demonstrated insensitivity to religion in DSM-III-R's glossary would further emphasize the already documented need for the mental health field to make a conscious effort to more accurately handle issues of religious commitment. Some members of the mental health field have already called for more sensitive handling of religious issues, particularly in clinical nosology (Lukoff et al. 1992; Post 1990, 1992), and the mental health field has responded to these calls by issuing guidelines for clinical care (American Psychiatric Association 1990) as well as education and training (Accreditation Council for Graduate Medical Education 1994). However, these recommendations will do little to improve the documented insensitivity to religion without adequate follow-up and attention by the field.

Given the publicity that has surrounded findings such as those discussed here, the field is to be commended for responding to concerns about the handling of religion in psychiatric nosology. Indeed, not only were negative inferences about religion removed from the glossary in the most recent version of the *Diagnostic and Statistical Manual of Mental Disorders*, DSM-IV (American Psychiatric Association 1994a), but a V code for "Religious or Spiritual Problems" was added as well. This new V code, included in a section entitled "Other Conditions That May Be a Focus of Clinical Attention," was included to address "distressing experiences that involve loss or questioning of faith, problems associated with conversion to a new faith, or questioning of other spiritual values" (Larson et al. 1993; Lukoff et al. 1992).

We hope that mental health professionals will continue to respond to concerns about religious insensitivity, whether found in psychiatric nosology, training, research, or care, and move beyond merely facilitating discussion to initiating more conscious and definitive action. Although the field has begun to recognize the clinical relevance of religion and allowed religion to "get a foot in the door," the time has come for mental health to begin to open the door all of the way and invite religion in from its present peripheral position. Only then will clinicians, educators, and researchers begin to understand the complex cultural impact that religion can have on their patients and respond to religious issues with more appropriate mental health care assessment and treatment.

Appendix I

Technical Terms Presenting Religion as Clinically Relevant

1. *Delusion:* "The belief is not one ordinarily accepted by other members of the person's culture or subculture (i.e. it is not an article of *religious faith*) [emphasis added]" (American Psychiatric Association 1987, p. 395).
2. *Delusion of Being Controlled:* "A delusion in which feelings, impulses, thoughts, or actions are experienced as being not one's own, as being imposed by some external force. This does not include the mere conviction that one is acting as an *agent of God,* has had a curse placed on him or her, is the victim of fate, or is not sufficiently assertive [emphasis added]" (p. 395).
3. *Delusion, Grandiose:* "A delusion whose content involves an exaggerated sense of one's importance, power, knowledge, or identity. It may have a *religious,* somatic, or other theme [emphasis added]" (p. 396).
4. *Hallucination:* "Hallucinations occurring in the course of an intensely shared *religious experience* generally have no pathological significance [emphasis added]" (p. 398).
5. *Illogical Thinking:* "Illogical thinking has psychopathological significance only when it is marked, as in the examples noted below, and when it is not due to cultural or *religious* values or to an intellectual deficit [emphasis added]" (p. 399).
6. *Mental Disorder:* "Neither deviant behavior, e.g. political, *religious,* or sexual, nor conflicts that are primarily between the individual and society are mental disorders unless the deviance or conflict is a symptom of a dysfunction in the person, as described above [emphasis added]" (p. 401).

Appendix II

Technical Terms Presenting Religion as Psychopathology

1. Quotations Made by the Patient:
   A. *Illogical Thinking:* "Examples: . . . In response to the question, 'Why did you go to Kingston?' a patient replied, "Be-

cause I believe in the King James Bible and my name is James. I went to Kingston to see the Queen' " (American Psychiatric Association 1987, p. 399).

B. *Incoherence:* "Example: Interviewer: 'Why do you think people believe in God?' Subject: 'Um, because making a do in life. Isn't none of that stuff about evolution guiding isn't true anymore now. It all happened a long time ago. It happened in eons and eons and stuff they wouldn't believe in Him. The time that Jesus Christ people believe in their thing people believed in, Jehovah God that they didn't believe in Jesus Christ that much' " (p. 400).

C. *Poverty of Content and Speech:* "Example: Interviewer: 'O.K. Why is it, do you think, that people believe in God?' Patient: 'Well, first of all because, he is the person that, is their personal savior. He walks with me and talks with me. And uh, the understanding that I have, a lot of peoples, they don't really know their own personal self. Because they ain't, they all just don't know their own personal self. They don't, know that He uh, seemed like to me, a lot of 'em don't understand that He walks and talks with them. And uh, show 'em their way to go. I understand also that, every man and every lady, is just not pointed in the same direction. Some are pointed different. They go in their different ways. The way that Jesus Christ wanted 'em to go. Myself, I am pointed in the ways of uh, knowing right from wrong, and doing it. I can't do anymore, or not less, than that' " (p. 403).

2. Descriptions of Patient Behavior, Thinking, or Language

A. *Affect:* "Example: A patient smiled and laughed while discussing demons who were persecuting him" (p. 391).

B. *Catatonic Posturing:* "Example: A patient may stand with arms outstretched as if he were Jesus on the cross" (p. 392).

C. *Delusion of Being Controlled:* "Examples: . . . [A] student believed his actions were under the control of a yogi" (p. 395).

D. *Hallucinations, Tactile:* "Examples: A man said he could feel the devil sticking pins into his flesh . . ." (p. 399).

E. *Hallucinations, Tactile:* "Examples: . . . another complained of experiencing pains, which he attributed to the Devil, throughout his body, although there was not evidence of any physical illness" (p. 399).

F. *Magical Thinking:* "Example: A man believed that if he said a specific prayer three times each night, his mother's death might be prevented indefinitely" (p. 401).

G. *Delusion:* "Example: . . . if someone claims he or she is the worst sinner in the world, this would generally be considered a delusional conviction" (p. 395).

References

Accreditation Council for Graduate Medical Education: Special requirements for residency training in psychiatry. Chicago, IL, Accreditation Council for Graduate Medical Education, 1994

American Psychiatric Association: Diagnostic and Statistical Manual of Mental Disorders, 3rd Edition. Washington, DC, American Psychiatric Association, 1980

American Psychiatric Association: Diagnostic and Statistical Manual of Mental Disorders, 3rd Edition, Revised. Washington, DC, American Psychiatric Association, 1987

American Psychiatric Association: APA guidelines regarding possible conflict between psychiatrists' religious commitments and psychiatric practice. Am J Psychiatry 147:542, 1990

American Psychiatric Association: Diagnostic and Statistical Manual of Mental Disorders, 4th Edition. Washington, DC, American Psychiatric Association, 1994a

American Psychiatric Association: Psychiatry and religion: a visit from Utah. American Psychiatric Association News 28:3,1994b

American Psychiatric Association Task Force on Religion and Psychiatry: Psychiatrists' Viewpoint on Religion and Their Services to Religious Institutions and the Ministry. Washington, DC, American Psychiatric Association, 1975

Amoateng AY, Bahr SJ: Religion, family, and adolescent drug use. Sociological Perspectives 29:53–73, 1986

Andreasen NJ: The role of religion in depression. Journal of Religion and Health 11:153–166, 1972

Bearon LB, Koenig HG: Religious cognitions and use of prayer in health and illness. Gerontologist 30:249–253, 1990

Bergin AE, Jensen JP: Religiosity of psychotherapists: a national study. Psychotherapy 27:3–7, 1990

Chu C, Klein HE: Psychological and environmental variables in outcome of black schizophrenics. J Natl Med Assoc 77:793–796, 1985

Cochran JK, Begley L, Bock EW: Religiosity and alcohol behavior: an exploration of reference group therapy. Sociological Forum 3:256–276, 1988

Comstock GW, Partridge KB: Church attendance and health. Journal of Chronic Disease 25:665–672, 1972

Craigie FC, Larson DB, Liu IY: References to religion in the Journal of Family Practice. J Fam Pract 30:477–480, 1990

Deikman A: Comments on the GAP report on mysticism. J Nerv Ment Dis 165:213–217, 1977

Elkins D, Anchor KN, Sandler HM: Relaxation training and prayer behavior as tension reduction techniques. Behavioral Engineering 5:81–87, 1979

Ellis A: Psychotherapy and atheistic values: a response to A. E. Bergin's "Psychotherapy and Religious Issues." J Consult Clin Psychol 48:635–639, 1980

Ellis A: Is religiosity pathological? Free Inquiry 8:27–32, 1988

Finney JR, Malony HN: An empirical study of contemplative prayer as an adjunct to psychotherapy. Journal of Psychology and Theology 13:284–290, 1985

Freud S: Civilization and its discontents (1930 [1929]), in The Standard Edition of the Complete Psychological Works of Sigmund Freud, Vol 21. Translated and edited by Strachey J. London, Hogarth Press, 1961, pp 59–145

Freud S: Obsessive actions and religious practices, in The Standard Edition of the Complete Psychological Works of Sigmund Freud, Vol 20. Edited by Strachey J. London, Hogarth, 1966

Gallup Report No 236. Religion in America. Princeton, NJ, Gallup Organization, May 1985

Gartner J, Larson DB, Allen GD, et al: Religious commitment and mental health: a review of the empirical literature. Journal of Psychology and Theology 19:6–25, 1991

Gorsuch RL, Butler MC: Initial drug abuse: a view of predisposing social psychological factors. Psychol Bull 3:120–137, 1976

Griffith EE, Mahy GE, Young JL: Psychological benefits of spiritual Baptist "mourning," II: an empirical assessment. Am J Psychiatry 143:226–229, 1986

Group for the Advancement of Psychiatry: Mysticism: Spiritual Quest or Mental Disorder? New York, Group for the Advancement of Psychiatry, 1976

Horton PC: The mystical experience: substance of an illusion. American Psychoanalytic Association Journal 22:364–380, 1974

Katkin S, Zimmerman V, Rosenthal J, et al: Using volunteer therapists to reduce hospital readmissions. Hosp Community Psychiatry 26:151–153, 1975

Koenig HG, Ford SM, George LK, et al: Religion and anxiety disorder. Journal of Anxiety Disorders 7:321–342, 1993

Koenig HG, George LK, Meador KG, et al: Religious affiliation and psychiatric disorder among Protestant baby boomers. Hosp Community Psychiatry 45:586–596, 1994

Kroll J, Sheehan W: Religious practices and beliefs among 52 psychiatric inpatients in Minnesota. Am J Psychiatry 146:67–72, 1989

Lannert J: Countertransference and spirituality. Journal of Humanistic Psychology 31:68–76, 1991

Larson DB, Wilson WP: Religious life of alcoholics. South Med J 73:723–727, 1980

Larson DB, Pattison EM, Blazer DG, et al: Systematic analysis of research on religious variables in four major psychiatric journals: 1978–1982. Am J Psychiatry 143:329–334, 1986a

Larson DB, Pattison EM, Blazer DG, et al: The measurement of religion in psychiatric research, in Psychiatry and Religion: Overlapping Concerns. Edited by Robinson LH. Washington, DC, American Psychiatric Association Press, 1986b, pp 155–177

Larson DB, Sherrill KA, Lyons JS, et al: Associations between dimensions of religious commitment and mental health reported in American Journal of Psychiatry and Archives of General Psychiatry: 1978–1989. Am J Psychiatry 149:557–559, 1992

Larson DB, Thielman SB, Greenwold MA, et al: Religious content in the Diagnostic and Statistical Manual, third edition—revised, appendix C: the glossary of technical terms. Am J Psychiatry 150:1884–1885, 1993

Larson DB, Sherrill KA, Lyons JS: Neglect and misuse of the r word: systematic reviews of religious measures in health, mental health, and aging, in Religion in Aging and Health. Edited by Levin J. Thousand Oaks, CA, Sage, 1994, pp 178–195

Lindenthal JJ, Myers JK, Pepper MK, et al: Mental status and religious behavior. Journal for the Scientific Study of Religion 9:143–149, 1970

Lukoff D, Lu F, Turner R: Toward a more culturally sensitive DSM-IV: psychoreligious and spiritual problems. J Nerv Ment Dis 180:673–682, 1992

Mandel AJ: Toward a psychobiology of transcendence: God in the brain, in The Psychobiology of Consciousness. Edited by Davidson RJ, Davidson JM. New York, Plenum, 1980

Morris PA: The effect of pilgrimage on anxiety, depression, and religious attitude. Psychol Med 12:291–294, 1982

Neuhaus RJ: Psychiatry's shrinking market. First Things 43:69, 1994

Post SG: Letter to the editor: DSM-III-R and religion. Am J Psychiatry 147:813, 1990

Post SG: DSM-III-R and religion. Soc Sci Med 35:81–90, 1992

Pressman P, Lyons JS, Larson DB, et al: Religious belief, depression, and ambulation status in elderly women with broken hips. Am J Psychiatry 147:758–760, 1990

Propst LR: The comparative efficacy of religious and nonreligious imagery for the treatment of mild depression in religious individuals. Cognitive Therapy and Research 4:167–178, 1980

Propst LR, Ostrom R, Watkins P, et al: Comparative efficacy of religious and nonreligious cognitive-behavioral therapy for the treatment of clinical depression in religious individuals. J Consult Clin Psychol 60:94–103, 1992

Sansone RA, Khatain K, Rodenhauser P: The role of religion in psychiatric training: a national survey. Academic Psychiatry 14:34–38, 1990

Sheehan W, Kroll J: Psychiatric patients' belief in general health factors and sin as causes of illness. Am J Psychiatry 147:112–113, 1990

Stark R: Psychopathology and religious commitment. Review of Religious Research 12:165–176, 1971

Steinfels P: Psychiatrists' manual shifts stance on religious and spiritual problems. The New York Times, February 10, 1994

Watters W: Deadly Doctrine: Health, Illness, and Christian God Talk. Buffalo, NY, Prometheus Books, 1992

Williams DR, Larson DB, Buckler RE, et al: Religion and psychological distress in a community sample. Soc Sci Med 32:1257–1262, 1991

Worthington EL Jr: Religious counseling: a review of published empirical research. Journal of Counseling and Development 64:421–431, 1986

Treatment Approaches

CHAPTER 11

Culture's Role in Clinical Psychiatric Assessment

CHARLES C. HUGHES, PH.D.[†]

SAMUEL O. OKPAKU, M.D., PH.D.

R ogler and Wohl provide the basis for this chapter:

> Culture in psychiatric diagnosis is an issue of scientific accuracy. (*Rogler 1993, p. 326*)

> Much of the time in the practice of psychotherapy, culture remains silent, part of a nonintrusive background, an invisible yet pervasive feature of the context of psychotherapy. . . . Psychotherapies differ as the cultures in which they were born and nurtured differ, and each bears the indelible imprint of its culture source. Psychotherapy and the human relationships that comprise both its subject matter and the medium in which it is performed have embedded within them values, rules, assumptions, myths, and rituals of a particular culture. Psychotherapy is thus inescapably bound to a particular cultural framework. (*Wohl 1989, p. 343*)

An extensive literature demonstrates the profound influence of socialization on a person's behavior and thought into a particular system of ideas (a culture) that pervasively programs intrapsychic as well as social behavior. That programming also provides not only value orientations but also intractable interpretations—*meanings*—of events experi-

---

[†]Charles Hughes died in August 1997.

enced by a person. Yet, until recently, the behavioral phenomena denoted by the concept of *culture* have been largely regarded as irrelevant in formal psychiatric assessments of pathology and consequent diagnoses. For example, *culture* was not indexed in the original *Diagnostic and Statistical Manual: Mental Disorders* (DSM-I) of the American Psychiatric Association (1952), nor in DSM-II (American Psychiatric Association 1968) or DSM-III (American Psychiatric Association 1980). Similarly, anything more than a passing reference to culture is seldom found in basic psychiatric texts.

But such dismissal of the relevance of cultural aspects of a patient's life is slowly changing—at least in a limited way. Indeed, DSM-III-R (American Psychiatric Association 1987) and DSM-IV (American Psychiatric Association 1994) admonish that the cultural dimension should be considered in the process of patient evaluation and diagnosis. The forward to DSM-III-R, for example, states that

> When the DSM-III-R classification and diagnostic criteria are used to evaluate a person from an ethnic or cultural group different from that of the clinician's, and especially when diagnoses are made in a non-Western culture, caution should be exercised in the application of DSM-III-R diagnostic criteria to assure that their use is culturally valid. It is important that the clinician not employ DSM-III-R in a mechanical fashion, insensitive to differences in language, values, behavioral norms, and idiomatic expressions of distress. (*American Psychiatric Association 1987, p. xxvi*)

But more than simply being sensitive to cultural differences, the clinician should hearken to operational directives:

> When applied in a non-Western-language community, DSM-III-R should be translated to provide equivalent meaning, not necessarily dictionary equivalence. The clinician working in such settings should apply DSM-III-R with open-mindedness to the presence of distinctive cultural patterns and sensitivity to the possibility of unintended bias because of such differences. (*American Psychiatric Association 1987, p. xxvi*)

DSM-IV has recognized the importance of including cultural factors in the database that informs an assessment and possible diagnosis.

Supported by a National Institute of Mental Health (NIMH) grant, a working committee of "cultural psychiatrists" and "psychiatric anthropologists" made a proposal to the DSM-IV task force charged with revising DSM-III-R, identifying a number of ways in which the cultural dimension is integral in shaping the behavior and thought that a patient presents to the clinician, data that are critical for a valid evaluation (Mezzich et al. 1993). However, an appraisal of the great bulk of clinical practice suggests that the success of these directives in informing clinicians' conceptualizations and procedures remains highly problematic; perhaps the appearance of DSM-IV will improve the situation.

Quite aside from scattered references to "the cultural dimension" in DSM-III-R and DSM-IV, there continue to be many exhortations found elsewhere in the psychiatric and behavioral science literature to the effect that cultural factors must be taken into account in patient assessment and diagnosis. Up to this point, however, the principal thrust of discussion about the importance of including cultural factors has focused on either an abstract, superficial level or fairly obvious cultural differences between social or ethnic groups—language, dress, behavior, expressed beliefs, and the like (essentially a tourist's experience of cultural differences). Although the intent may be to go deeper than that—somehow to penetrate the culturally different person's phenomenologic world (mind)—an assessment of most of the published literature dealing with cultural sensitivity forces one to the conclusion that there is usually a major gap between the earnest plea (and sincere commitment) vicariously to enter the other person's lived world and the ability to find effective modes of entry into that domain.

Further, a major—indeed, a critical—fallacy arising from a too-ready, nonthinking assent that cultural factors should be considered is that a focus on only the obvious differences results in the failure to recognize that a generic cultural process shapes *all* therapeutic encounters, even when the clinician and patient are of the same ethnic background. For one thing, regardless of cultural setting, a social class difference often exists between clinician and patient, and such a difference in social status is a major factor shaping the worldview of both. Indeed, in its influence in creating a person's structure of values, expectations, and norms for behavior, social class membership (no matter where it is found) operates as a subculture within a larger social whole (Hughes 1993).

Wohl has highlighted another usually overlooked yet very important aspect of the therapeutic encounter:

> When culture is a background factor, as is usually the case, which is to say, when no obvious cultural differences are apparent, it presents few if any problems. Paradoxically it may provoke problems where extraordinary cultural closeness between patient and therapist prevails. Two people of the same culture, or subculture, say Boston Irish-American or New York Jewish-American, are locked in a therapeutic venture. Because of the mutually identified ethnic similarity, the therapist may make assumptions about the patient that are not justified, or may ignore and fail to explore certain material because it seems self-evident. . . . Thus, even when differences are minimized, culture can be an intrusive factor in treatment. Clearly in such a situation it is possible that assumptions held by each party about the other because of the recognized ethnic similarity can be wrong. Similarity is not identity; each person carries a unique version of the ostensibly same culture. *There is always a difference in the understanding and internalization of a culture. For this reason it can be said that all psychotherapy is transcultural or cross cultural. There is always a cultural gap to be traversed* [emphasis added]. (*Wohl 1989, pp. 343–344*)

H. B. M. Murphy (1977), one of the pioneers in cultural psychiatry, argued in the same fashion almost 20 years ago in an editorial article entitled "Transcultural Psychiatry Should Begin at Home."

However, even while accepting the importance of culture as an integral part of the database that the clinician should review for arriving at an assessment, the critical question is how he or she can employ culturally relevant insights and observational skills in the interview situation itself without being an expert in specific cultural knowledge relevant to that patient. If not already ethnographically skilled, can the clinician learn anything on-the-job, so to speak, formulating from such primary encounter data new insights into the psychological and cultural construction of the patient's own world? How can the time-pressed clinician operationalize the exhortations to take cultural factors into account in the course of an intake interview?

It has been suggested that the clinician self-direct a process of introspective analysis of the data presented by the patient, that he or she conduct an inner mental dialogue to explore different perspectives and meanings of observations made about the patient's appearance and manner of presenting data about the problem that occasioned the visit (Hughes 1993). Also, Kleinman and colleagues (1978) have advised that the "patient's explanatory model" of the affliction be explored through the use of questions that invite a response in the patient's own cultural framework rather than that of the clinician.

Why not, therefore, demand the same of the clinician—that is, that he or she turn the critical eye of analysis selfward, inward, to assess the data that would lead to examinable hypotheses about the presence of pathology?

Although both of these techniques take steps toward developing insights into the cultural-psychological dynamics that constitute the patient's world, they may still be too abstract and unfamiliar to be useful. The need to develop other approaches has been stressed by a number of clinicians and other professionals as a preventive measure against a premature and incompletely informed (and thereby possibly misleading) application of the clinician's own categories that may be insensitive to, or incongruent with, the patient's construction of his or her world and the forces that move it.

Are there other insights that could be used to examine the primary data on which psychiatric inferences and formulations are based? Some have suggested a need to go back to the observed particulars, the level of primary observation, of symptoms and their presentation (Costello 1992; Finestein 1957; Meyer 1951, 1957; Persons 1986; Simons 1985). The challenge is to cut through established cultural filters (the clinician's as well as the patient's) and reach as fresh an apprehension as possible of the current psychodynamics. This approach requires, during the course of the interview, constant self-monitoring of one's own behavior as well as that of the patient—questions asked, replies (and nonreplies) received, nonverbal behavior or motoric "language," and interpretations or proto-assessments being developed. It is best to use as nonprestructured a view as possible, one in which the power of one's own culturally structured categories is minimized and that facilitates formulation of alternate hypotheses and a fruitful conceptualization of the problem and its analysis in culturally relevant and appropriate terms.

The primary data of the psychiatric interview is a dialogue between a clinician and a patient. A well-recognized yet flexibly standardized format is commonly used to elicit basic data from a patient presenting with a complaint of a possibly psychiatric nature. The general categories comprising that format are usually considered culture free.

But the assumption of the culture-free status of such a format has been critically questioned: first, by anthropologists as an instinctive part of their agenda of inquiry into any aspect of human behavior, and secondly by an increasing number of psychiatrists themselves who have gone behind the implicit assumptions of such a format and in an explicit and focused way looked at the role of culture in shaping and giving meaning to behavior.

We discuss in this chapter how selected portions of that format are employed in initial data gathering. The clinician needs to enlarge his or her perspective on the varieties of normal-yet-different patterns of behavior found in a patient population (Hughes 1993). The intent of this chapter is to provoke a thought experiment, a self-conscious, introspective, questioning-of-assumptions process in the clinician him- or herself in the clinical context (Hughes 1993).

The format suggested by Nicoli (1988) for the psychiatric examination is of course familiar to every clinician, since it is covered in the first year of residency. Although there is no question of its relevance, what may well be problematic is the way the categories are operationalized in the course of clinical assessment (Hughes 1993). Depending on the meanings assigned when interpreted by a clinician, such data may not indicate pathology but rather normal culturally based behavior and thoughts that are different from the clinician's own culturally derived appropriate behavior and meanings.

Nicoli's categories are general appearance, attitude, motor behavior, speech, affective states, thought processes, thought content, perception, intellectual functioning, orientation, memory, and judgment. Are these categories to be accepted uncritically and culturally unexamined? For example, such a critical and often emotionally laden attribute of a person as personal name is not mentioned in Nicoli's list of categories.

A practicing clinician's response to this observation may be, "Obviously the clinician asks the name first . . . or is told the name by the receptionist." But why should that be taken for granted? And why should there be no thought given to questions such as "Is this the 'true' name?" And what is the meaning, to the person uttering it, of the name given? Are there particular customs about the bestowal and use of personal names in the patient's cultural group that would be important to know—such as any religiously or supernaturally interpreted meaning of a personal name for the person whose character, personality, or dimensions of self it may influence? Or the importance to the person him- or herself of a nickname such as "Red," "Shorty," or "Chuck"? How are these accepted—enthusiastically or begrudgingly—by the person on whom they were bestowed by social usage? Were they suggested by that person him- or herself? It makes a difference.

We will be creative for a moment now and ask how such a standardized, Western-science-based psychiatric procedural format might play out in a setting that brings together two persons from different sociocultural backgrounds, one a specialist from Western biomedicine and the other a patient from a very different cultural background.[1] This hypothetical example of a patient interview offers lines of dialogue followed by explanation and analysis.

Scene

A mental health outpatient clinic in a remote part of the Navajo Reservation.

Characters

Psychiatrist (newly assigned by the National Health Service Corps to the Navajo Reservation)
Patient (an elderly Navajo male who speaks little English)
Young man (presumably Navajo)

---

1. Although based in ethnographic fact, a specialist on Navajo culture will find flaws in this sketch. It is, however, a heuristic exercise to highlight the often subtle and covert aspects of the cultural structuring of behavior that are not likely to be considered by a reader who has not had an in-depth experience in another culture.

Nurse (a white female who, to judge by her clothing and insignia, has had many years of experience working in mental health on the reservation)

Dialogue

Therapist: "What is your name?"

Norms of etiquette in human societies vary in such issues as indicating the purpose of an interaction immediately rather than taking time to establish an appropriate interpersonal climate for what happens next. To avoid souring the tone of the interaction, the clinician should work with the patient, being attentive to the individual's culture, to establish the purpose of the meeting. Navajo cultural norms would regard the American-style, abrupt, getting-down-to-business approach displayed by the clinician as highly impolite.

The courteous approach is for people (outsiders included) to engage in some small talk, or chitchat, before entering into the reason for the conversation. Although Navajos have had many years of experience with the ways of Anglos, they have had to learn to be tolerant, however rude they consider Anglos' behavior to be in this regard (Adair et al. 1988).

[Young man translates the question]

Patient: "Ben Begay."

A Navajo has several personal names. The patient here has given a commonly used form—one based on a kinship term (*begay* derives from the term meaning "his son" [i.e., Ben's son]). In small, face-to-face communities there is no need to be more specific. Consequently, in Navajoland there are many people with the surname "Begay," and the outsider should not conclude that they are necessarily of the same family or even extended family. In this regard, researchers in the Navajo-Cornell public health project familiar with modern Navajo culture comment:

Today most Navajo carry an Anglo or Spanish name or an anglicized version of a Navajo name. Until quite recently such names were arbitrarily assigned by traders, government personnel, or missionaries. A further complication arises from the Navajo reluctance to abandon what they consider a perfectly functional naming system. The result of this, especially in dealing with older people, is often an unwillingness or actual inability to "name" the members of one's family. *(Adair et al. 1988, p. 116)*

And quite apart from the patient's use of the name "Ben Begay," very likely he also has a unique and secret name "known only to one's family and perhaps by a medicine man. It should never be used either to refer to the person or to call him by except in certain ritual situations and in times of great danger. This name . . . is considered part of the person [and] almost a part of his being, and he could become ill or weakened if it were used indiscriminately" (Adair et al. 1988, p. 115). The importance of keeping accurate patient records for such activities as the Navajo-Cornell project, and the difficulty of doing so when naming patterns are based on different rationales and social usages, is considerable.

This example also illustrates the diversity in naming patterns found in human societies (Alford 1988). The substantial ethnographic literature on the topic raises questions about the implications a name may have for the concept of self. The Yoruba of Nigeria provide an illustration, with the personal name Abiku (meaning "death was merciful") being given to a child who is purportedly the reincarnation of a parent (Lawson 1987, p. 14). This example is similar to the traditional Eskimo pattern of bestowing the name-soul of a deceased upon a newborn infant, the "name" believed to be not simply a name but the embodiment of the personality characteristics of the deceased (Marsella et al. 1985).

The clinician, therefore, should always consider that there may be other names or commonly used designations such as nicknames or pseudonyms. Obtain the most complete data possible on the person's name. And remember that a given name is not simply a name; it has affective connotations and implications for concept of self and self-image. "Word-magic" occurs here: through common usage the personal name fuses with the person's self-concept.

Therapist: [Young man translates] "Are you called by any other name?"
Patient: "White Moustache."

Giving a nickname based on personal appearance is common usage among the Navajos.

Therapist: "Have you been to this clinic before?"
Patient: "Yes."
Therapist: "How old are you?"
Patient: [No answer]
Therapist: "When were you born?"
Patient: [Does not answer; appears to be thinking about how to answer the question]
Therapist: "Can you remember what the old people said was happening about the time you were born?"

This response is an excellent way to elicit the desired data. The Navajo people, like those in so many other societies, have a "space-time vagueness" with regard to specific dates (D. C. Leighton and Kluckhohn 1947, pp. 108ff). In the Cornell-Aro mental health project in Nigeria, a similar impasse was reached in our attempt to obtain detailed demographic data. After asking—and not receiving answers to—questions directed at specific dates of birth, we developed a checklist of well-known and important local historical events, such as the crowning of the tribal king or the occurrence of a severe drought, that the informant could use to match against significant personal events.

Patient: "The old people in my tribe told me that it was about the time when the government came and killed off many horses and sheep."

As part of a drastic stock reduction program to prevent overgrazing and erosion of the land, in the mid-1930s the federal government killed many horses and sheep owned by the Navajos. Done precipitously and without consultation with Navajo leaders, it resulted in long-lasting resentment and distrust of the federal government and its policies.

Therapist: [Continuing the attempt to obtain demographic data] "Are you married?"
Patient: "No."

Therapist: "Were you ever married?"

Patient: "Yes."

Therapist: "What happened?"

Patient: "I was married, but my wife died."

Therapist: "I am sorry about your wife's death. I'm sure that was very difficult for you. When did she die?"

Patient: [No answer; patient avoids eye contact]

Therapist: "You must miss your wife very much."

Patient: [Long silence. Even the therapist begins to feel uncomfortable. Introspectively he asks, "What's going on here?"]

Therapist: "Do you have any children?"

Patient: "Yes."

Therapist: "How many?"

Patient: "Six."

Therapist: "Do they live near you?"

Patient: "No."

Therapist: "Where do they live?"

Patient: "My three sons live far away, with their wives' outfits. My daughter lives near me."

The Navajo are a matrilineal society; that is, children belong to the clan of their mother. The traditional—and still-prevalent—residence pattern is for the husband to marry a woman from a different clan and usually move out of his local area and live with his wife's family. This system is called matrilocal or uxorial residence in anthropological jargon.

Therapist: "What about the other two children?"

Patient: "They passed on."

Therapist: "How did they die?"

Patient: [No answer; eyes averted]

Therapist: [Sensing reluctance to continue] "It is very difficult to lose children."

Patient: [No answer; stares at floor]

Therapist: "Have you talked with anyone about your children's deaths?"

Patient: "Not really."

Therapist: "This is one of the things we can talk about. Is there some other reason you are here today?"

Patient: [No response; period of silence; no eye contact with the clinician; eyes averted, gazing at the floor]

The language of eye-to-eye contact (gaze) is culturally elaborated in
many different ways in diverse societies to indicate social ranking including gender relations, respect, amorous intent, and other types of social situations and meanings. Particular patterns of gaze can also be interpreted as malevolent, such as the "evil eye" (*mal ojo*), widely found
in a range of societies. For example, in Mediterranean and Hispanic
cultures, sometimes the sickness of a child is explained as caused by an
adult having stared intently at the person and, through that action,
stolen his or her soul. In the case of Ben Begay as patient, though, such
avoidance of eye contact usually would be considered normal and simply polite behavior. However, in this particular instance it might also be
interpreted very differently. The clinician is asking about the patient's
dead relatives (wife and children). While trying to show a compassion-
ate interest (as well as gather important data), he has ventured into an
enormously frightening area for the Navajos—the dead and the ghosts
of the dead, who can return to this earth and cause great misfortune.
Therefore, for the psychiatrist to continue to press the issue of eliciting
important data about the patient's family in this manner is to create
strong anxiety and even intense fear in the patient, because ghosts can
return to the world of the living and cause accident, sickness, misfortune, and death. As noted in a classic ethnographic report, the import
of which continues even today, "Talking about ghosts increases the
danger from them, hence the reluctance of the Navajo to impart information about them to the ethnologist [or psychiatrist]" (Wyman et al.
1942, p. 24).

Note Nicoli's second category—attitude—and its operational definition:

What is the patient's attitude toward his illness, toward the interview, and toward the doctor? If ill, is he aware that he is ill? Is he
cooperative or evasive, arrogant or ingratiating, aggressive or submissive, outgoing or withdrawn? Does he express feelings freely or
does he avoid them obviously? These observations give clues to

the patient's main defense mechanisms as well as to patterns of relating to people generally. *(Nicoli 1988, p. 35)*

Therapist: [After waiting, perplexedly, for a response] "Is something bothering you?"

Whether the patient's behavior should be interpreted as pathologic in this instance should be appraised in the context of a culturally stereotypic response to perceived threat (or interpreted threat) in an unfamiliar social environment. Jewell's classic case study (1952) details how one "normal" Navajo young man, relatively unacculturated, was confined to a mental hospital with the diagnosis of schizophrenia (hebephrenic type) after displaying behavior similar to the patient's. He continued to show such symptoms for 8 months until discovered by a clinical psychologist with some knowledge of Navajo culture. Therefore, it is important not to rush to conclusions. Continue listening, gathering data for alternate hypotheses.

Patient: [Finally says something—in Navajo]

Young man: "He says he stepped on a tree branch that had been struck by lightning and that his body is hurting all over."

Therapist: [Pondering what to make of this exotic association. What does stepping on a tree branch that had been struck by lightning have to do with one's body feeling "hurt" all over? After all, the patient himself was not struck by lightning. . . . Something strange, some superstitious belief occurring here maybe?]

Young man: "He also says that yesterday morning he saw some strange tracks around his hogan, tracks not like any others that he knows."

An extensive body of beliefs exists among the Navajo regarding the avoidance of numerous kinds of dangerous objects or situations (*báhádzid*, meaning "dangerous to do"), such as contact with a tree or anything struck by lightning, seeing a coyote, or entering a hogan (traditional dwelling) where someone has died. As put by one expert, the Navajo are "morbidly fearful of death and anything associated with it." Further, the reference to "strange tracks" could indicate that a malevolent agent dressed in skins (a witch) had been near the hogan and the grandfather was understandably very frightened (in terms of cultural belief) at that possibility. Remember that many people around the world believe in taboos—things to do or not to do. In contemporary industrialized United States society, compare not stepping under a ladder for fear of bad luck, carrying a rabbit's foot for good luck, and many hotels in the United States omitting a 13th floor. So, in this case, ask the young man why the patient believes that stepping on the lightning-struck tree would make him feel sick.

Therapist: [At this point, not wanting to pick up directly on the patient's intriguing reference to "tracks," he asks instead] "Is there anything else troubling your grandfather?"

For the first time the clinician notices the patient's manner of dress and appearance. The patient has long hair, uncut and hanging to his shoulders. Is this "normal"? Also, the patient is dressed in the type of clothing and jewelry the clinician has seen in innumerable Hollywood and television movies portraying "Indians." "Specific idiosyncratic characteristics of dress and grooming ought to be noted, as well as posture, gait, facial expression, and gestures. The interviewer should note any distinctive feature that would identify the individual immediately" (Nicoli 1988, p. 35).

Young man: "My grandfather also says that he's very frightened by all of the sickness and deaths that have been happening lately—lots of people (especially the young people) are dying from the flu. And some of the bilagáana [Navajo term for whites or Anglos] are saying that it comes from the mice. . . . My grandfather thinks that maybe the ʔáda´nǐí [witches] also are causing some of those deaths. . . ."

The driving concept at the core of Navajo culture is harmony and order. Sickness occurs when the person is out of harmony with the universe—for whatever reason—and the function of traditional ceremonies is to restore that harmony among humankind, nature, and the universe. This concept is still firmly adhered to among most Navajos. In the summer of 1993, for example, following the outbreak of the "mysterious new disease" (as it was called), Navajo Singers (medicine men) met to try to divine the cause, and they indicated that the Navajos' changing from the old ways had broken the harmony among humans, nature, and the universe and the Hanta Virus disease was a consequence (McGraw 1993).

Therapist: "Ask him to tell me more about the witches." [Here obviously pursuing the possibility of delusions]

Whereas ghosts—the shades of departed living people—are considered malevolent and predisposed to doing destructive things to the living, witches are conceived to be still-living humans who, like ghosts, also have the power to cause illness, death, and accident. Being potentially omnipresent, their influence is used to explain all kinds of misfortune.

Patient: [Translated] "There are witches everywhere." [Reluctance to continue]
Therapist: "Do other people think that there are witches everywhere?"

This is a very important question, since it gets at the issue of whether the patient's belief in witches is idiosyncratic and therefore possibly pathologic. If it is a shared culturally based belief about the structure of the world, its status as a straightforward symptom of disorder is called into question. But if it functions in the economy of the personality as an omnipresent explanation for misfortune and frustration, one may begin to suspect it as having pathologic significance.

In the Cornell-Aro psychiatric study in Nigeria, for example (A. H. Leighton et al. 1963), a Yoruba village member said of one of his neighbors who had been diagnosed by Nigerian and American psychiatrists as exhibiting delusional disorder, "Yes, we all know that there are witches around. But he doesn't even plant his crops, and then says the witches made bad magic to cause them to fail."

Patient: "Yes; everybody knows that."
Therapist: "Now I would like to ask you some other questions. Who is the President of the United States?"

Patient: [No response; silence]
Therapist: [Moving into a different area] "What is the color of the sky?"
Patient: [Navajo word . . .]
Therapist: "What color are the leaves of a tree?"

Although the question is well intentioned to check mental status, asking it so straightforwardly creates a confusing semantic field in the mind of the patient. The interviewer is assuming that a singular and exclusive color term is applied to what in mainstream Anglo society is called *blue* or *green* on the color spectrum. When referring to color, better to say something such as the following: "Tell me what it is like" (Adair et al. 1988, p. 139).

The Navajo language does not differentiate between what are called *blue* and *green* in English; in fact, there is no generic term for *color,* and differentiations among hues are made on the basis of specific instances (Adair et al. 1988, p. 139ff). Color nomenclature varies significantly in societies around the world, and a clinician should not infer disorientation on the basis of such a response. The clinician tries to ask a question that is relevant to the patient, to check mental status and orientation.

Therapist: "How far is it from here to Shiprock?"
Patient: [No response]
Therapist: "When did you last go there?"
Patient: "Maybe last month."
Therapist: "How long did it take?"
Patient: "Maybe six hours."

Mileage is only one measure of distance; another is the time required for travel between two places, which takes into account road conditions, weather, and other relevant real-world factors. In this case—unknown to and not asked by the clinician—was the fact that the patient lived in a part of the reservation away from paved roads and had to be brought by a relative in a pickup truck over dirt roads that often became impassable after snows or the occasional thunderstorm outbursts. Hence, the functional definition of time includes such conditions (Hall 1959).

Not all cultural groups in the world are rigidly focused (as is typical of industrialized societies) on an exact specification of time or of guiding their behavior by an internalized sense that the "time" as a rigid structure external to the self must be rigidly adhered to (Hall 1959).

Therapist: [Still wanting to evaluate the patient for orientation, the clinician thinks of attempting the Serial Sevens. But reflecting on the language problem and the serious cultural difference that is becoming apparent, decides against pursuing it further (Paulos 1989, pp. 1, 16).]

Nurse: [Turning to the therapist and whispering something to him]

Therapist: [With a look of surprise on his face, asks the nurse in a lowered voice: "What do you mean, a ceremony?" She whispers something more, and the clinician thinks about it for a few minutes.]

Therapist: [Addressing his question to the young man]:   "Has your grandfather talked to a medicine man about the things that are bothering him?"

Young man: "No. The people in the hospital told me to bring him to you at this clinic."

Therapist: "I would be glad to talk with him at any time. But first I suggest that you take your grandfather to a . . . [at this point the nurse whispers something to the psychiatrist] hat 'ha 'athli [Navajo word for medicine man, or Singer] and ask him to help you. You are welcome at any time to return here and let me help you with white man's medicine."

In recent years, cooperation rather than rejection has existed between Western medical practitioners and the Navajo healers, the Singers. The Navajo themselves recognize that some diseases (e.g., those requiring surgery and infectious disease) are better treated by Western medicine than indigenous medicine and will refer to the hospitals and clinics. On the other hand, Navajos also believe that Western treatment is only part of the restoration of harmony with the universe, and ritual treatment by a Singer is required for critical conditions (Adair et al. 1988; Dajer 1989).

Conclusions

Rogler (1993) has suggested a tripartite scheme depicting the several ways in which culture is involved in psychiatric assessment and diagnosis. The first level pertains to the symptoms themselves, in which "[c]ulture is relevant to endogenous experiences of distress . . . and to subjective information from which distress is inferred. . . . [I]t is relevant also to the willingness of respondents to divulge symptoms" (pp. 325–326).

The second level addresses ethnopsychiatric diagnostic patterns and the "syndromization" of symptoms into patterns that include but are not limited to the familiar culture-bound syndromes found in various societies.

Finally,

> the third level focuses on the interpersonal situation of the diagnostic interview. Cultural factors intervene to affect diagnostic outcomes in the bicultural pairing between diagnostician and client, and in the client's familiarity with the language of the diagnostic interview. . . . The general hypothesis is that therapeutic situations that increase the cultural distance between diagnostician and client increase diagnostic error in assessing the type and severity of illness. *(Rogler 1993, p. 326)*

Coming, then, full circle from Rogler's assessment at the beginning of the chapter,

> Culture sees all levels of the diagnostic hierarchy so that from level 1 to level 3, diagnostic errors either due to the neglect of culture or arising from misconceptions about culture cumulatively increase. *(Rogler 1993, p. 326)*

References

Adair J, Deuschle KW, Barnett CR: The People's Health: Medicine and Anthropology in a Navajo Community. Albuquerque, NM, University of New Mexico Press, 1988

Alford RD: Naming and Identity: A Cross-Cultural Study of Personal Naming Practices. New Haven, CT, HRAF Press, 1988

American Psychiatric Association: Diagnostic and Statistical Manual: Mental Disorders. Washington, DC, American Psychiatric Association, 1952

American Psychiatric Association: Diagnostic and Statistical Manual of Mental Disorders, 2nd Edition. Washington, DC, American Psychiatric Association, 1968

American Psychiatric Association: Diagnostic and Statistical Manual of Mental Disorders, 3rd Edition. Washington, DC, American Psychiatric Association, 1980

American Psychiatric Association: Diagnostic and Statistical Manual of Mental Disorders, 3rd Edition, Revised. Washington, DC, American Psychiatric Association, 1987

American Psychiatric Association: Diagnostic and Statistical Manual of Mental Disorders, 4th Edition. Washington, DC, American Psychiatric Association, 1994

Costello CG: Research on symptoms versus research on syndromes: arguments in favour of allocating more research time to the study of symptoms. Br J Psychiatry 160:304–308, 1992

Dajer T: Medicine man. Discover, July 1989, pp 47–51

Finestein AR: A critical overview of diagnosis in psychiatry, in Psychiatric Diagnosis. Edited by Rakoff VM, Stancer HC, Kedward HB. New York, Brunner/Mazel, 1977, pp 189–206

Hall ET: Space speaks, in The Silent Language. Edited by Hall ET. Greenwich, CT, Premier Books, 1959, pp 19–29, 146–164

Hughes CC: Culture in clinical psychiatry, in Culture, Ethnicity, and Mental Illness. Edited by Gaw AC. Washington, DC, American Psychiatric Press, 1993, pp 3–41

Jewell DP: A case of "psychotic" Navaho Indian male. Human Organization 1:32–36, 1952

Kleinman A, Eisenberg L, Good B: Culture, illness, and care: clinical lessons from anthropologic and cross-cultural research. Ann Intern Med 88:251–258, 1978

Lawson ED (compiler): Personal Names and Naming: An Annotated Bibliography. New York, Greenwood, 1987

Leighton AH, Lambo TA, Hughes CC, et al: Psychiatric Disorder Among the Yoruba: A Report From the Cornell-Aro Mental Health Research Project in the Western Region, Nigeria. Ithaca, NY, Cornell University Press, 1963

Leighton DC, Kluckhohn C: Children of the People: The Navaho Individual and His Development. Cambridge, MA, Harvard University Press, 1947

Marsella AJ, DeVos G, Hsu FLL (eds): Culture and Self: Asian and Western Perspectives. New York, Tavistock, 1985

McGraw D: A desert killer, a culture clash. U.S. News and World Report, June 14, 1993, pp 30–31

Meyer A: The Collected Papers of Adolf Meyer, Vol 3. Edited by Winters E. Baltimore, MD, Johns Hopkins University Press, 1951

Meyer A: Psychobiology: A Science of Man. Springfield, IL, Charles C Thomas, 1957

Mezzich JE, Kleinman A, Fabrega H, et al: Revised Cultural Proposals for DSM-IV. Submitted to the DSM-IV Task Force by the Steering Committee, NIMH-Sponsored Group on Culture and Diagnosis, 1993

Murphy HBM: Transcultural psychiatry should begin at home. Psychol Med 7:369–371, 1977

Nicoli AM (ed): The New Harvard Guide to Psychiatry. Cambridge, MA, Belknap Press of Harvard University Press, 1988

Paulos JA: The odds are you're innumerate. The New York Times Book Review, January 1, 1989, pp 1, 16

Persons JB: The advantages of studying psychological phenomena rather than psychiatric diagnoses. Am Psychol 41:1252–1260, 1986

Rogler LH: Culture in psychiatric diagnosis: an issue of scientific accuracy. Psychiatry 56:324–327, 1993

Simons RC: Sorting the culture-bound syndromes, in The Culture-Bound Syndromes: Folk Illnesses of Psychiatric and Anthropological Interest. Edited by Simons RC, Hughes CC. Dordrecht, Reidel, 1985, pp 25–381

Wohl J: Integration of cultural awareness into psychotherapy. Am J Psychother 43:343–355, 1989

Wyman L, Hill WW, Ósanai I: Navajo Eschatology. University of New Mexico Bulletin 4: 1942

CHAPTER 12

Somatization and Psychologization
Understanding Cultural Idioms of Distress

LAURENCE J. KIRMAYER, M.D., F.R.C.P.C.
THI HONG TRANG DAO, M.D., F.R.C.P.C.
ANDRÉ SMITH, M.S.W.

In this chapter we consider what is known about cultural variations in somatization and in its obverse, psychologization (White 1982). The term *somatization* is used clinically in several conceptually distinct ways (Kirmayer 1984): to refer to a family of psychiatric disorders (somatoform disorders in DSM-IV [American Psychiatric Association 1994]); to refer to a process of transforming or transducing psychological conflict into bodily symptoms (often including medically unexplained and functional somatic symptoms); and to describe a pattern of illness behavior, especially a style of clinical presentation, in which somatic symptoms are presented to the exclusion or eclipse of emotional distress and social problems. These different uses of the term are not equivalent and involve varying degrees of inference about underlying processes that are, at present, unmeasurable. In research studies, somatization has been operationalized in three main ways (Kirmayer and Robbins 1991): 1) as medically unexplained somatic symptoms (e.g., in the somatization disorder module of the Diagnostic Interview Schedule [Escobar et al. 1989]); 2) as hypochondriacal worry or somatic preoccupation (Barsky 1992); and 3) as somatic clinical presentations of affective, anxiety, or other psychiatric disorders (Goldberg and Bridges 1988).

Although somatization is often thought to be characteristic of specific ethnocultural groups, recent evidence shows that somatization is common in all cultural groups and societies. Differences among groups may reflect cultural styles of expressing distress (idioms of distress) that are influenced not only by cultural beliefs and practices but also by familiarity with health care systems and pathways to care. Many immigrants and ethnocultural groups are unfamiliar with psychiatric diagnosis and treatment or associate it only with severe mental disorder. Accustomed to receiving health care in a primary care setting, where the focus is usually on physical illness, and concerned to avoid psychiatric stigmatization, they deemphasize the psychosocial aspects of their distress. In most cases, this presentation does not mean that patients do not experience emotional and psychological symptoms, only that they are very reluctant to make them the focus of the clinical encounter. Clinical work with such patients requires a negotiation of appropriate goals and strategies based on knowledge of the personal and cultural meanings of illness.

In the first section, we discuss the place of culture in the current nosology of somatoform disorders. Despite efforts to incorporate cultural considerations into the DSM-IV text, important issues remain in the application of this nosology cross-culturally. This section reviews some ethnocultural variations in somatization and its relationship to culture-bound syndromes and idioms of distress. A cultural perspective can also be applied to psychiatric theory itself, which raises basic questions about what somatic symptoms mean—that is, when they are to be taken as symbolic communications and when they are simply indications of pathology, the topic of the second section. Next, we illustrate a cultural perspective on somatization with a clinical case. Finally, we discuss the implications of a cultural perspective for working with patients with somatic distress. Much clinical work is aimed at reinterpreting bodily distress in terms of personal and social conflict. This approach can be helpful or harmful, depending on the fit of such psychologizing with local ways of expressing, legitimating, and managing distress.

Cultural Issues in the Nosology of Somatoform Disorders

The notion that somatization is more common or characteristic of patients from certain non-Western cultures, particularly Asians and

Africans, has become well entrenched. For example, in a recent compendium (Gaw 1993), virtually all of the chapters that mention somatization concern Asian groups. In fact, research suggests that somatization is ubiquitous—although its prevalence and specific features vary considerably across cultures; the processes of focusing on, amplifying, and clinically presenting somatic distress are universal; and somatic symptoms are the most common expression and clinical presentation of emotional distress worldwide (Kirmayer 1984).

Although somatization covers a broader territory than the somatoform disorders per se, official nosology has a powerful effect on clinicians' thinking and the practice of psychiatry. Accordingly, it is important to consider the relevance of existing nosology to cultural variations in somatization. In a review of the literature for the National Institute of Mental Health (NIMH) working group on cultural considerations for DSM-IV, Kirmayer and Weiss (1997) identified three basic problems with existing nosology for cross-cultural work: 1) the overlap between somatic, affective, and anxiety disorders renders the whole concept of somatoform disorders misleading; 2) a wide range of culture-specific somatic symptoms and syndromes fall outside existing nosology; and 3) the use of somatic symptoms in idioms of distress may lead to excessive pathologizing of patients who are using cultural codes of communication to express subclinical levels of distress or social concerns.

The confluence of somatoform, affective, and anxiety disorders. Human suffering is cut from one cloth: when people are miserable they tend to be miserable in every sphere. Somatic distress is a normal feature of any perturbation of the person's adaptation (any state of ill health) and regularly accompanies both major psychiatric disorders and milder levels of emotional distress. The psychodynamic claim that an either-or relationship exists between somatic and emotional symbolic expressions of distress is not borne out by clinical, laboratory, and community epidemiological studies. Somatic and emotional symptoms were highly intercorrelated in the epidemiologic catchment area (ECA) study data (Simon and Von Korff 1991). In fact, somatic symptoms are generally viewed as nonspecific indicators of psychiatric distress, and somatic symptom checklists are a useful screening technique for a broad range of psychiatric disorders in primary care, not only in India (Srinivasan and Suresh 1991) and Africa (Gureje and Obikoya 1992) but throughout the world.

The very existence of a discrete nosological category (or genus) of somatoform disorders implies a separation of affective, anxiety, dissociative, and somatic symptoms that is not reflected in the co-occurrence of these symptoms in syndromes worldwide. This separation largely reflects the persistent mind-body dualism of Western medicine: psychiatric disorders are perceived as mental disorders, notwithstanding their prominent somatic symptoms. Other medical conditions are physical, although they may cause mental symptoms as a by-product of disturbed physiology or difficulty coping with their burden. The somatoform disorders are then a residual category lying between the somatic and the psychic, used to make the nosological system complete. This function is particularly relevant in consultation-liaison psychiatry, in which clinicians are called on to diagnose patients whose problems do not fall neatly into either category. The label of somatization then serves to fit the recalcitrant patient and problem into the overall system of medicine (even if it offers little in the way of clarity) (Kirmayer 1988, 1994).

In other parts of the world, and in the experience of patients from many ethnocultural groups, the sharp distinction between psychological and somatic symptoms is far from obvious. As a result, certain diagnostic categories that combine somatic and psychological symptoms have continued to be popular in other countries; for example, neurasthenia remains a common diagnosis in China (Kleinman 1986; Lee 1994; Ware and Weiss 1994). Although DSM-III-R (American Psychiatric Association 1987) and DSM-IV largely eliminated diagnostic hierarchies, there is still an implicit hierarchy based on therapeutic efficacy and strategies, in which, for example, major depression should be diagnosed over neurasthenia, since it leads to a specific and often efficacious treatment with antidepressants. Of course, the prominence and centrality of somatic symptoms in depression challenges the notion that it is essentially a mental disorder. It is possible to conceive of depression as a somatic syndrome of energy depletion and slowing down in which demoralization and other psychological symptoms sometimes accompany what is essentially a physical disease. The phenomenological basis for viewing disorders as somatic is of course distinct from arguments about their underlying biology; however, it serves to show how arbitrary the broad distinctions among types of disorder in DSM-IV remain, the more so from a cross-cultural perspective.

Culture-specific symptoms and syndromes. In an attempt to expand its coverage of cultural issues, DSM-IV includes a glossary of culture-related syndromes. Many of these syndromes have predominately somatic symptoms and so might be viewed as forms of somatization (e.g., bilis or colera, *hwa-byung,* brain fag, *dhat, shenkui,* falling-out, *koro, shenjing shuairuo,* and neurasthenia). However, consistent with the point made earlier, in most cases somatic symptoms coexist with and are even attributed to emotional distress and psychosocial stressors.

The Korean syndrome *hwa-byung,* for example, is viewed as a somatic manifestation of suppressed anger or rage (Kim 1993; Lin 1983; Lin et al. 1992; Pang 1990). In the United States, *hwa-byung* has been described predominantly among lower-socioeconomic-level, married Korean women immigrants after middle age. Common symptoms include feelings of heaviness, burning, or mass in the epigastric region; headaches; muscular aches and pains; dry mouth; insomnia; palpitations; and indigestion. But *hwa-byung* also includes depressive symptoms (i.e., sadness, negative thinking, loss of interest, regret, guilt, and suicidal ideas), anxious mood, irritability, tendency to lose one's temper, and absentmindedness. It is thought by sufferers to be due to the suppression of feelings of anger and resentment, which form a sort of mass in the chest. Korean psychiatrists relate *hwa-byung* to the culturally distinctive sociomoral sentiment of *haan*—accumulated anger, resentment, and despair at historical, collective, and individual victimization. Patients can usually readily identify interpersonal and social problems that give rise to the anger, suppression of which then leads to physical illness. Clinicians unfamiliar with the social meanings of *hwa-byung* may focus exclusively on the somatic dimensions and so contribute to patients' bodily preoccupations.

In eastern Africa and Nigeria, brain fag is a common syndrome involving sensations of heaviness, or heat, in the head associated with the effort of studying. It may occur in conjunction with major depression, anxiety disorders, or adjustment disorders (Guinness 1992; Jegede

1983; Morakinyo 1980; Prince 1960). Typically, it has been found among students who are the first in their families to become literate and who, in the process, have experienced both geographical and psychological separation from their families and communities of origin. Symptoms of hot or "peppery" feelings in the head or sensations of worms crawling in the head are common throughout equatorial Africa and Asia and may be associated with a similarly wide range of disorders (Ebigbo 1986; Makanjuola 1987).

In south and east Asia, a great variety of physical and psychological symptoms may be attributed to loss of vital essence through semen. In India, this disorder takes the form of *dhat* syndrome (Bhatia and Malik 1991; Paris 1992). As evidence of semen loss, patients may report turbid urine or express concern about nocturnal emissions or masturbation. Treatment of a coexisting anxiety or depressive disorder may be effective in alleviating symptoms of *dhat* (Bhatia and Malik 1991).

Episodes of loss of consciousness are found in the syndromes of falling-out or blacking-out among some Afro-Caribbean and other groups (Lefley 1979; Weidman 1979) and *indisposition* among Haitians (Philippe and Romain 1979). Such conversion symptoms may inflate epidemiological estimates of the prevalence of somatization disorder in these populations. Similarly, *ataques de nervios,* a syndrome of agitation, screaming, and "loss of control" (found in Puerto Rico and throughout Latin America) may be interpreted as a dissociative symptom and contribute to the overdiagnosis of somatoform disorders in this group (Guarnaccia 1993; Oquendo et al. 1992).

The presence of these culture-related symptoms and syndromes means that conventional clinical inquiry into somatic distress based on the symptom lists of DSM-IV may fail to inquire about or misinterpret significant areas of concern. When such symptoms are elicited, clinicians unfamiliar with their cultural prevalence and meaning may view them as bizarre and indicative of severe pathology (e.g., sensations of worms crawling in the head may be reminiscent of formication hallucinations in cocaine intoxication or interpreted as frankly psychotic).

Although these folk illnesses are often described as culture-bound (or better, culture-related) syndromes, the term is misleading because, in many cases, the lay terms do not name syndromes but rather explanations or attributions for distress. For example, while *dhat* is commonly associated with the symptom of loss of semen in the urine, this symptom perception is clearly an interpretation based on cultural beliefs. Even in the absence of specific symptoms, *dhat* functions as an explanation for a host of somatic and psychological problems.

It is most accurate, then, to understand these syndromes as idioms of distress: modes and methods of communicating a wide range of personal and social concerns and forms of distress in a way that is acceptable, or at least intelligible, to others.

Somatic idioms of distress. As noted previously, higher levels of medically unexplained somatic symptoms have been found in community studies of some ethnocultural groups. To an unknown extent, this greater prevalence may reflect the use of somatic symptoms as part of local cultural idioms of distress (Nichter 1981). As idioms of distress, somatic symptoms or illness attributions serve to communicate distress in a locally intelligible and legitimate fashion. As such, somatic symptoms may come to be experienced and expressed in response to relatively low levels of emotional distress or interpersonal conflict. Clinicians may then overdiagnose somatoform disorders in situations in which patients are simply using the best available language to signal their predicament and mobilize support.

The use of somatic idioms of distress runs counter to Western folk psychological norms for explicit talk about emotions and relationships and so may lead to patients being labeled as pathologically deficient in their capacity for psychological self-understanding. This perspective ignores the way in which somatic symptoms are commonly understood, in many cultures, not just as bodily events but as direct reflections— both indices of, and metaphors for—events of personal and social significance (Kirmayer 1987). In a seminal paper, Good (1977) showed how the idiom of heart distress among Iranians could be understood as a culturally prescribed way of talking about a host of personal and social concerns primarily related to loss and grief. Throughout the Middle East references to the heart are commonly understood not just as potential signs of illness but also as natural metaphors for a range of emotions. Similar metaphors grounded in bodily sensations and ethnophysiological notions are found in the complaints of chest tightness among Turkish women (Mirdal 1985) and the corresponding Greek symptom of *stenohoria*.

Certain common ethnophysiological ideas serve to link diverse bodily symptoms and behaviors within a system that has both hygienic and moral dimensions. For example, *nervios* (Mexican-American), *nevra* (Greek), and other syndromes of "nerves" are common as somatized forms of anxiety and depression (Davis and Whitten 1988; Guarnaccia 1993; Lock and Wakewich-Dunk 1990; Low 1994). Similarly, notions of blood as central to health are found among many peoples and may tie together diverse symptoms in syndromes such as *sangue dormido* or "low blood" among Afro-Caribbeans (Laguerre 1987; Sobo 1993).

Fatigue syndromes (e.g., *shenjing shuairuo*, neurasthenia, chronic fatigue syndrome, and myalgic encephalitis in Britain) remain common around the world, although with varying degrees of use and legitimacy within local systems of biomedicine (Cathébras 1994; Kitanishi and Kondo 1994; Starcevic 1994; Ware and Weiss 1994; Wessely 1994). Notions of chronic fatigue in Hong Kong actually center on headache and insomnia rather than weakness or fatigue per se (Lee 1994). But when patients talk about fatigue, headache, insomnia, or heart distress, they are more or less explicitly pointing to life circumstances that they find difficult or overwhelming. This circumstance is made clear in Kleinman's (1986) account of neurasthenia in China, where, despite the persistence of Confucian values and the threat of state surveillance of clinical encounters, patients nonetheless weave the facts of personal trauma, loss, and emotional suffering into their illness narratives.

It is fair to ask, then, who is somatizing. Is somatization primarily a failure of clinicians to understand and accept somatic modes of expression as culturally valid means of expressing feelings and predicaments or an unwillingness to face, together with patients, those same predicaments? This question points to the need for a broader view of the meaning of bodily distress in psychiatric practice than that implicit in the diagnostic nosology of DSM-IV.

The Meaning of Somatic Symptoms

Somatic symptoms can be interpreted, and hence have meaning attached to them, in several different ways. Depending on the clinician's interpretive stance, somatic symptoms may be treated as 1) an index of disease or disorder, 2) an indication of psychopathology, 3) a symbolic condensation of intrapsychic conflict, 4) an idiomatic expression of distress, 5) a metaphor for experience, 6) a form of social commentary or protest, and 7) an act of positioning within a local world. These levels of meaning are not mutually exclusive. Which level of meaning predominates may differ for patient, family, employer, clinician, and researcher. The choice of a level of meaning to emphasize, however, has important implications for clinical strategies. This section considers each of these modes of interpretation in turn.

Different disciplines have tended to privilege one or another of these forms of symptom meaning. There is a tendency in biomedicine to reduce all symptom reports to more or less accurate signs (or indices) of disease. When no disease can be found, the symptom report is suspect, and the patient is seen as having illness without disease (e.g., the worried well, hypochondriasis, and somatoform disorders). In psychodynamic psychiatry, the tendency has been to reduce all symptom reports to symbolic communications, reflective of intrapsychic conflict, whether as metaphors for experience or more extended narratives of self. The tendency in social anthropology and ethnography has been to reduce all symptom reports to collective representations (instances of explanatory models), commentary on social conditions or predicaments, social action (protest or contestation), or positioning (Harré and Van Langenhove 1991).

Somatic symptoms as indices of disease.   As an index of disease or disorder, somatic symptoms follow automatically from disturbed physiology. Emotional distress and social stress readily give rise to physiological disturbances with specific somatic symptoms. This situation does not imply, however, that the meaning of somatic symptoms can be entirely subsumed by the inciting emotion or social event. Even where emotions or social stressors can be unequivocally identified as causal agents, they may work through psychophysiological mechanisms that have their own dynamics. For example, there is some evidence that selective disturbance of stage IV non-REM sleep can give rise to symptoms of diffuse muscular pain and tender points characteristic of fibromyalgia (Moldofsky 1986). Sleep disturbance may also contribute to symptoms of irritable bowel and a wide range of symptoms attributed to chronic fatigue syndromes (van Diest and Appels 1994).

Physical symptoms then may simply be an index of psychosocial problems, independent of the individual's cognitive schema of such problems. Since many cultures have notions of sociosomatics in which social events are understood to lead directly to physical illness, it is often helpful for patients to receive this type of explanation in terms of their own ethnophysiological beliefs. Of course, once symptoms occur, they may be differentially focused on and interpreted in ways that contribute to either successful coping or catastrophic amplification of distress (Kirmayer 1990; Wickramasekera 1988).

Somatic symptoms as manifestations of psychopathology. Somatic symptoms may also be interpreted as evidence of a specific type of psychopathology. Some evidence suggests that certain individuals have an amplifying somatic style that leads them to experience and report more distressing somatic symptoms (Barsky 1992). Certain personality traits may predispose individuals to experience and focus on physical distress (Kirmayer et al. 1994a). Childhood events that reinforce somatic illness as a legitimate means of seeking help from others and of resolving conflict may also lead to somatization (Craig et al. 1993).

In the case of many physical symptoms, current psychodynamic theory argues that the symptoms occur because of deficits in the capacity to symbolically express and resolve emotional conflict and distress, a problem sometimes referred to as alexithymia. Alexithymia, however, seems more strongly related to pain and dysphoria, which occupy consciousness and occlude awareness, thus making it difficult to discriminate nuances of feeling and elaborate symbolism and fantasy (Kirmayer and Taillefer 1997).

Medically unexplained symptoms are extremely common in the community, but most do not lead to help seeking and probably do not indicate any psychiatric disorder. Somatization disorder requires so many medically unexplained symptoms that it is likely to identify individuals who are globally distressed (and who, in fact, suffer from depression, anxiety, and a wide range of other psychiatric disorders including severe personality disorders [Kirmayer et al. 1994a]); however, the milder forms of somatization involving just a few unexplained symptoms (which are far more common) may not be psychiatric disorders per se but rather represent functional disturbances of normal physiology, aggravated by psychiatric disorders when (and if) they co-exist. This effect of psychiatric disorders on functional somatic syndromes may occur in two main ways: first, the autonomic arousal that accompanies strong emotion may result in more somatic symptoms; and second, cognitive-emotional changes accompanying depression, anxiety, or other disorders may lead to amplification of somatic distress through processes of symptom perception, attention, attribution, and interpretation. Most functional somatic symptoms in the community probably are handled by taking home remedies or by normalizing and ignoring them. When a stressful life event or a major psychiatric disorder supervenes, the combination may be sufficient to prompt medical help seeking. Thus the frequent observation of high rates of psychiatric morbidity in clinical samples of patients with medically unexplained or functional somatic syndromes may be an artifact of help seeking.

Although it is always possible to find some emotional distress or life event on which to pin somatic symptoms, the attribution is not equally easy to confirm, and some authorities remain skeptical of the facile interpretation of somatic syndromes as stress-related disorders (Merskey 1993). Further, while depression can lead to chronic pain, pain can lead to depression, and the latter direction of causality actually appears to be somewhat stronger in the general population (Magni et al. 1994).

In fact, somatization and somatoform disorder diagnoses tend to function as residual categories invoked whenever other medical explanations cannot be found (Kirmayer 1994). Indeed, which symptoms are considered to be medically unexplained depends in part on current fashion. Many common somatic symptoms can be attributed to such syndromes as fibromyalgia, irritable bowel syndrome, and chronic fatigue, which have varying degrees of credibility as disorders or diseases and which lack definitive diagnostic methods and standards. Physiological explanations can be found for many somatic symptoms (e.g., hyperventilation, muscle tension, and sleep disturbance), moving them from the realm of somatization to a position as bona fide disease aggravated by stress (Sharpe and Bass 1992). Somatization would then be limited to the situation in which patients ignore, minimize, or deny any role for psychosocial stressors.

Somatic symptoms as symbolic condensations. Classic conversion symptoms are said to express the individual's conflict and so function as symbolic condensations or displacements of specific interpersonal and intrapsychic conflicts. The evidence suggests, however, that conversion symptoms tend to more closely follow cultural and local models than specific conflictual themes (the more so, since, as the later discussion on metaphor suggests, any theme can be grafted onto any symptom).

Since plausible explanations usually can be generated for medically unexplained symptoms, it is a matter of preference or prejudice whether one explains an unexplained symptom in terms of disturbed sleep, stress, tension, or emotional conflict. Where one stops in this chain depends, at present, on pragmatic-therapeutic considerations more than on any possibility of diagnostic certainty (Kirmayer 1994).

Somatic symptoms as cultural idioms of distress. As we have argued, somatic symptoms can also be understood as reflecting cultural models or idioms of distress. Cultural models work more generally to supply not just symptoms but also attributions and ways of explaining and situating distress. As an idiom of distress, somatic symptoms may be used simply to express discomfort or low levels of distress in ways that are intelligible to others.

The notion of idiom of distress may be misleading, however, for two clinically important reasons: 1) *idiom* implies a well-structured, codified, conventional way of expressing distress when in fact culturally mediated forms of distress are often fragmentary, tentative, and contradictory; and 2) most somatic symptoms, even those that fit the idiom, are not consciously intended as communications (Kirmayer and Young, in press).

The explanatory model approach of medical anthropology has tended to view idioms of distress as the result of a schema or template for understanding the label, cause, course, consequence, treatment, and outcome of problems (Good and Good 1980; Kleinman 1980). Explanatory models are elicited by asking patients direct questions about their illness beliefs. This approach assumes that people are lay scientists with detailed knowledge about indigenous illness categories. Although this is sometimes true, it has been exaggerated in the medical anthropological literature, because people who can give such accounts make good informants who contribute to good ethnographic texts. In clinical situations, it is more common for people to be incompletely familiar with their own cultures' illness models or idioms of distress and unable to describe an explanatory model in explicit detail. Instead, patients' illness narratives are based on other knowledge structures, specifically prototypical experiences (giving rise to idiosyncratic images, metaphors, and analogies) and chain complexes (giving rise to procedural knowledge) (Young 1982). Prototypes are based on salient personal experiences or cultural exemplars. They make idiosyncratic features of events central to the definition of a problem or behavior. Other events are then related by family resemblance through metaphors or analogies based on sensory, affective, or more abstract similarities. Chain complexes are knowledge structures in which events follow in sequences that can be reproduced by the person but usually not explicitly articulated. Chain complexes are learned like skills, through body practices. Like the steps to a familiar recipe, they can be shown but not readily described. They link events through contiguity in space or time rather than by causal implication.

As a result of these complex origins of illness narratives, multiple strategies are necessary to unpack the meaning of distress (Kirmayer et al. 1994b). Prototypes can be elicited by asking whether the patient or anyone else he or she knows has ever experienced anything like the present symptom or illness episode and then following up on all of the idiosyncratic particulars of the recollected case. Chain complexes can be elicited by asking patients about sequences of events associated with the symptom. Each of these methods of eliciting illness meanings will obtain additional information that may be unavailable when patients are asked directly for an explanatory model.

Somatic symptoms as metaphors for experience. An extension of the notion of idioms of distress considers the sense in which somatic symptoms provide metaphors for experience (Kirmayer 1992). Metaphors may be dead, fixed, or conventional figures of speech. Used to express strong emotion, however, metaphors can come alive again to engender some of the same bodily sensations or experiences from which they were originally derived. When a patient speaks of heart distress, he or she may simultaneously be speaking of physical sensations attributed to the heart and employing an evocative metaphor conveying specific emotional meaning. Similarly, sensations of tightness in the chest among Turkish immigrant women in Europe provide a means of pointing to social and interpersonal dilemmas faced by disadvantaged migrants (Devisch 1985; Mirdal 1985). This metaphoric use of bodily symptoms can occur regardless of whether the symptoms are actually experienced and whether they are, in fact, signs of cardiovascular disease, costochondritis, or simply muscle tension.

Metaphors allow the generation of new meanings that can contain, or create, anxiety (Kirmayer 1994). Metaphor serves to propose new meanings to others, some of which may be unintended by the patient. As a result of this social embedding, we can understand the meaning of symptoms in terms of presentation rather than representation; that is, symptoms come to have meaning when they are used in a specific social context (Kirmayer 1992).

Somatic symptoms as social commentary or contestation. Somatic symptoms function as communication whether or not they are so intended. The social origins of somatic distress are apparent to most, and so the simple declaration of ill health raises questions about the adequacy and legitimacy of existing social structures and arrangements. Whether used consciously and strategically or inadvertently, somatic symptoms then may present a commentary on social circumstances. At times, they may serve as a form of protest, challenge, or contestation of social conditions (Lock 1993).

Somatic symptoms as positioning. The processes of help seeking, adaptation, and disablement, initiated in response to somatic symptoms, can serve to reconfigure family relationships and other social roles. In a larger sense, then, symptoms can be understood as having meaning as moves within a local system of power. Symptoms attributed to oppressive circumstances can be used as a means of protest or contestation. However, even when made by sufferers themselves, this attribution does not mean that symptoms are willful, intentional, or conscious. Indeed, somatic symptoms may function as social moves or positioning, whether or not the individual is aware of this process.

This attribution is most obviously true for oppressed women and for other groups or individuals subject to racism and economic disadvantage (Lewis 1971; Lock 1993). In this case certain symptoms have been understood as forms of resistance or weapons of the weak used to call attention to injustice and undermine otherwise unassailable power structures. The dilemma created by this view is that by attributing more power and consciousness to the oppressed than they themselves experience, it may delegitimate the very means they have stumbled on for protest. This danger would urge caution in interpreting somatic symptoms as willful or purely strategic.

The fundamental indeterminacy of clinical diagnosis means that the "correct" interpretation (and the conflicting agendas represented by these different modes of interpretation) cannot be completely resolved in each case (Kirmayer 1994). The choice of interpretation is then not simply a matter of truth, since there are many partial truths available, but a strategic choice of what will be of most benefit to the patient.

The value of this perspective is that it puts emphasis where it belongs: not on manufacturing closed and coherent clinical narratives for consumption by colleagues or to shore up psychiatric authority but on finding creative solutions to patients' predicaments. It also encourages us to look critically at the goals that motivate (and subtend) our diagnostic and therapeutic choices.

The Pain of Dislocation

To see how the different levels of potential meaning of somatic symptoms pertain to the clinical situation, consider the following case. Mrs. Tran (a pseudonym) is a 57-year-old Vietnamese woman who came to North America 15 years ago. She is referred to psychiatric emergency services by her family doctor because of suicidal ideation. Six months earlier, she had suffered a knee injury that required surgery. Subsequently she developed recurrent pain and loss of mobility, making it difficult for her to care for herself. She has seen three different orthopedic specialists, who have told her that there is nothing wrong with her knee now and that she should be able to walk. She finds their reassurance confusing, since it is obvious to her that something is terribly wrong because she is in constant pain and cannot walk.

Mrs. Tran felt better 3 months ago, during a period when she was visiting a daughter who lives in another province, but, on her return home, her pain worsened, and she has become progressively more despondent. Over the last 3 months, she has been crying almost daily, feeling helpless and hopeless, wanting to die, and thinking of strangling herself. She has been unable to take pleasure in her usual activities and has had anorexia, with a 2- to 3-kilogram weight loss. She sleeps 3–4 hours a night with both initial insomnia and early morning wakening. She reports no previous episodes of chronic pain or suicidal ideation and no previous personal or family psychiatric history.

Mrs. Tran was widowed 20 years ago, at age 37. She came to Canada to live with her three sons. Two have moved out to establish their own households, and she now lives with her oldest son, who is unmarried but works long hours and is rarely home. She has little contact with extended family, friends, or neighbors.

On mental status examination, Mrs. Tran is a well-kempt woman who appears somewhat older than her stated age. Her sensorium is clear and cognitive functions intact. She displays some psychomotor retardation and walks very slowly with the aid of a cane. She looks worried and in pain. At the mention of her apparent sadness, she begins to cry. She speaks openly of suicidal thoughts but denies any intention to act on them. She acknowledges that she is lonely and discouraged but sees her dysphoric mood and suicidal thoughts entirely as a reaction to her knee pain and not as problems in their own right.

Mrs. Tran completed the Vietnamese version of the Hopkins Symptom Checklist 25 (HSCL-25 [Mollica et al. 1997]). She received scores of 1.8 on both the anxiety and depression scales, just above the suggested symptomatic threshold. The symptoms she reported most intensely were a pounding or racing heart and crying easily. She reported no feelings of worthlessness and specified that her feelings of hopelessness applied only to her knee condition.

The diagnostic impression was as follows: Axis I: 1) major depression with suicidal ideation, 2) pain disorder; Axis II: no diagnosis; Axis

III: history of knee injury; Axis IV: moderate stress; and Axis V: moderate level of functioning. She was referred to the psychiatric crisis service for follow-up.

Mrs. Tran is a typical patient with somatization: despite obvious indicators of severe depression with suicidal ideation, she sees her problem as primarily one of physical injury and pain. Although she did suffer an injury and had surgery on her knee, her doctors can find nothing physically wrong with her now to account for her persistent pain. Accordingly, they view her complaints of pain and her depression as the "real" problem and suggest psychiatric consultation and treatment. Both Mrs. Tran and her family are very unsatisfied with this characterization of her problem and do not believe it will lead to any resolution of her predicament. The clinical problem for the psychiatrist is how to understand and interpret Mrs. Tran's illness experience and negotiate a successful clinical outcome.

Although originally caused by a knee injury, Mrs. Tran's persistent pain was viewed as medically unexplained by her physicians and attributed to her personality (a "difficult" patient), social circumstances (an isolated immigrant), or to a major depression. These explanations did not fit Mrs. Tran's own view of her illness and, in any event, did not lead to effective treatment. Mrs. Tran's emphasis on somatic explanations for her distress makes sense in terms of the levels of meaning described earlier. First, it fits with the observation that persistent pain can indeed lead to depression. Second, it fits cultural explanatory models that link bodily illness to family and social disharmony. From this perspective, the pain signals an ongoing predicament in her life world: her dependence on her oldest son, while appropriate in traditional Vietnamese society, grows more problematic over time, as they both face the problem of adaptation to North American cultural values. Third, her pain becomes part of a process of renegotiating relationships, because it requires her son to participate more actively in her care and justifies visits to her daughter in a distant city.

The fundamental values of Vietnamese culture include a conservatism that maintains the stability of society by perpetuating traditions and sacred beliefs and a conformism that maintains the uniformity of the community by placing great pressure to conform on anyone with marginal beliefs, attitudes, or behaviors. As a result, each person must blend into his or her family, social, and spiritual environment, regardless of personal need or desire. In Vietnam, the values of conservatism and conformism are in synchrony. When an immigrant community is large enough to recreate traditional extended families and kinship networks, these cultural values may be maintained. For immigrants whose families are fragmented, isolated, or reduced to a small nucleus, however, there is a potential contradiction, in which conservatism dictates holding on to cultural traditions while conformism mandates fitting in with the host society (Kibria 1993). Disharmony within the family may occur when a few family members are successful in acculturating through integration or assimilation while others hold onto traditional values and ways of life. Mrs. Tran's family situation is uncommon in Vietnam but, unfortunately, more the norm for Vietnamese immigrants to industrialized countries.

Although Vietnamese folk and medical concepts of health and illness are influenced by Chinese medicine, important differences exist between the traditions (D. M. Nguyen 1985). The central principle of Chinese medicine is that illness arises from disharmony between the patient and the cosmos. Treatment aims to restore the balance of energies (yin and yang) in the body and hence its harmony with the larger world. Remedies consist of decoctions of natural ingredients gathered from precise, often remote locations in China; grown at a specific season; combined according to traditional recipes; and dosed in exact proportions. Traditional Vietnamese medicine also attributes illness to imbalance but usually in terms of local and personal "winds." Symptoms of depression are commonly viewed as an imbalance of "winds," with predominately somatic manifestations (Eisenbruch 1983). Vietnamese medicine aims to restore harmony between the "wind" of the patient and the local "wind" but seeks the cure in the immediate habitat of the patient. The patient consults a knowledgeable traditional doctor or medicates him- or herself with raw herbs or roots growing in the same geographical area and at the same season as the onset of the illness. As a result, when the environment is unfamiliar (as it is for immigrants), the local remedies are still unexplored, and the proper course of treatment may be unclear. In such a situation, the immigrant from rural Vietnam would consult a Vietnamese or Chinese physician, preferably one with traditional training, for advice. The concept of illness resulting from a disharmony between the local environmental "wind" and the personal or familial "wind" would be the equivalent of the North American concept of illness as a result of family dysfunction and might be better accepted by some Vietnamese patients.

In general, Vietnamese place a high value on the self-control of emotions. This trait influences both their ability to cope with distress and their interactions with health care providers. For example, D. M. Nguyen (1985) notes that Vietnamese often give affirmative answers to interviewers even when faced with delicate or embarrassing questions in order to prevent confrontations that could lead to the expression of strong emotions. Expression of such strong emotion is considered to be a "weakness of the mind." The expression of pain, distress, and unhappiness is also frowned upon since such feelings are viewed as part of life's normal burden. Lack of control over one's emotions is described as "losing *lien*," which is akin to losing face (D. M. Nguyen 1985). To maintain *lien* is to demonstrate that one has control over one's moral character, for example, by smiling even when feelings of sadness and despair are intense. To say that someone has lost *lien* is the greatest insult that can be made in the Vietnamese culture (Eyton and Neuwirth 1984). Hence, it is understandable that in clinical settings some Vietnamese patients will smile and not complain, even when desperately depressed (Tran 1981).

This cultural emphasis on the control and containment of emotion is frequently mentioned as a contributor to somatization among Vietnamese and other Southeast Asian groups. Several studies report that Vietnamese refugees with depressive symptomatology score high on somatic symptom inventories including respiratory-, gastrointestinal-, skin-, and central nervous system–related symptoms (Kinzie et al. 1982; Westermeyer et al. 1989). Common somatic complaints include headaches, insomnia, chest pain, fatigue, dizziness, fainting, and palpitations (Nguyen 1982). However, some authors have questioned the commonly accepted implication that high levels of somatic symptoms imply difficulty expressing emotional distress. For example, Lin and colleagues (1979) found that Vietnamese had no reluctance to express psychological symptoms on various self-report questionnaires. It is possible that Vietnamese express emotions more freely in a "neutral" or nonstigmatizing context such as an anonymous questionnaire, especially when it is administered to them in English. A similar phenomenon was observed by Chan (1985) with Hong Kong Chinese university students completing the General Health Questionnaire (GHQ) (Goldberg 1987). The same respondents were willing to endorse more psychological symptoms in English than in their native tongue, suggesting that it was easier for respondents to achieve distance from threatening affect when expressing distress in another language.

In any event, it should be clear that a lack of overt emotional expression does not indicate a lack of significant emotional experience. This circumstance does not mean, however, that such hidden emotions are the "real," underlying, or essential features of depression or other problems among Vietnamese. Somatic distress may be the most intense and salient aspect of "depression" for both physiological and cultural reasons. As a result of ethnophysiological notions, Vietnamese commonly report problems with specific body organs (e.g., liver) in addition to specific bodily symptoms. A wide range of common idioms for social or emotional distress invoke organ systems, especially the abdomen and gastrointestinal tract.

In the development of a Vietnamese Depression Scale, Kinzie and colleagues (1982) identified several culture-related symptoms, including feeling *nhuc nha* ("shameful and dishonored") and *muon dien len* ("going crazy"). Feeling shameful and dishonored is not simply equivalent to the Western notion of guilt, since for the Vietnamese there is seldom an element of personal responsibility in determining the events that could precipitate such feelings. Rather, the feeling stems from an inability of the depressed person and his or her family to properly attend to obligations of the ancestral past. Ancestral spirits play a key role in confirming the correctness of present actions and ensuring the continuity and benevolent future of the family (Kibria 1993). The ancestor cult, along with other Confucian ideals, reinforces the importance of the family over the individual and may lead patients to suppress their own suffering or to focus on those aspects that have the greatest impact on other family members.

The feeling of "going crazy" is not typically part of the Western definition of depression, but for Vietnamese it stems from the experience of extreme discomfort with the affective and physical aspects of the disorder. This lack of comfort with strong emotion may lead to a higher threshold for reporting any depressive symptoms.

Gold (1992) suggests that many Vietnamese immigrants lack the cultural prerequisites for psychodynamic psychotherapy such as the willingness to confide, a belief in the unconscious, and the ability to openly criticize their parents. Vietnamese refugees also have difficulty understanding the usefulness of psychotherapy and perceive mental health problems as a source of shame and embarrassment (Chan and Lam 1983).

Lower rates of utilization of mental health services by Vietnamese have also been linked to the structure of the health care system. Most Southeast Asian immigrants have previously experienced a health care system that is crisis oriented and where appointments are not needed, diagnostic tests are fewer, and drugs are administered along with traditional medicines in injectable form rather than in oral preparations (Hoang and Erickson 1985). The notion of a thorough inquiry into personal and social difficulties as a form of medical treatment may seem distinctly peculiar.

These observations clarify why Mrs. Tran would tend to emphasize the somatic aspects of her distress, namely, to avoid psychiatric stigma, focus on a clear-cut somatic problem appropriate for acute medical treatment, and deflect attention from emotional difficulties that are embarrassing to her and her family. Indeed, Mrs. Tran's presentation must be understood not just as reflective of her own illness beliefs and behaviors but also as a response to family expectations. When Mrs. Tran was interviewed with her son as an interpreter, he filtered and interpreted various questions to minimize her emotional distress. Both Mrs. Tran and her son were concerned to avoid any implication that she had a psychiatric disorder or required antidepressant medication.

In the process of completing the Vietnamese HSCL-25, it was easy to see Mrs. Tran weighing where to situate herself on the scales and choosing to minimize her distress; for several items she gave a higher rating at first and then revised it downward, sometimes in response to the prompting of her son. They both insisted that her depression was entirely secondary to her knee pain, which, in turn, was simply the consequence of an injury. When the possibility of taking medication for her pain and depression was raised, Mrs. Tran proposed the alternate idea of visiting her daughter again, a plan supported by her son. This appeal to family resources was culturally consonant and fit with the family dynamics.

Clinical Strategies

Although there is no universally agreed upon treatment approach, several authors have outlined useful strategies for working with somatizing patients (Creed and Guthrie 1993; Goldberg et al. 1989; Sharpe et al. 1992; Wickramasekera 1989). These have in common careful attention to the patient's initial somatic complaints and the application of cognitive-behavioral techniques for reattributing somatic symptoms to benign causes, improving coping with distress and conflict, and reducing disability through graded increases in physical and social activity.

McDaniel and colleagues (1989, 1992) discuss the management of "somatically fixated" patients from a family therapy perspective. They divide treatment into three overlapping phases. In the early phase of treatment, the clinician works within a medical idiom or metaphor to focus on symptoms, listen to the illness narrative, collaborate with family, explore family structure and history, and identify illness-related role changes (McDaniel et al. 1992). In the middle phase, the aim is to negotiate a problem label and definition, introduce emotion language, reinforce activity and engagement in therapy, intervene in family structure and process, and help the identified patient and family members acquire more effective coping skills. The late phase of treatment works to consolidate changes and prevent relapses. This phase may require the therapist to predict setbacks, write a prescription for steps to take if illness recurs, reattribute success to the patient, and plan a gradual ending with "fading" of the therapist's presence.

A cultural approach would combine these methods with the attention to meaning and context outlined earlier in the following way: 1) understanding the potential and effective meaning of somatic symptoms; 2) joining the patient by eliciting and employing his or her own explanatory models, attributions, and metaphors; 3) applying behavioral medicine interventions to achieve some symptomatic improvement; 4) broadening the context of illness through considering its impact on the patient's daily life and social network; and 5) intervening in the social context that sustains distress through culturally responsive methods.

In working with somatizing patients, many psychodynamically trained clinicians err in moving too quickly from assessment of physical symptoms to a focus on emotional experience. From an interpersonal perspective, it could be argued that explicit talk about emotions can serve as a more effective way of drawing attention to personal needs. Where emotion conveys information about interpersonal conflicts, it may also serve to address problems in relationships and motivate others to change. Although emotions are quintessentially social constructions, psychological talk about emotions tends to situate problems entirely within the individual and so may work against the ability of emotion to point to social problems or inequities.

A sociocultural perspective might accept all of the potential benefits of emotion talk but insist that each depends to some degree on a particular cultural concept of the person and a corresponding way of life. Each of these theories fits well with certain aspects of the American concept of the person, particularly with the values of expressive individualism (Bellah et al. 1985; Kirmayer 1989). The implicit norms of professional psychiatric practice assume that people will be healthier if they talk openly about their emotions and relationships and that when an internal or interpersonal conflict exists it should be resolved in favor of the autonomy of the individual. In North America, the mental health practitioner is viewed as an appropriate person to whom to present all manner of problem—emotional, social, and moral as well as physical.

These assumptions ignore minority and immigrant groups' experiences with different models of problem resolution and systems of health care. For people from many cultures, the harmony of the family and the group is more important than individual autonomy. The cultural concept of the person is based on the social and communal embedding of the individual, who is rarely conceived of as a freestanding unit (Marsella et al. 1985; Shweder 1991; Triandis et al. 1988). Hence, emotional containment and adaptation to social circumstances are viewed as signs of maturity (Weisz et al. 1984; Wikan 1990). Fostering individualism through psychotherapy may put people from such cultures further at odds with their families and local worlds and so undermine both social support and their own sense of self-worth (Kirmayer 1989). As a result, solutions that make sense from the perspective of Euro-American psychiatry and health psychology may involve trade-offs for some ethnocultural groups that mitigate even the presumptively universal mechanisms of catharsis and healing.

As a counter to the individual-centered bias of much psychotherapy, a family- or social network–oriented approach is often of great utility, because it lays bare the social context and contingencies that may contribute to persistent somatic distress at the same time as it makes available to the clinician the cultural knowledge and coping resources of a more extended network. It requires careful attention to cultural variations in family structure to identify appropriate ways to enter and join with the family to effect change (Ho 1992).

Awareness of the diverse levels of potential meaning of somatic symptoms allows the clinician to understand the patient's distress in terms of psychophysiology, personal history, the struggle for power and position within a family and local world, and the creative and misprisoning effects of larger cultural ideologies and practices. The initial focus on the somatic symptom and the application of specific behavioral medicine techniques or pharmacological treatments to reduce distress allow the clinician to build a relationship with the patient based on evidence that therapy can be of help (Mayou et al. 1995). This narrow focus on somatic symptoms can be broadened both in assessment and treatment by inquiring into the impact of illness on everyday life. In this way, psychosocial issues can be explored without implying that they are more real or important than the somatic distress. Questions about how the patient copes, limitations of activity, and response of the family all situate the problem in a larger social context. Cognitive-psychological, family, and social network interventions can then be designed to reverse the contingencies that contribute to persistent somatic distress. Symptoms that patients perceive as out of their control and that are aggravated by anxious efforts to reestablish control can be relieved by reattribution therapy (Kirmayer 1990).

Symptoms that serve as expressions of power and protest within troubled relationships can be subverted by reframing them as voluntary (Madanes 1981). However, this form of confrontation delegitimates patients' suffering and runs the risk of damaging or destroying the therapeutic alliance. More helpfully, where somatic symptoms serve as protest or positioning within interpersonal relationships and a local world, patients can be guided to develop other means of obtaining and using power. Assertiveness training and related techniques are individual-focused methods suitable for patients who subscribe to the values of American individualism. Couple, family, and social network interventions are more flexible and broadly applicable, since they allow the clinician to both assess the resources available for change and plan interventions that are consonant with shared values and beliefs and that therefore have a far better chance of success.

These steps do not form a rigid sequence. They interact and must be returned to in a cyclical process many times in the course of treatment. For example, understanding the meaning of symptoms allows joining; joining, in turn, leads to greater understanding of the meaning of symptoms. Joining allows initial behavioral medicine interventions to be applied, and, when such interventions prove helpful, the alliance with the patient is strengthened. In this way, the clinician's knowledge of the cultural and personal meanings of somatic distress grows in parallel with the patient's own capacity to cope with illness and its associated social predicaments.

James and Melissa Griffith (1994) have written a sensitive book on the treatment of somatization through individual and family therapy from a systemic and constructivist perspective. Although not explicitly directed to problems of cultural diversity, their work closely parallels recent perspectives in medical anthropology that emphasize the role of patients' metaphors and illness narratives in bodily experience and the construction of local social worlds (Kirmayer 1992, 1993, 1994; Kleinman 1988). Their clinical methods involve careful inquiry into patients' experiences of their bodies and their local worlds. Such inquiry reveals how certain illness narratives construct the clinical problem or impasse. In many cases, they find that somatizing patients have developed disabling symptoms because they have not been able or allowed to speak openly about terrible traumas and family predicaments. Patients are helped to tell their story and to construct new narratives of the self that free the body from the burden of communicating what otherwise cannot be said. Although not found in every somatizing patient, the oppressive family circumstances they recount certainly have their counter-parts in cross-cultural work. The situation of immigrants and disadvantaged minorities adds another form of potential silencing, not from within the family but by the larger society. The Griffiths' thoughtful and empathic work provides an integrative framework for therapy (including psychopharmacology) that can be readily adapted to cross-cultural work with somatizing patients.

Conclusions

Somatization is a concept that reflects the dualism inherent in the Western cultural concept of the person. Within biomedicine this dualism is both epistemological and ontological. Epistemologically, biomedicine separates objective evidence of disease through physical signs and laboratory testing from patients' subjective reports of distress. Patients who complain of somatic symptoms in the absence of physiological confirmation are then suspect. This difference in the source and credibility of information supports a more radical ontological distinction between physical disease and psychological disorder. Notwithstanding the current biological turn in psychiatry, the pervasive dualistic concepts of the person lead to a sharp contrast between "real" diseases, for which one is not responsible and to which the various rights and duties of the sick role accrue, and "imaginary" illness, in which one occupies a gray zone of hysteria, hypochondriasis, histrionic exaggeration, and malingering. Nosological attempts to make sharp distinctions among the latter categories do not prevent these patients from all being tarred with the same brush (Kirmayer 1988, 1994).

Fabrega (1991) has pointed out that in most of the great traditions of medicine (e.g., Ayurveda, Chinese medicine), the same sharp ontological distinction between the mental and the physical as two fundamentally different types of medical problem did not occur. In the case of Chinese medicine, he argues that there was no ontological notion of disease at all; medicine was based on symptom clusters or syndromes, reflecting imbalances in bodily systems that were also aligned with aspects of larger social and ecological systems. This difference does not mean that Chinese medicine, or other traditions, dissolved the mind-body dualism of Western medicine: they never created it in the first place. The holism of Chinese medicine does not develop psychology as a separate realm of discourse. Instead, in conformity with the Confucian ethos, attention is paid to disharmony in relationships as a potent cause of illness; however, this disharmony is to be understood not in terms of interpersonal conflict and struggles for independence but in terms of contraventions of Confucian ideals of hierarchical social order.

Each medical tradition, then, has its own languages of illness and healing and its own version of holism. None can lay claim to integrating all of the different aspects of human misery. Indeed, it seems clear that Western psychological notions, while they may at times be causes of certain forms of suffering (e.g., narcissism or alienation due to excessive individualism), are also powerful analytic tools for understanding relationships and opening up new possibilities for change. Nevertheless, introducing psychological language as a way of understanding a problem is also introducing a culture-specific concept of the person that may conflict with the values and perspectives of the patient's culture of origin and so create new dilemmas for the individual. Psychiatric diagnosis and treatment—and even the prescription of medication—must then be understood not simply as technical interventions but also as interpretive actions that contribute to cultural and sociomoral change (Kirmayer 1989).

References

American Psychiatric Association: Diagnostic and Statistical Manual of Mental Disorders, 3rd Edition, Revised. Washington, DC, American Psychiatric Association, 1987

American Psychiatric Association: Diagnostic and Statistical Manual of Mental Disorders, 4th Edition. Washington, DC, American Psychiatric Association, 1994

Barsky AJ: Amplification, somatization, and the somatoform disorders. Psychosomatics 33:28–34, 1992

Bellah RN, Madsen R, Sullivan WM, et al: Habits of the Heart: Individualism and Commitment in American Life. Berkeley and Los Angeles, CA, University of California Press, 1985

Bhatia MS, Malik SC: Dhat syndrome: a useful diagnostic entity in Indian culture. Br J Psychiatry 159:691–695, 1991

Cathébras P: Neurasthenia and chronic fatigue syndrome in France. Transcultural Psychiatric Research Review 31:259–270, 1994

Chan KB, Lam L: Resettlement of Vietnamese-Canadian refugees in Montreal: some socio-psychological problems and dilemmas. Canadian Ethnic Studies 15:1–17, 1983

Craig TKJ, Boardman AP, Mills K, et al: The South London Somatisation Study, I: longitudinal course and the influence of early life experiences. Br J Psychiatry 163:579–588, 1993

Creed F, Guthrie E: Techniques for interviewing the somatising patient. Br J Psychiatry 162:467–471, 1993

Davis DL, Whitten RG: Medical and popular traditions of nerves. Soc Sci Med 26:1209–1211, 1988

Devisch R: A therapeutic self-help group among Turkish women. Dertlesmek: "the sharing of sorrow." Psichiatria e Psicoterapi Analitica 4:133–152, 1985

Ebigbo PO: A cross-sectional study of somatic complaints of Nigerian females using the Enugu somatization scale. Cult Med Psychiatry 10:167–186, 1986

Eisenbruch M: "Wind illness" or somatic depression? a case study in psychiatric anthropology. Br J Psychiatry 143:323–326, 1983

Escobar JL, Rubio-Stipec M, Canino G, et al: Somatic Symptom Index (SSI): a new and abridged somatization construct. J Nerv Ment Dis 177:140–146, 1989

Eyton J, Neuwirth G: Cross-cultural validity: ethnocentrism in health studies with special reference to the Vietnamese. Soc Sci Med 18:447–453, 1984

Fabrega H: Somatization in cultural and historical perspective, in Current Concepts of Somatization: Research and Clinical Perspectives. Edited by Kirmayer LJ, Robbins JM. Washington, DC, American Psychiatric Press, 1991, pp 181–199

Gaw AC: Culture, Ethnicity, and Mental Illness. Washington, DC, American Psychiatric Press, 1993

Gold SJ: Refugee Communities: A Comparative Field Study. Newbury Park, CA, Sage, 1992

Goldberg D: The general health questionnaire, in Measuring Health: A Guide to Rating Scales and Questionnaires. Edited by McDowell I, Newell C. New York, Oxford University Press, 1987, pp 139–151

Goldberg DP, Bridges K: Somatic presentations of psychiatric illness in primary care setting. J Psychosom Res 32:137–144, 1988

Goldberg DP, Gask L, O'Dowd T: The treatment of somatization: teaching techniques of reattribution. J Psychosom Res 33:689–695, 1989

Good BJ: The heart of what's the matter: the semantics of illness in Iran. Cult Med Psychiatry 1:25–58, 1977

Good B, Good MJD: The meaning of symptoms: a cultural hermeneutic model for clinical practice, in The Relevance of Social Science for Medicine. Edited by Eisenberg L, Kleinman A. Dordrecht, Reidel, 1980, pp 165–196

Griffith JL, Griffith ME: The Body Speaks: Therapeutic Dialogues for Mind-Body Problems. New York, Basic Books, 1994

Guarnaccia PJ: Ataques de nervios in Puerto Rico: culture-bound syndrome or popular illness? Med Anthropol 15:157–170, 1993

Guinness EA: Profile and prevalence of the brain fag syndrome: psychiatric morbidity in school populations in Africa. Br J Psychiatry 160:42–52, 1992

Gureje O, Obikoya B: Somatization in primary care: pattern and correlates in a clinic in Nigeria. Acta Psychiatr Scand 86:223–227, 1992

Harré R, Van Langenhove L: Varieties of positioning. Journal for the Theory of Social Behavior 21:393–407, 1991

Ho MK: Differential application of treatment modalities with Asian American youth, in Working With Culture: Psychotherapeutic Interventions With Ethnic Minority Children and Adolescents. Edited by Vargas LA, Koss-Chioino JD. San Francisco, CA, Jossey-Bass, 1992, pp 182–203

Hoang GN, Erickson RV: Cultural barriers to effective medical care among Indochinese patients. Annu Rev Med 36:229–239, 1985

Jegede RO: Psychiatric illness in African students: "brain fag" syndrome revisited. Can J Psychiatry 28:188–192, 1983

Kibria N: Family Tightrope: The Changing Lives of Vietnamese Americans. Princeton, NJ, Princeton University Press, 1993

Kim LIC: Psychiatric care of Korean Americans, in Culture, Ethnicity, and Mental Illness. Edited by Gaw AC. Washington, DC, American Psychiatric Press, 1993, pp 347–376

Kinzie JD, Manson SM, Vinh DT, et al: Development and validation of a Vietnamese-language depression rating scale. Am J Psychiatry 139: 1276–1281, 1982

Kirmayer LJ: Culture, affect, and somatization. Transcultural Psychiatric Research Review 21:159–188, 237–262, 1984

Kirmayer LJ: Languages of suffering and healing: alexithymia as a social and cultural process. Transcultural Psychiatric Research Review 24:119–136, 1987

Kirmayer LJ: Mind and body as metaphors: hidden values in biomedicine, in Biomedicine Examined. Edited by Lock M, Gordon D. Dordrecht, Kluwer, 1988, pp 57–92

Kirmayer LJ: Psychotherapy and the cultural concept of the person. Santé, Culture, Health 6:241–270, 1989

Kirmayer LJ: Resistance, reactance, and reluctance to change: a cognitive attributional approach to strategic interventions. Journal of Cognitive Psychotherapy 4:83–104, 1990

Kirmayer LJ: The body's insistence on meaning: metaphor as presentation and representation in illness experience. Med Anthropol Q 6:323–346, 1992

Kirmayer LJ: Healing and the invention of metaphor: the effectiveness of symbols revisited. Cult Med Psychiatry 17:161–195, 1993

Kirmayer LJ: Improvisation and authority in illness meaning. Cult Med Psychiatry 18:183–214, 1994

Kirmayer LJ, Robbins JM: Three forms of somatization in primary care: prevalence, co-occurrence, and sociodemographic characteristics. J Nerv Ment Dis 179:647–655, 1991

Kirmayer LJ, Taillefer S: Somatoform disorders, in Adult Psychopathology, 3rd Edition. Edited by Turner S, Hersen M. New York, Wiley, 1997, pp 333–383

Kirmayer LJ, Weiss MG: Cultural considerations for somatoform disorders, in DSM-IV Sourcebook. Edited by Widiger TA, Frances AJ, Pincus HA, et al. Washington, DC, American Psychiatric Press, 1997, pp 933–941

Kirmayer LJ, Young A: Culture and somatization: clinical, epidemiological, and ethnographic perspectives. Psychosom Med (in press)

Kirmayer LJ, Robbins JM, Paris J: Somatoform disorders: personality and the social matrix of somatic distress. J Abnorm Psychol 103:125–136, 1994a

Kirmayer LJ, Young A, Robbins JM: Symptom attribution in cultural perspective. Can J Psychiatry 39:584–595, 1994b

Kitanishi K, Kondo K: The rise and fall of neurasthenia in Japanese psychiatry. Transcultural Psychiatric Research Review 31:137–152, 1994

Kleinman A: Patients and Healers in the Context of Culture. Berkeley and Los Angeles, CA, University of California Press, 1980

Kleinman A: Social Origins of Distress and Disease. New Haven, CT, Yale University Press, 1986

Kleinman A: The Illness Narratives. New York, Basic Books, 1988

Laguerre M: Afro-Caribbean Folk Medicine. South Hadley, MA, Bergin & Garvey, 1987

Lee S: The vicissitudes of neurasthenia in Chinese societies: where will it go from the ICD-10? Transcultural Psychiatric Research Review 31:153–172, 1994

Lefley HP: Prevalence of potential falling-out cases among the black, Latin, and non-Latin white populations of the city of Miami. Soc Sci Med 13B:113–114, 1979

Lewis IM: Ecstatic Religion: An Anthropological Study of Spirit Possession and Shamanism. London, Penguin Books, 1971

Lin K-M: Hwa-Byung: a Korean culture-bound syndrome? Am J Psychiatry 140:105–107, 1983

Lin K-M, Tazuma L, Masuda M: Adaptational problems of Vietnamese refugees. Arch Gen Psychiatry 36:955–961, 1979

Lin K-M, Lau JKC, Yamamoto J, et al: Hwa-byung: a community study of Korean Americans. J Nerv Ment Dis 180:386–391, 1992

Lock M: Cultivating the body: anthropology and epistemologies of bodily practice and knowledge. Annual Review of Anthropology 22:133–135, 1993

Lock M, Wakewich-Dunk P: Nerves and nostalgia: expression of loss among Greek immigrants in Montreal. Can Fam Physician 36:253–258, 1990

Low S: Embodied metaphors: nerves as lived experience, in Embodiment and Experience: The Existential Ground of Culture and Self. Edited by Csordas T. Cambridge, Cambridge University Press, 1994, pp 139–162

Madanes C: Strategic Family Therapy. San Francisco, CA, Jossey-Bass, 1981

Magni G, Moreschi C, Rigatti Luchini S, et al: Prospective study on the relationship between depressive symptoms and chronic musculoskeletal pain. Pain 56:289–297, 1994

Makanjuola ROA: "Ode Ori": a culture-bound disorder with prominent somatic features in Yoruba Nigerian patients. Acta Psychiatr Scand 75:231–236, 1987

Marsella AJ, DeVos G, Hsu FLK: Culture and Self: Asian and Western Perspectives. New York, Tavistock, 1985, pp 185–230

Mayou R, Bass C, Sharpe M: Treatment of Functional Somatic Symptoms. Oxford, Oxford University Press, 1995

McDaniel SH, Campbell T, Seaburn D: Somatic fixation in patients and physicians: a biopsychosocial approach. Family Systems Medicine 7:5–16, 1989

McDaniel SH, Hepworth J, Doherty WJ: Medical Family Therapy. New York, Basic Books, 1992

Merskey H: Chronic muscular pain: a life stress syndrome? Journal of Musculoskeletal Pain 1:61–69, 1993

Mirdal GM: The condition of "tightness": the somatic complaints of Turkish migrant women. Acta Psychiatr Scand 71:287–296, 1985

Moldofsky H: Sleep and musculoskeletal pain. Am J Med 81:85–89, 1986

Mollica FR, Wyshak G, de Marneffe D, et al: Indochinese version of the Hopkins Symptom Checklist—25: a screening instrument for the psychiatric care of refugees. Am J Psychiatry 144:497–500, 1987

Morakinyo O: A psychophysiological theory of a psychiatric illness (the brain fag syndrome) associated with study among Africans. J Nerv Ment Dis 168:84–89, 1980

Nguyen DM: Culture shock: a review of Vietnamese culture and its concepts of health and disease. West J Med 142:409–412, 1985

Nguyen SD: Psychiatric and psychosomatic problems among Southeast Asian refugees. Psychiatric Journal of the University of Ottawa 7:163–172, 1982

Nichter M: Idioms of distress: alternatives in the expression of psychosocial distress: a case study from India. Cult Med Psychiatry 5:379–408, 1981

Oquendo M, Horwath E, Martinez A: Ataques de nervios: proposed diagnostic criteria for a culture specific syndrome. Cult Med Psychiatry 16:367–376, 1992

Pang KYC: Hwabyung: the construction of a Korean popular illness among Korean elderly immigrant women in the United States. Cult Med Psychiatry 14:495–512, 1990

Paris J: Dhat: the semen loss anxiety syndrome. Transcultural Psychiatric Research Review 29:109–118, 1992

Philippe J, Romain JB: Indisposition in Haiti. Soc Sci Med 13B:129–133, 1979

Prince R: The brain fag syndrome in Nigerian students. Journal of Mental Science 106:559–570, 1960

Sharpe M, Bass C: Pathophysiological mechanisms in somatization. International Review of Psychiatry 4:81–97, 1992

Sharpe MJ, Peveler R, Mayou R: The psychological treatment of patients with functional somatic symptoms: a practical guide. J Psychosom Res 36:515–529, 1992

Shweder R: Thinking Through Culture: Expeditions in Cultural Psychology. Cambridge, MA, Harvard University Press, 1991

Simon GE, Von Korff M: Somatization and psychiatric disorder in the NIMH epidemiologic catchment area study. Am J Psychiatry 148:1494–1500, 1991

Sobo EJ: One Blood: The Jamaican Body. Albany, NY, State University of New York Press, 1993

Srinivasan TN, Suresh TR: The nonspecific symptom screening method: detection of nonpsychotic morbidity based on nonspecific symptoms. Gen Hosp Psychiatry 13:106–114, 1991

Starcevic V: Neurasthenia in European psychiatric literature. Transcultural Psychiatric Research Review 31:125–136, 1994

Tran MT: Indochinese refugees as patients. Journal of Refugee Resettlement 1:53–60, 1981

Triandis HC, Bontempo R, Villareal MJ, et al: Individualism and collectivism: cross-cultural perspectives on self-in-group relationships. J Pers Soc Psychol 54:323–338, 1988

van Diest R, Appels AWPM: Sleep physiological characteristics of exhausted men. Psychosom Med 56:28–35, 1994

Ware NC, Weiss MG: Neurasthenia and the social construction of psychiatric knowledge. Transcultural Psychiatric Research Review 31:101–124, 1994

Weidman HH: Falling-out: a diagnostic and treatment problem viewed from a transcultural perspective. Soc Sci Med 13B:95–112, 1979

Weisz JR, Rothbaum FM, Blackburn TC: Standing out and standing in: the psychology of control in America and Japan. Am Psychol 39:955–969, 1984

Wessely S: Neurasthenia and chronic fatigue: theory and practice in Britain and America. Transcultural Psychiatric Research Review 31:173–208, 1994

Westermeyer J, Bouafuely M, Neider J, et al: Somatization among refugees: an epidemiologic study. Psychosomatics 30:34–43, 1989

White GM: The role of cultural explanations in "somatization" and "psychologization." Soc Sci Med 16:1519–1530, 1982

Wickramasekera I: Enabling the somatizing patient to exit the somatic closet: a high risk model. Psychotherapy 26:530–544, 1989

Wickramasekera IE: Clinical Behavioral Medicine: Some Concepts and Procedures. New York, Plenum Press, 1988

Wikan U: Managing Turbulent Hearts: A Balinese Formula for Living. Chicago, IL, University of Chicago Press, 1990

Young A: Rational men and the explanatory model approach. Cult Med Psychiatry 6:57–71, 1982

Acknowledgment

Preparation of this chapter was supported by a grant from the Fonds de la recherche en santé du Québec. Parts of this chapter are drawn from Kirmayer and Young (in press).

CHAPTER 13

The Therapeutic Alliance Across Cultures

IRMA J. BLAND, M.D.
IRVIN KRAFT, M.D., P.A.

Many types of psychotherapy exist, generally differentiated by the particular therapeutic strategy (activity and role of the therapist) and by the overall treatment goals. Common to all psychodynamic, insight-oriented, or supportive-expressive psychotherapies is the development of a therapeutic process. One of the most critical agents in this process is the therapeutic alliance. Although it may be difficult theoretically as well as clinically to distinguish among a weak therapeutic alliance, ego resistance, and negative transference, a patient's distinctly positive experience with a therapist is predictive of a favorable outcome (Piper et al. 1991). Patients who have positive experiences with their therapists are more likely to develop a therapeutic alliance that sustains their involvement in therapy. Staying in therapy has been directly correlated with interactive factors between the patient and therapist (Orlinsky and Howard 1986), even as early as the screening interview (Mohl et al. 1991).

In this chapter we examine issues in the therapeutic alliance from a psychoanalytic theoretical perspective. Although equally effective with racial or ethnic minority patients, traditional psychoanalytic psychotherapy may not be the practical, clinically appropriate, or preferred treatment of choice in all circumstances. This theoretical perspective, however, provides an in-depth understanding of issues that can lead to early recognition of problems in the therapeutic alliance, regardless of the particular psychotherapeutic modality utilized.

The therapeutic alliance was first described by Zetzel (1956, 1958), although it was earlier referred to by Freud (1913/1958) as the "effective transference" or the proper rapport with the patient. It is the collaborative, working relationship (Greenson 1965) that develops between the patient and the therapist, a relationship based on a sense of trust and in which the participants work together toward a common goal (Ursano et al. 1991). By virtue of his or her availability, sensitivity, affirming and nonjudgmental attitude, and accurate and empathic understanding, the therapist gains the power and authority to contain the patient's anxieties. This result facilitates communication, self-disclosure, and evolution of the transference. The psychotherapeutic situation provides an opportunity for the patient to feel "at one," or in union, with the therapist, and this identification becomes a means to a relationship. Within this relationship, transference develops—that is, the patient reenacts and displaces old unresolved feelings, thoughts, and behavior (from early relationships), causing distortions and misperceptions of the therapist. The therapist's accurate interpretation of this transference in the context of the patient's sense of relatedness to him or her ultimately leads to modification or alleviation of symptoms and pathological processes that interfere with adaptive functioning and personality development (Moore and Fine 1990). In other words, the relationship makes treatment possible.

In the cross-cultural context, the patient and the therapist differ in some substantial way and perceive themselves as being at a distance from each other. This difference may be based on racial or ethnic identity, gender, religion, age, socioeconomic class, family background, or other major sociocultural influence. The perception of distance and the lack of commonality (whether real or imagined), inevitable in the cross-cultural context, may generate anxiety in the patient and therapist. The protective defenses erected by both patient and therapist and the associated anxiety clutter the psychotherapeutic field. These reactions impede identification and an empathic connection, both critical in the establishment of the therapeutic alliance.

The establishment and maintenance of the therapeutic alliance, critical in fostering therapeutic process and directly related to successful treatment outcome, is considered one of the most challenging tasks for the therapist (Horvath and Luborsky 1993; Piper et al. 1991). Both intrapsychic resistances and external reality factors have the potential to interfere. The challenge to bridge the gap across cultures is even greater (Jones and Gray 1986; I. Yamamoto et al. 1967). Yet a difference of culture by no means precludes the establishment of a therapeutic alliance. The work to establish the therapeutic alliance across cultures, however, requires an open attitude, self-awareness, cultural sensitivity, and astute clinical skills on the part of the therapist (Bland and Martin 1994).

Empathy in the Cross-Cultural Context

Empathy, defined as a way of knowing and understanding another person (i.e., "feeling into" their psychological state), is neither mystical nor transcendent. Rather, it results from the therapist's evenly suspended attention and autonomy of his or her work ego. These factors allow the therapist to resonate with the patient's emotional state and use his or her self-introspection to permit an easily reversible trial identification with the patient. The integration of this neutral, nonjudgmental, empathic data with other objective information leads to an accurate perception and understanding of the patient's feelings and needs and to appropriate therapeutic responses (Moore and Fine 1990).

J. Yamamoto and Steinberg (1981) reviewed the literature, calling attention to problems with empathy, establishment of the therapeutic alliance, and its impact on treatment outcome in the context of cross-cultural issues as related to race or ethnicity and class. They presented evidence suggesting that patients from racial or ethnic minority groups or lower social class were less likely to be selected for psychodynamic psychotherapy, or, once selected, had higher attrition rates. This finding raised questions about difficulties in the effective establishment of the cross-cultural therapeutic alliance based on race or ethnicity and class. These patients were seen as having inappropriate treatment needs and expectations and as unsuitable for dynamic psychotherapy. Middle-class therapists from the majority group had difficulties identifying with patients across their cultural boundaries. Tremendous diversity across different cultural groups and heterogeneity within groups exist in a multicultural society. Differences persist across cultural groups in the use of language and ways of communicating, such as the expression of emotions. Conceptual ideas regarding interpersonal relatedness, ego boundaries, and autonomy versus dependence also vary. Different internal and external points of reference that determine what is important and how things are perceived usually exist. When theory and therapeutic technique are compelled by the premises of a dominant culture (without consideration of other points of view), the tendency is to dichotomize into good-bad, superior-inferior, right-wrong, and so forth, with the dominant culture as the standard of reference (Bell et al. 1983). Individual variations and the associated differences in internal and external frames of reference go unrecognized. This oversight results in the failure of empathy and ultimately the inability to facilitate establishment of the therapeutic alliance across cultures.

Knowledge about essential differences across cultures is helpful in improving communication and the accuracy of one's perceptions and understanding in a cross-cultural context. At the same time, simplistic notions about these differences can be misapplied and may be alienating and destructive (Blue and Gonzalez 1992). Although helpful, overemphasis on the mere accumulation of specific knowledge about different cultural groups can perpetuate stereotyped notions, lead to an array of "culturally specific" techniques, and bring premature closure to the task of empathic understanding and the establishment of the therapeutic alliance.

The Therapeutic Dyad

The bond between patient and therapist in the therapeutic situation constitutes the therapeutic dyad. The nature and quality of this dyadic relationship, determined by the quality of the alliance, is contributed to by both intrapsychic and reality aspects of both patient and therapist. Regardless of the particular psychotherapeutic modality, it is within this dyadic relationship that the patient is able to recognize and work out old conflicts (to various degrees), gaining a more objective perception of self and learning new and more adaptive ways of relating. A positive, sturdy therapeutic alliance is necessary for the patient to remain connected within this dyad despite recrudescence of old conflicts and the associated uncomfortable feelings that may be generated. Pine (1988) considers the therapeutic dyad to be a new, "corrective" object relationship, modeled on the parent-child dyad but permitting new integrations to occur (as a result of the interpretive work of the therapist) and, with it, progressive ego mastery. Kohut (1971, 1977, 1984) further elucidated the reparative effects of being empathically understood and valued and, through the patient's experience of the therapist as an idealized object, on the experience and sense of the self.

The matched therapeutic dyad.   When patient and therapist share some easily perceived or identifiable characteristic (e.g., race or ethnicity, gender, religion, age, or background), a matched therapeutic dyad is created. No controlled studies have been undertaken to demonstrate the relative superiority of the matched therapeutic dyad. However, clinical experience, as well as the teaching and supervision of trainees, demonstrates the ease of engagement, development of rapport and communication, more natural establishment of empathy, and lessened negative countertransference in the matched therapeutic dyad.

The matched dyadic constellation may catalyze an immediate identification of the patient with the therapist and the development of an idealizing transference in an attempt to gratify narcissistic wishes. This event can have therapeutic effects. Through this idealizing transference, the patient achieves a sense of affirmation of self and identity that facilitates conscious acknowledgment of previously repressed need states and conflict and their working-through and resolution (Foulks et al. 1995). At the same time, it may be erected as resistance against depression, anxiety, erotic or aggressive wishes, and memories of painful and disappointing experiences in early object relationships in the past. If the therapist overidentifies with the patient or overresonates with particular areas of conflict (Comas-Diaz and Jacobsen 1991) the potential for countertransference enactments increases. The matched therapeutic dyad may be of more importance in the maintenance of the therapeutic alliance and the progression of the therapy with patients who exhibit high levels of mistrust, narcissistic issues, identity conflicts, or extreme tentativeness in their commitment to therapy.

The cross-matched therapeutic dyad.   We all would like to hold to the ideal that regardless of difference (race or ethnicity, gender, or other real and imagined differences), the therapist's education, training, and skill (particularly the awareness, understanding, and effective management of countertransference) can effectively bridge this gap. The cross-matched therapeutic dyad, however, challenges the resilience of the therapeutic alliance in distinctly different ways (Draguns 1981; Shechter 1992).

The cross-matched therapeutic dyad will more likely precipitate changes in the patient's (or therapist's) perceptions, usual way of communicating, behavior, or emotional reactions, cluttering the therapeutic field and obscuring the nature of the core issues in therapy. These results are due to the threat to the sense of self, security, dignity, or historical continuity in the context of what is perceived or anticipated to be a nonmirroring or nonaffirming self object. The cross-matched therapeutic dyad is more likely to be problematic when there is inadequate integration and consolidation of the sense of self and identity along cultural parameters.

In his analysis of "cross-cultural passages" (cultural relocation, transformation, and acculturation), Antokoletz (1993) provides a model from a self psychology point of view, helpful in understanding issues in the cross-cultural interface. Whether an individual on the journey to a permanent relocation and cultural transformation or in the temporary interface of patient and therapist in the cross-cultural therapeutic dyad, the need for a "transitional zone" of experience exists (Winnicott 1953). Within this zone, patient and therapist must come together despite their different points of reference.

In the cross-cultural therapeutic dyad, the patient must create the illusion and experience of commonality and sameness of experience in which the true self is acceptable. For this development to occur, the therapist must be able to transcend his or her own cultural boundaries and empathically bond with the patient. This approach requires self-awareness on the part of the therapist and an understanding of his or her culture-bound feelings, perceptions, and expectations and how they differ from those of the patient (Wintrob and Harvey 1981). By avoiding intrusion of his or her stereotyped notions and countertransference reactions, the therapist, better able to recognize the patient's emotional needs, can respond within the patient's cultural context and experience, validating the legitimacy of those emotional needs. Thus the therapist gains credibility with the patient.

Common Problems in the Therapeutic Alliance Across Cultures: Clinical Methods for Resolution

Common problems in a faulty therapeutic alliance across cultures include the failure of engagement, miscommunication, mistrust, and the patient's failure to disclose, which leads to false assumptions by the therapist (see Table 13–1). Without a sense of engagement and encumbered by his or her own anxiety and countertransference reactions, the therapist more likely fails to acknowledge the patient's real and imagined concerns and ultimately is unable to work beyond the cross-cultural boundaries. No empathic bonding occurs between the patient

Table 13–1. **Failed therapeutic process: cross-cultural context**

Engagement

Patient notices difference	*Therapist notices difference*
Perceives social distance	Perceives social distance
Assumes therapist will not understand	Disacknowledges importance
Fears being judged	Sees patient as stereotype
Exhibits increased anxiety	Does not address anxiety or mistrust

Therapeutic alliance

Patient	*Therapist*
Does not develop rapport	Exhibits countertransference anxiety
Feels misunderstood	Does not understand patient
Shows increased mistrust	Fails to respond to mistrust
Exhibits decreased self-disclosure	Sees patient as unmotivated and not psychologically minded

Outcome

Patient	*Therapist*
Exhibits anxiety and frustration	Shows anxiety and frustration
Cancels session	Exhibits misalliance; misdiagnoses
Fails to show	Perceives faulty treatment planning
Terminates therapy prematurely	Observes failed outcome

and the therapist, and the therapeutic process becomes stalled. This stasis inevitably results in a failed therapeutic outcome manifested by misdiagnosis, premature termination, and faulty treatment planning, with pronouncements of the patient as unworkable, unmotivated, and unpsychologically minded.

In an examination of interactive factors between patients and therapists, Mohl and colleagues (1991) identified a number of specific factors that differentiated (as early as the screening interview) early dropouts from patients who continued in therapy. Early dropouts experienced a less-positive "helping alliance" (Luborsky 1984; Luborsky et al. 1980, 1985). They saw the therapist as less helpful, more passive, and not insightful. The patients did not feel respected, liked, or understood by the therapist. In general, the psychotherapeutic process was experienced as less potent. Different effects were seen with different therapists, despite the similarity of the patient demographics, diagnosis, and disposition.

As the authors concluded, these data suggest that something in the interaction is susceptible to influence by the therapist. Specific actions on the part of the therapist clearly can affect the patient's experience of and participation in the therapeutic process. This interaction is particularly critical in the cross-cultural context, in which there is both real and perceived distance and with it the high potential for negative perceptions and expectations. Both the patient and the therapist may be prone to such perceptions.

The quality of the therapeutic alliance is critical to a successful therapeutic process. The parallel process that must occur between patient and therapist to facilitate a successful outcome is illustrated in Table 13–2. Although obstacles may be inevitable in the cross-cultural context, they do not preclude the establishment of the therapeutic alliance. First and foremost, the therapist must be able to see the patient as unique rather than based on stereotyped notions. Such a perception conveys to the patient the therapist's interest and openness to understand the patient wholly as an individual in his or her cultural context. This perspective helps the therapist to remain aware of and able to manage his or her own potential countertransference.

The therapist's sensitivity to and acknowledgment of the patient's discomfort and mistrust lead to a beginning engagement and establish-

Table 13–2. **Successful therapeutic process: cross-cultural context**

Engagement	
Patient	*Therapist*
Perceives distance	Sees patient as unique and has some knowledge and much interest and curiosity about patient's cultural context
Is mistrustful	Perceives patient's mistrust
Hesitates to self-disclose	Acknowledges the cross-cultural context; conveys an open attitude and genuine desire to understand patient (including in a cultural context); addresses concerns, perceptions, fears, and expectations; is aware of and manages potential countertransference

Therapeutic alliance	
Patient	*Therapist*
Senses rapport, comfort, and trust	Perceives alliance deepening
Increases self-disclosure	Learns about patient's sense of self and life experiences
Feels empathically understood	Uncovers core issues (e.g., patient's wishes, fears, and conflicts)
Works purposefully in therapy	Moves therapeutic process forward, helps patient to understand feelings in relationship to other issues in his or her life, and so forth

Outcome	
Patient experiences	*Therapist observes*
Decreased emotional pain	Improved affect
Increased insight	Positive behavioral change
Increased self-esteem and sense of identity	Improved interpersonal relatedness
Increased ego resourcefulness	Clearer resolution of problems

ment of the therapeutic alliance. This development allows the patient to settle in with somewhat less apprehension and to increasingly self-disclose, which affords the therapist the opportunity to better understand the patient's core conflictual issues and defensive patterns. The patient works purposefully in therapy, and the therapist moves the therapeutic process forward, helping the patient to understand feelings and the relationship to other issues in the patient's life. This mutual involvement ultimately leads to a very successful therapeutic outcome. The patient experiences decreased emotional suffering, increased ego resourcefulness and functioning, and a more integrated sense of self and identity, evidence that patient and therapist have come together in an effective, collaborative working relationship, providing a new opportunity for the patient to move toward wholeness (Bland and Martin 1994).

Conclusions

Although obstacles inevitably occur in the engagement, establishment, and maintenance of the therapeutic alliance across cultures, differences in cultures do not preclude the possibility of the development of rapport, deepening engagement, and durable alliance. No effective alliance occurs, however, without receptivity, empathic bonding, sensitive collaboration, and the therapist's awareness and management of his or her own cultural biases and countertransference potential.

Each configuration of patient and therapist in the therapeutic dyad has its own unique way of catalyzing, facilitating, or potentially encumbering the therapeutic process. What psychotherapy requires of us in general, as well as in regard to particular patients, is the ability to "feel into" the total world and psychological experience of our patients (including their cultural experience) and the effective application of the psychotherapeutic process. It requires the acceptance of diversity (rather than the premise of a dominant culture), a thorough evaluation and empathic understanding of the patient in his or her cultural context and experience, awareness and working through of one's own potential countertransference issues (across cultures), and knowledge and skill in working through troubled transactions (Marziali and Alexander 1991) that threaten the durability of the therapeutic alliance. Common problems in the therapeutic alliance across cultures, and thus the parallel process that must occur with the therapist to resolve them, have been presented.

References

Antokoletz JC: A psychoanalytic view of cross-cultural passages. Am J Psychoanal 53:35–54, 1993

Bell C, Bland IJ, Houston E, et al: Enhancement of knowledge and skills for the psychiatric treatment of black populations, in Mental Health and People of Color. Edited by Chunn J, Dunston PJ, Ross-Sheriff F. Washington, DC, Howard University Press, 1983

Bland IJ, Martin WF: The Cross-cultural Therapeutic Alliance: The African-American Patient. Produced by Magerkurth P, Rovaris M. Topeka, KS, Menninger Video Productions, 1994

Blue HC, Gonzalez CA: The meaning of ethnocultural difference: its impact on and use in the psychotherapeutic process. New Dir Ment Health Serv 55:73–83, 1992

Comas-Diaz L, Jacobsen FF: Ethnocultural transference and countertransference in the therapeutic dyad. Am J Orthopsychiatry 61:392–402, 1991

Draguns JG: Counseling across cultures: common themes and distinct approaches, in Counseling Across Cultures. Edited by Pedersen PB, Draguns JG, Lonner WJ, et al. Honolulu, HI, University Press of Hawaii, 1981, pp 3–21

Foulks EF, Bland IJ, Shervington D: Psychotherapy across cultures, in Annual Review of Psychiatry, Vol 14. Edited by Oldham JM, Riba M. Washington, DC, American Psychiatric Press, 1995

Freud S: On beginning the treatment (1913), in Standard Edition of the Complete Psychological Works of Sigmund Freud, Vol 12. London, Hogarth Press, 1958, pp 123–144

Greenson R: The working alliance and the transference neurosis. Psychoanal Q 34:155–181, 1965

Horvath AO, Luborsky L: The role of the therapeutic alliance in psychotherapy. J Consult Clin Psychol 61:561–573, 1993

Jones BE, Gray BA: Problems in diagnosing schizophrenia and affective disorders among blacks. Hosp Community Psychiatry 37:61–65, 1986

Kohut H: The Analysis of the Self. New York, International Universities Press, 1971

Kohut H: The Restoration of the Self. New York, International Universities Press, 1977

Kohut H: How Does Analysis Cure? Edited by Goldberg A with the collaboration of Stepansky PE. Chicago, IL, University of Chicago Press, 1984

Luborsky L: Principles of Psychoanalytic Psychotherapy: A Manual for Supportive-Expressive Treatment. New York, Basic Books, 1984

Luborsky LR, Mint J, Auerbach A, et al: Predicting the outcome of psychotherapy: findings of the Penn psychotherapy project. Arch Gen Psychiatry 37:471–481, 1980

Luborsky L, McLellan AT, Woody GE, et al: Therapist success and its determinants. Arch Gen Psychiatry 42:602–611, 1985

Marziali E, Alexander L: The power of the therapeutic relationship. Am J Orthopsychiatry 61:383–391, 1991

Mohl PC, Martinez D, Ticknor C, et al: Early dropouts from psychotherapy. J Nerv Ment Dis 179:478–481, 1991

Moore BE, Fine BD: Psychoanalytic Terms and Concepts. New Haven, CT, Yale University Press, 1990

Orlinsky DE, Howard KI: Process and outcome in psychotherapy, in Handbook of Psychotherapy and Behavior Change, 3rd Edition. Edited by Garfield S, Bergin A. New York, Wiley, 1986, pp 283–329

Pine F: On the four psychologies of psychoanalysis and the nature of the therapeutic impact, in How Does Treatment Help? On the Modes of Therapeutic Action of Psychoanalytic Psychotherapy. Edited by Rothstein A. Madison, CT, International Universities Press, 1988, pp 145–155

Piper WE, Azim HFA, Joyce AS, et al: Transference interpretation, therapeutic alliance, and outcome in short-term individual psychotherapy. Arch Gen Psychiatry 48:946–953, 1991

Shechter RA: Voice of a hidden minority: identification and countertransference in the cross-cultural working alliance. Am J Psychoanal 52:339–349, 1992

Ursano RJ, Sonnenberg SM, Lazar SG: Concise Guide to Psychodynamic Psychotherapy. Washington, DC, American Psychiatric Press, 1991

Winnicott DW: Transitional objects and transitional phenomena. Int J Psychoanal 34:89–93, 1953

Wintrob RM, Harvey YK: The self-awareness factor in intercultural psychotherapy: some personal reflections, in Counseling Across Cultures (revised and expanded edition). Edited by Pedersen PB, Draguns JG, Lonner WJ, et al. Honolulu, HI, University Press of Hawaii, 1981, pp 108–131

Yamamoto I, Janes QC, Bloombaum M, et al: Racial factors in patient selection. Am J Psychiatry 124:630–636, 1967

Yamamoto J, Steinberg AL: Ethnic, racial, and social class factors in mental health. J Natl Med Assoc 73:231–240, 1981

Zetzel ER: Current concepts of transference. Int J Psychoanal 37:369–376, 1956

Zetzel ER: The therapeutic alliance in the analysis of hysteria, in The Capacity for Emotional Growth. Edited by Zetzel E. London, Hogarth Press, 1958, pp 182–196

CHAPTER 14

Commonsense Reasoning in the Transcultural Psychotherapy Process

JURG SIEGFRIED, PH.D.

This chapter is a theoretical contribution to cross-cultural research and therapy. It suggests that cross-cultural psychotherapy is in need of a shift of paradigms. Traditional scientific paradigms and those used in practice (e.g., psychoanalysis) focus mainly on *inner* mechanisms governing human behavior and change. I argue for a shift from traditional paradigms to more adequate paradigms, focusing exclusively on the *external* sociocultural practice of human communication. Scientists and practitioners who work in this manner consider cross-cultural dialogue as a more useful object of psychotherapeutic investigation and change. I substantiate my arguments with a short section on the necessary preconditions for cross-cultural psychotherapy, define common sense and commonsense reasoning, proceed to an analysis of the patterns of reasoning in psychotherapy with an Indian patient, report an experiment with Tibetan subjects regarding the pattern of commonsense reasoning in the context of emotions, and discuss consequences of commonsense reasoning for transcultural psychotherapy.

Necessary Preconditions for Cross-Cultural Psychotherapy

Cross-cultural psychotherapeutic models, theories, practical experience, and good research share at least one common characteristic: they all aim to reduce ordinary experience to a few core characteristics and easily explain psychological phenomena. Personality, depression, culture, society, ego functioning, and genetic predisposition are just a few conceptual examples labeling the reduction of a large number of individual-, context-, and situation-bound experiences to some assumed underlying function of our patients (Leighton 1993).

Kant showed two centuries ago how such reduction of individual experiences to unifying concepts is a necessary precondition for any human experience to occur at all. If unifying conceptual reduction did not occur, we simply would not be able to have any experience at all, because for experience to happen, it is necessary for one to compare present with past impressions. Only such comparison in time will allow a cross-culturally acceptable typification and reduction of actual sensual impressions of an object, say a computer. Reduction of sensual information thus is a necessary condition of experience.

Because the comparison is made with actual sensory impressions, every unifying concept has to have a clear empirical basis in ordinary experience; otherwise, it is a metaphysical concept without any real meaning. Mathematics, physics, geometry, chemistry, and the like are clearly rooted in ordinary experience. However, most theological and many psychological concepts are not.

An empirical basis in ordinary experience is established when competent language users share a verifying strategy for a particular concept. That is, I and any other competent language user who has learned the word *computer* (or any other synonymous concept of that object in another language) know the particular verification strategy for the object *computer*. We know we can look upon this object, ask other people, check our eyes or brains when in doubt, touch it, and work with it.

Fortunately, many linguistic concepts share the same verifying strategies across languages and cultures. Consequently, we can make ourselves understood across cultures and grasp what others of different ethnic backgrounds have to say. For example, probably in all human languages, touching, looking, sharing of experience, and working with it are correct strategies for the verification of the object *computer*.

But how should expert concepts (e.g., in physics or psychology), with unfamiliar concepts of other cultures and with differently used concepts in particular sociocultural groups, be handled? How are we able to understand them at all when we lack the corresponding verifying strategy? Clearly, the fully verifying strategies of concepts are available in this case only from competent language users understanding the concepts in question. Further, if we lack a corresponding verifying strategy, we only partly know what to do with the concept and do not know in this case exactly how to use the unfamiliar concept in language. We need to learn its verifying strategy first (and not only the concept) to understand its meaning. For example, DSM-IV (American Psychiatric Association 1994) lists diagnostic criteria teaching the reader in part how to verify disorders, such as obsessive-compulsive disorder. This approach allows others to understand what is meant by the term. However, DSM-IV does not give criteria to verify that someone is behaving or thinking in a certain manner. Verifying strategies for these commonsense concepts, of course, are taken for granted.

In cross-cultural psychotherapy, unfamiliar concepts and reasoning strategies are frequently met. In order to communicate, there is no other choice but to learn continuously the communicative practices of our patients and know how they and their culture reason before attempting to convince them of the need for change. There are three preconditions for such learning:

1. A necessary reduction of the many ordinary experiences to concepts (typification).
2. A necessary similarity of verifying strategies across languages (structure identity).
3. A clear relation of all verifying strategies to ordinary, shared empirical experience in a given society or culture (nonideation).

In short, the most important precondition for cross-cultural psychology is a similar structure of commonsense languages and communicative practices in all cultures, together with the grounding of every sensible communicative structure in the ordinary empirical experiences in a given culture. Only based on this common ground is sensible cross-cultural psychotherapy possible at all.

When these preconditions are met, cross-cultural differences in behaviors, attitudes, emotions, morals, practical life, nursing, cultural events, music, and the like can be important sources for understanding the patient's basic assumptions and can eventually inspire possible changes within a patient's commonsense understanding of the world. Only then will a suggested behavioral change make sense to a patient and inspire him or her to take action for change. Thus, the basis of cross-cultural psychotherapy is the therapist's understanding of a patient's socioculturally formed commonsense language. Successful cross-cultural psychotherapy consists in changing patients' communicative and social practices when necessary. Cross-cultural therapy, as any other therapy, in this sense becomes a rhetorical enterprise, attempting to convince the patient of a particular attitude, way of looking at things, or need to take specific action.

Common Sense and Commonsense Reasoning

Common sense can be defined as a shared socioculturally determined pattern of attributions, categories, and values leading to a successful mutual appreciation of others' attitudes, behaviors, and actions. Commonsense reasoning, on the other hand, can be defined as individually available attributing strategies when dealing with a particular topic.

Common sense and commonsense reasoning, in this view, in principle cannot be wrong. For example, a causal attribution of problematic behavior, labeling it as problematic behavior in a given society or culture, and classifying it as being problematic behavior is part of one's appreciation and understanding of the other's actions or attitudes. This appreciation is a prerequisite of understanding and making sense of the world or form of life of the other. In this respect common sense and commonsense reasoning are not only the basis of every communication and understanding but also of scientific research on human behavior and change. Ignoring this common sense, calling it raw and most of the time wrong, is in fact doubting the validity of the basis for communication and mutual understanding itself. Even further, it questions the whole of the sociocultural education we have gone through and thus does not make sense (Schuetz 1953).

This principal acceptance of common sense, of course, does not mean that all judgments, perceptions, memories, lay explanations of behaviors, and emotions are unmistaken and correct. Numerous studies have demonstrated, for example, the limitations of human judgments and the like (Kahneman and Tversky 1973; Nisbett and Wilson 1977; Stegmuller 1969). However, it is in the nature of common sense to assimilate and accommodate a new accessible expert or other information and correct itself again and again when the need arises. Communication with others or the world thus may be seen as a process of eliminating misunderstandings and doubts. And it is this interactive attempt to make sense of the other's talk, behavior, or masses of sensory input by continuously eliminating false hypotheses that in principle cannot be wrong. When sufficient information is given, individuals usually succeed in finding common ground, enabling them to share experiences and understand each other. In the case of insufficient information or time, the obviously best guess can serve as a working hypothesis for interacting with the world (Antaki 1994; Toda and Higuchi 1994).

This view of common sense and commonsense reasoning offers a perspective from which to investigate more fully patients' patterns of reasoning and actions and thus better understand processes of attributions, classifications of external and internal phenomena, and evaluations of behaviors of others and oneself. Transcultural psychotherapy based on common sense emerges as an inquiry into useful, possible, and mutually acceptable transformations of patients' categorizations (Rosch and Lloyd 1978), evaluations, attributions, prototypes of emotions, and other behaviors (Lakoff 1987).

Commonsense Reasoning in Therapeutic Encounters in India

For some time, I worked with an Indian psychiatrist and Indian psychotherapist. My friendship with the psychiatrist, Dr. Khanna, who lived at the foothills of the Himalayas, lasted for the 2 years I was conducting cross-cultural research in the community of Dharamsala in Himachal Pradesh. The community is mixed exile-Tibetan and Indian and one of the main areas in India where Tibetans were settled after the

Chinese invasion of Tibet. The Indian population is generally of rural background, owning small businesses, and of Hindu tradition, frequenting temples and shrines of various gods and goddesses (Shiva, his consort Durga, Kali, Ganesa, and the like). The households usually are matriarchally structured, with grandmothers often making final decisions. The Tibetan population consists of Tibetans in exile, originating from either central, eastern, or southern Tibet. Most of the adult population is government employed, and many have an academic background. Virtually all Tibetans believe strongly in Buddhism. Households have different organizations, some being centered around the father, others around the mother.

With this background established, I now describe a 19-year-old patient who consulted with my psychiatrist friend. As usual in this setting, the female patient did not come alone to her appointment; she was accompanied by her female employer. The employer and patient had previously consulted a traditional Indian healer, but this tactic had not seemed to help the patient's situation. Eventually, the well-educated employer decided that a psychiatrist should be consulted. As protocol required, the young female patient spoke rarely. Rather, we were told by her employer about the patient's unfortunate marriage to an Indian man that had lasted 2 months and during which she was beaten. She left after 2 months and returned to her employer's home as a servant. There, she said, she had been well treated. However, since her return, symptoms of hyperventilation and tremendous fears had been occurring frequently to the point that the patient was no longer able to work properly. At the times of her attacks, she was reported as lying on the floor, sweating, and having difficulty in breathing.

While listening to the account of these occurrences, we sat in an office where people went in and out, some asking the psychiatrist questions, others bringing tea, and others waiting for their turn to discuss their problems. Nobody seemed to care about the confidentiality of the material presented to us. The interactions of all participants, including the patients, made clear their readiness to share this problem with the community and to ask specialists in the community for help. The ease with which the patient acknowledged the accounts of her employer made it clear that psychotherapy in India is a social event and that an individual's sickness is a problem rooted within the whole of the community and passed on to persons with expert knowledge to whom the problem is described and accounted for. Thus even the setting itself illustrates how the patient's present difficulty is constructed as a problem within the particular society. Its treatment, too, clearly has a social dimension. This situation is similar to that encountered in scientifically based Western psychotherapy. There, too, telling one's troubles (Lee 1995) is basically a social event, even if it is hidden behind the privacy of closed doors.

Further, a deeper look at the Indian commonsense accounts and reasonings reveals a second characteristic, that of their intrinsic contextuality. The course of the employer's commonsense reasoning implied two things. First, that the patient's emotional psychic problem was not causally related in any way to the employer's treatment of the patient during work and leisure. On the contrary, she asserted again and again that she treated the patient well. Secondly, she was keen to offer what she obviously thought to be a plausible explanation of the problem as caused by the patient's unfortunate marriage. It is important to note that according to Indian (as well as Western) commonsense reasoning, unfortunate marriages seem to be socially acceptable causes for a mental problem we might call hysteria.

A third characteristic of the description is what Stich (1983) has called a typical causal history of the problem account. The employer described at length how she constructed the problem of the patient by basically explaining her language use of the problem descriptors, her attributions, and ways she selected a topic and made it relevant in the context of her account. For example, she made us understand that her first hypothesis about the origin of the problem was rooted in her belief in spirits and other harmful forces. Consequently, she had consulted an expert in traditional healing who seemed to know the necessary rituals for elimination of these forces. Because this strategy did not help, she continued to try to solve the problem by declaring it physical in nature. In the hospital again, she was directed to a psychiatrist, because the resident medical doctor considered the problem's psychological aspects more important than its physical aspects. In the course of her actions, the employer eliminated a number of hypotheses (i.e., the spirit hypothesis and the medical hypothesis). As the situation developed, her belief in the psychological nature of the problem obviously strengthened.

Of course, this belief was also nourished by our own expert problem construction. With our educational background, both I and the Indian psychiatrist definitely agreed to view the problem as something at least in part psychological. The interaction between the employer's explanations and her typical causal history of the problem, together with our own trained attributions and experiences, allowed us to label it as a problem type by eliminating the immediate context and situation from the problem description. This typification allowed us to construct our own typical causal history of the problem. Consequently, the employer was informed that the patient was probably suffering from hysteria, with repressed elements of a sexual nature as causal agents for the problem. Treatment would consist, we informed her, in working through this repressed material. The patient and her employer were told to make another appointment at the office.

However, the employer chose not to return to the office because of difficulties in traveling and other obligations. She obviously did not share our understanding of a psychological treatment and hoped for an easy and quick solution in the form of an injection or the like. Thus, despite her readiness to consider causal explanations of a psychological nature, she was not willing to share the experts' social construction of psychological treatment. Western psychological treatment is socially constructed in a way that usually implies at least a few regular consultations, using problem-related discourse between patient and therapist as a means of producing behavioral change. However, Western-style direct, confrontational, and nonconfessional discourse in a setting excluding others was clearly alien to the patient and her employer. Further, the mere thought of speaking directly to a person in authority was unthinkable for the patient. For her to reveal anything of her sexual experiences during marriage to an unknown male who had no relation whatsoever to her own family was, in rural India, an almost absurd expectation. The patient probably had expected a sort of group treatment in which the expert and the persons present would engage in a one-time collaborative effort to control and eliminate the problem. Collective, effective, one-time action, and not lengthy causal explanation and working through, was the patient's expectation during treatment. These expectations were not met by the psychiatrist. Instead, the psychiatrist introduced alien, noncommonsensible expert explanations. Therefore, this part of therapeutic discourse between psychiatrist and patient failed; misunderstanding, disbelief, and even mistrust resulted. Such a result is frequently encountered in our commonsense experience. When attempts in communication fail, patients frequently drop out of therapy.

Common Sense, Discourse Analysis, and Cross-Cultural Research

What can be learned from this example of an attempt to introduce Western-type psychotherapy sessions and alien, noncommonsensible expert reasoning into an Indian context? If we attempt to generalize from this example by considering it an epistemologically relevant social situation (Siegfried 1994), six important observations can be readily made. The first observation is the social construction of psychotherapeutic talk and the nature of psychotherapy itself. Psychotherapy is obviously practiced within a particular sociocultural background. This sociocultural background consists of values, causal connections, commonsense reasons, socially relevant attributions, and explanations of patient and therapist that are specific to a particular society (Winch 1978). For this reason, the acceptance of treatments is dependent on the time and sociocultural context and is relevant only within a particular context. The validity of Westernized expert reasoning in our example was threatened by the obvious differences in commonsense reasoning in the Indian culture (Kuppuswamy 1985; Sinha 1986; Singh 1977). Some of these differences may arise from the fact that people in India are more group oriented, have different topicalizations of problems (e.g., the concept of improper, shameless behavior that is obviously rooted in the moral background of Indian culture) (see Singh 1977 for traditional diagnostic systems in India and Lee 1995, for topicalization in problem talk), and have different values (as shown by the patient's unwillingness to talk directly to people of authority).

Although such cultural differences are well-known, they still lack due attention when designing empirical studies in psychotherapy. Cultural differences manifest only in communication and discourse. Discourse is context dependent, and its understanding is possible only through grasping the typical causal history of explanations given in a particular discourse.

However, empirical research in psychotherapy is aimed at generalizing its results. Generalization is dependent on context and time independence and on typifications (e.g., through a diagnostic system). Thus traditional psychotherapy research necessarily reduces patients' causal explanations and therapeutic discourse to a relatively small number of acultural and ahistorical segments in order to effect change (Siegfried 1996). In the process, cultural background, social events, and contexts, as well as typical causal histories, are necessarily lost. Consequently, relatively culture-free models of human behavior and change result. Such models are important for proving the effectiveness of particular therapies but do not give any indication of how and why people from different socioeconomic backgrounds change.

Traditional researchers, for this reason, are not in a position to give adequate consideration to patients' and therapists' cultural backgrounds. What methodology meeting the criteria of replication and validity, then, is more suitable for cross-cultural research?

According to the reasons provided, there are obvious advantages for empirical research in psychology to be discourse related (Labov and Fanshel 1977; Potter and Wetherell 1987). Discourse-related research succeeds in maintaining the particularities of reasoning and attribution strategies of patients with their particular sociocultural backgrounds and gives adequate consideration to different categorizations (Rosch and Lloyd 1978), to topicalizations of problem talk (Lee 1995), and to specific socializations of researchers and patients. Discourse analysis and its culture-fair application have been described elsewhere (Parker 1995; Siegfried 1995b).

Discourse analysis is analysis of culture-specific natural language, taking context, commonsense reasoning, and variability fully into account. Discourse includes all forms of communication, whether verbal or nonverbal, aimed at facilitating a mutual understanding between two individuals. Discourse is not only written text. However, although there is plenty of variation, culture-specific discourse still follows a clear organizational structure starting with specific ways of categorization (e.g., how the category of the self is constituted in the Maori) (Harre 1983), prototypicalization (e.g., emotions having a clear pattern of arousal ranging from specific physical reactions to cognitive and behavioral patterns, and sequential organization. Discourse analysis is an attempt to understand this organization by comparing the viewpoints of the participants, their different language uses, and the construction of their social worlds.

Secondly, culture-specific research must take common sense fully into account. Allowing for common sense, including commonsense reasoning, beliefs, and sociocultural practices, enables one to understand what people of a specific sociocultural background think and why they think the way they do. It also tells us what means of changing problematic behavior are available in a given society.

Discourse-related research is still rare in cross-cultural clinical psychology. However, a number of promising empirical results are available. For example, in a more extensive research project, I asked Tibetan subjects what counteractions they used against the frequently topicalized problem of anger and jealousy in the Tibetan society. Table 14–1 gives the average proportions of subjects considering the particular cure as being a treatment of excessive anger and jealousy.

Table 14–1 lists three categories of counteractions against anger and jealousy. First are traditional Tibetan medical cures such as taking herbal medicine to balance what are believed to be "winds" (similar to mental energies) in the body. Unbalanced "winds" are said to cause mental disturbances such as anger and jealousy. Further, in a cure called moxa, small portions of herbal medicine are burned at specific spots on the skin of the body where mental energies are believed not to flow smoothly.

Besides traditional medical cures, a number of Buddhist religious practices are used. Foremost is the practice of patience for anger and jealousy. In traditional Tibetan psychology and religion, a great number of techniques are given for the practice of patience (Shantideva 1981), and more than 93% of our 100 subjects seem to apply them in daily life or at least consider them useful.

Surprising in Western eyes is the heavy reliance on guidance and support from friends. In Tibetan society, a lama or elder person is often consulted if problems of excessive anger and jealousy arise. The topicalization of a problem and attempts to minimize anger and jealousy may

Table 14–1. **Tibetan medical cures and behavioral counteractions to anger and jealousy (N = 100)**

Tibetan counteractions to anger	Mean proportions	Tibetan counteractions to jealousy	Mean proportions
Medical cures		*Medical cures*	
Diet	.67*	Diet	.38*
Cures for "wind" disorders	.69*	Cures for "wind" disorders	.40
Medicine	.60	Medicine	.34*
Moxa	.43	Moxa	.27*
Medicinal ointment	.53	Medicinal ointment	.32*
Massage	.55	Massage	.18*
Religious practices		*Religious practices*	
Practice of the 10 moral principles	.93*	Practice of the 10 moral principles	.95*
Accumulation of merits	.86*	Accumulation of merits	.87*
Offering and confession	.90*	Offering and confession	.91*
Patience	.95*	Patience	.93*
Meditation on emptiness	.91*	Meditation on emptiness	.90*
Meditation on nature of mind	.89*	Meditation on nature of mind	.89*
Rituals	.69	Rituals	.54
Guidance		*Guidance*	
Guidance	.90*	Guidance	.94*
Advice	.96*	Advice	.90*
Social activities		*Social activities*	
Cultivating of friendship	.97*	Cultivating of friendship	.84*
Lifestyle changes	.84*	Lifestyle changes	.73*
Diversion of attention	.73*	Diversion of attention	.67*
Drinking and dancing	.73*	Drinking and dancing	.44
Sexual relations	.65*	Sexual relations	.36*

*Significant deviation from random answering (P = .50).

be responsible for the generally gentle character of the Tibetans. The social support system together with tradition may facilitate gentle interaction.

The remedies against anger and jealousy found in Table 14–1 are all available coping strategies according to Tibetan common sense and ready to be used in commonsense reasoning. They are obviously part of culturally acceptable coping strategies. Expert coping strategies may add to these ordinarily available methods. However, the introduction of such "new" methods to the individual often requires elaborate rhetoric to convince the patient to use them.

Practical Implications

Theoretical issues remain useless unless they involve strategies for psychotherapeutic practice. What, then, are the practical applications of the theoretical issues mentioned? I believe there are four: 1) the need to understand patients' sociocultural backgrounds, 2) the need to explore whether individual behavior is in accordance with or departs from the society and culture's rules and norms by 3) using a culture-specific system of analysis, and 4) the need to explore and use individually available strategies to cope with problem behavior.

In practices involving other sociocultural groups, therapists need to have a good understanding of their patients and their cultures. Indeed, therapists must understand acceptable and unacceptable modes of living within a particular culture and society. In the case of the Indian patient, a potential therapist needed to understand the Indian caste system, the special Indian constructs of an employer-employee relationship, Indian marriages and the consequences of divorce, and the status of healers in Indian society, to name only a few. Needless to say, all of these concepts and practices vary between India and Western societies.

This need to understand patients' sociocultural backgrounds is a consequence of the concept of psychotherapeutic change used in this chapter. According to this view, therapists' attempts for changing patient behavior are communicative rhetorical acts based on conceptual clarifications and other verbal and nonverbal discursive elaborations between patient and therapist.

With such an understanding of the importance of the sociocultural context of psychotherapy, therapists have secondly to explore whether a patient's problem-related behavior is in accordance with ordinary sociocultural practices. Further, they must explore how symptoms related to deviance might arise. Such deviance must be searched for with the knowledge that problem behavior is not problematic per se. Rather, problematic behavior is necessarily related to an identified and specific sociocultural reference group. Necessity here stems from linguistic use of the term *problem behavior* and not from logic or any other ultimately given norms. That is, the term *problem behavior* can be understood only with implicit reference to the unproblematic behavior of a larger body of subjects.

Furthermore, it is important to use a culture-specific system of analysis for the identification of problem behaviors. Sociocultural-specific categorizations of problem behaviors are crucial for a society's definitions of problematic behavior. In traditional India, problems such as overindulgence in erotic impulses, pleasure, and enjoyment (*Rajas*); evil (*Tamas*) and neglect of goodness and misuse of the senses (neglect of *Sattav*) (Singh 1977); anger; hatred; jealousy; attachment; and the like clearly are problems deserving of treatment by health specialists. On the other hand, lack of self-efficacy, self-assertiveness, and so forth are typical Western forms of problematic behavior.

Others have erroneously taken Western categories of the DSM or ICD type to describe problem behavior in India. Kulhara and Chandiramani (1988) have tried to conduct epidemiological studies of schizophrenia in India. Clearly, schizophrenia, maturity, stress, and hysteria are all Western concepts applicable within a particular sociocultural environment. In some other cultures, such concepts do not even make sense. Their application in such a context, in fact, creates an illusion of referring to similar patterns of facts or behaviors that Western people usually associate with these concepts. In India, for example, problem behavior is not topicalized in the same way as in Western cultures. One sees this difference in the fact that tolerance for not being able to work is much greater in India. For some, it is even prestigious not to work. Older people are expected to retire from worldly activities, leading what Westerners would call a disorderly life, and are often treated as persons of worship. Transvestites, at least in parts of India, are persons of special blessing and are readily provided with food and shelter. Hallucinations are not necessarily seen as problematic. Rather, what Westerners would call hallucinations may in India be perceived as memories of past lives, superior knowledge, and special abilities to foresee the future.

In short, categories of problem behavior are structured quite differently in India and in the West. In the West, the inability to work, hallucinations, withdrawal, lack of self-assertiveness, and inability to express one's feelings and desires are topicalized as problems; in India topics of problematic value are emotional imbalances of anger, hatred, attachment, and the like. A series of experiments have shown that even if problem topics are shared between two cultures, the weight given to them may be completely different. For example, empirical results indicate that jealousy has a much greater problem weight in the United States than in the Tibetan culture, where anger is seen as the more disturbing problem.

Understanding the sociocultural background and analyzing deviances with locally available classifications of problematic behavior still do not give any indication of the therapeutic steps to be taken. As Table 14–1 shows, an understanding of the individually available methods for changing human behavior is crucial. Guidance, traditional medical cures, religious practices, and particular social activities appear to be readily available tools for changing human behavior in our patients' Indo-Tibetan community. These individually available commonsense tools for changing problem behavior have received attention only recently (Furnham 1988; Rippere 1981). However, especially in cross-cultural therapies in which therapists of different ethnic origin are usually forced to rely on only their rough knowledge of patients' cultural backgrounds, it is even more important to ask patients about their available methods for changing behavior.

Preliminary Treating Heuristics for the Indian Patient's Psychotherapeutic Treatment in an Indian Context

Behavioral problems are working, ontologically established mechanisms within the individual. In our treatment of the Indian patient, it was thus important to fit into her basic understanding of the world and treatment expectations in order to be able to share her problem definition.

In cross-cultural psychology, the first heuristic one is forced to use in establishing a mutual understanding is to meet patients' basic expectations and conform with patients' sociocultural norms. In respect to the Indian patient, this meant accepting her employer as her representative and offering an immediate remedy to her problem. Therefore, my Indian psychiatrist friend tried to apply relaxation techniques, giving both patient and employer some advice on how to deal with the problem and eventually providing the patient with a Western tranquilizer to be taken at critical times. In this way the psychiatrist performed the Indian medical doctor's socioculturally established ritual for treating a patient.

The second heuristic is to establish a therapeutic plan that meets the patient's basic expectations of what constitutes effective treatment. The Indian patient and her employer had some rather clear-cut expectations of how an Indian psychiatrist would deal with the problem. They obviously expected a causal explanation of the problem by the psychiatrist, some advice regarding further measures to be taken, advice of how to prevent recurrence of the problem, and future involvement of expert help for treating the problem. The Indian psychiatrist explained the problem as being rooted in the unsuccessful marriage of the patient; however, because he was educated in Western psychological methods, he asked the patient to relate the experiences of the marriage to him. By using this approach, he not only failed to conform to the expectations of the patient but also disregarded her sociocultural background. Treating problems by talking about them is a typical Western approach based on the idea of catharsis. Because catharsis was not one of the patient's treatment options, she consequently refused to relate her marital experiences to the psychiatrist. The psychiatrist then asked the patient to hyperventilate and was thus able to trigger a state of hysteria followed by nausea. He then gave her a tranquilizer to be used when such states recurred. In addition, he asked the patient to return for more treatment sessions. When the patient refused, the psychiatrist finally suggested a checkup scheduled in 2 weeks. This appointment was welcomed by the patient and her employer.

A third useful heuristic for the treatment of the Indian patient was to link her problem to her religious beliefs. The psychiatrist suggested that she make offerings of food and flowers to a number of Shiva temples and urged her to pray for her quick recovery. She gladly accepted this advice, because this therapeutic action, regardless of its effectiveness, was congruent with her cultural heritage and part of her own repertoire for treating problems in life.

Fourth, because the patient was seeking expert help, it was obvious that her own coping strategies were insufficient for effectively resolving her problem. Thus the patient had to either learn a number of more effective coping strategies or make environmental changes of some kind (e.g., searching for another employer or attempting to get more education). These were the goals of effective treatment. The challenging task for the therapist was using acceptable language to persuade the patient (Billig 1985, 1987; Shotter 1994) to introduce one or a few new elements into her life and socioculturally determined system of thought. Because the therapist's task is primarily rhetorical in nature, knowledge of patients' assumptions and thoughts, doubts, conditions for attitudinal and behavioral change, available options in life, and the like is essential. Patients' resistance to change is thus merely an expression of therapists' insufficient knowledge of patients' assumptions and conditions for stimulating a process of change and not an occult, hidden, unconscious mechanism preventing conscious change. Because the Indian psychiatrist was unable to obtain a thorough understanding of the Indian patient's commonsense reasonings and conditions under which she would change in the short time available, he was unable to alter her situation.

These four guiding heuristics for the Indian psychiatrist (meeting patient expectations, establishing a treatment plan, using sociocultural practices familiar to the patient in treatment, and adding a number of new behavioral alternatives or reasoning strategies to the patient's available cognitive or behavioral options) were worked out with the psychiatrist retrospectively by reviewing his experience of the encounter with the patient. Although these guidelines are not empirically verified and do not cover a wide range of psychiatrists' actions in India, they are useful principles supporting the need to take into close consideration patients' assumptions, attitudes, commonsense reasonings, coping strategies, and so forth to deal with such a problem.

Conclusions

Case histories and empirical research in alien cultures are especially suitable means of reflecting on the assumptions of research strategies needed to take cultural differences into account. I have argued that cultural aspects of psychotherapy can be adequately incorporated into valid research strategies only if these strategies include ways of dealing with context, socioculturally supported definitions of problem areas, and typical causal histories, as well as the common sense of the particular group under investigation. Discourse analysis and empirical research based on common sense are seen to be promising methods of advancing psychotherapy research involving patients of different cultural, ethnic, and racial backgrounds. Problems of reliability and validity have still to be met with new research strategies allowing for comparisons of results across studies. However, even though we are still far from meeting most of the challenges of cross-cultural research in psychotherapy, research strategies based on the assumptions suggested in this chapter allow more comprehensive consideration of sociocultural differences.

Acknowledgments

This project was supported in part by the Swiss National Science Foundation, grant no. 8210–025979.

I would like to thank two anonymous reviewers of earlier drafts of the chapter for their constructive critique and suggestions and Dr. Sam Okpaku for his comments and valuable discussions.

Dr. Khanna is a practicing psychiatrist in Dharamsala, India. Between 1990 and 1991, during my research activities in India in relation to my research grant from the National Science Foundation of Switzerland, he kindly integrated me into his practice for many days by giving me the opportunity to see his patients and discuss the cases with him. By this gesture he allowed me to gain insight into psychotherapeutic procedures in India. Professor Singh, former director of psychology at Hardwar University in India, also gave me the opportunity to gain more knowledge about traditional psychotherapy originating from the Vedas.

These traditional psychotherapeutic strategies *(Kakar)* are still practiced today.

References

Antaki C: Commonsense reasoning: arriving at conclusions or traveling towards them?, in The Status of Common Sense in Psychology. Edited by Siegfried J. Norwood, NJ, Ablex, 1994, pp 169–182

Billig M: Prejudice, categorization, and particularization: from a perceptual to a rhetorical approach. European Journal of Social Psychology 15:79–103, 1985

Billig M: Arguing and Thinking: A Rhetorical Approach to Social Psychology. Cambridge, Cambridge University Press, 1987

Furnham A: Lay Perspectives: Everyday Understanding of Problems in the Social Sciences. Oxford, Pergamon Press, 1988

Harre R: Personal Being: A Theory for Individual Psychology. Oxford, Blackwell, 1983

Kahneman D, Tversky A: On the psychology of prediction. Psychol Rev 80:237–251, 1973

Kulhara P, Chandiramani K: Outcome of schizophrenia in India using various diagnostic systems. Schizophr Res 1:339–349, 1988

Kuppuswamy B: Elements of ancient Indian psychology. Delhi, Vikas, 1985

Labov W, Fanshel D: Therapeutic Discourse. New York, Academic Press, 1977

Lakoff G: Women, Fire, and Dangerous Things: What Categories Reveal About the Mind. Chicago, IL, University of Chicago Press, 1987

Lee JRE: The trouble is nobody listens, in Therapeutic and Everyday Discourse as Behavior Change: Towards a Micro-Analysis in Psychotherapy Process Research. Edited by Siegfried J. Norwood, NJ, Ablex, 1995

Leighton AH: Recollections of Personality and Culture. Rockport, MA, Society for the Study of Psychiatry and Culture, 1993

Nisbett RE, Wilson TD: Telling more than we can know: verbal reports on mental processes. Psychol Rev 84:231–259, 1977

Parker I: Everyday behaviorism and therapeutic discourse: deconstructing the ego as verbal nucleus in Skinner and Lacan, in Therapeutic and Everyday Discourse as Behavior Change: Towards a Micro-Analysis in Psychotherapy Process Research. Edited by Siegfried J. Norwood, NJ, Ablex, 1995

Potter J, Wetherell M: Discourse and Social Psychology. London, Sage, 1987

Rippere V: Depression, common sense, and psychosocial evolution. Br J Med Psychol 54:379–387, 1981

Rosch E, Lloyd B: Cognition and Categorization. Hillsdale, NJ, Earlbaum, 1978

Schuetz A: Common sense and scientific interpretation of human action. Philosophy and Phenomenological Research 14:1–38, 1953

Shantideva: A Guide to the Bodhisattva's Way of Life. Dharamsala, Library of Tibetan Works and Archives, 1981

Shotter J: Is there a logic in common sense?, in The Status of Common Sense in Psychology. Edited by Siegfried J. Norwood, NJ, Ablex, 1994

Siegfried J: From virtual to systematic replication, in Reconstructing the Mind: Replicability in Research on Human Development. Edited by van der Veer R, van Ijzendoorn M, Valsiner J. Norwood, NJ, Ablex, 1994

Siegfried J: Technical terms versus ordinary language use, in Towards a Micro-Analysis in Psychotherapy Process Research. Edited by Siegfried J. Norwood, NJ, Ablex, 1995a

Siegfried J: Therapeutic and everyday discourse as behavior change, in Towards a Micro-Analysis in Psychotherapy Process Research. Edited by Siegfried J. Norwood, NJ, Ablex, 1995b

Siegfried J: Microgenesis of re-learning: a new view on the process of psychotherapy, in The Structure of Learning Processes. Edited by Valsiner J, Voss HG. Norwood, NJ, Ablex, 1996

Singh HG: Psychotherapy in India. Meerut, Punjabi Press, 1977

Sinha J: Indian Psychology. Delhi, Motilal Banarsidass, 1986

Stegmuller W: Scientific Explanation and Proof-Structure. Berlin, Springer-Verlag, 1969

Stich S: From Folk Psychology to Cognitive Science: The Case Against Belief. Cambridge, MA, MIT Press, 1983

Toda M, Higuchi K: Common sense, emotion, and chatting and their roles in interpersonal interactions, in The Status of Common Sense in Psychology. Edited by Siegfried J. Norwood, NJ, Ablex, 1994, pp 208–246

Winch P: Was heisst "eine primitive Gessellschaft verstehen?" [What does it mean to understand a primitive society?], in Magic: Sozialwissenschaftliche Kontroverse ueber das Verstehen fremden Denkens [Magic: A Social Scientific Controversy on the Understanding of Alien Thought]. Edited by Kippenberg H, Luchesi B. Frankfurt, Suhrkamp, 1978

Recent Research
and Special Topics

CHAPTER 15

Somatization Patterns in Mediterranean Migrants

Myriam M. M. P. Van Moffaert, M.D., Ph.D.

The expression of mental distress in patients who have migrated from Mediterranean rural communities to northwestern Europe constitutes a special challenge in psychiatric diagnosis and treatment. Generally the extent and nature of their somatization of psychological problems or psychiatric disorders lead to an overuse of psychiatric labels such as hysteria and hypochondriasis. The message conveyed by the somatic symptom patterns in Mediterranean psychiatric patients cannot be properly understood unless the cultural background is taken into account. Simply diagnosing the somatization as belonging to somatoform disorders, such as conversion disorder, or interpreting dramatized symptom presentation as the expression of a histrionic personality is not justified.

The northwestern European psychiatric approach, which relies mainly on verbal interaction between patient and psychiatrist, must be better attuned to the body language of the Mediterranean patient, who is inclined to communicate nonverbally, regardless of whether he or she is mentally ill. The correct interpretation of somatization, although mandatory, is in itself insufficient. It must engender the extension of therapeutic management with somatopsychic principles and techniques. Psychiatrists, psychologists, and physicians who fail to focus on the somatic symptoms will often be considered inadequate by their Mediterranean patients and consequently lose their patients' confidence. Even when Mediterranean patients demand therapy for purely psychogenic problems (such as insomnia due to stress or tension headaches), somatic action should accompany the psychotherapy. The use of medication, particularly in the form of injections, often helps, because it suggests a strong medical commitment. Belgian psychiatrists who treat Mediterranean migrant patients must be prepared to extend their usual psychiatric means of psychotherapy, social measures, and psychotropic drugs with the therapeutic procedures that belong to ethnomedicine (Gailly 1982) and to cooperate with other health workers such as transcultural health personnel (bridging persons), Mediterranean health nurses, and local healers.

The psychological treatment of biculturally educated Mediterranean adolescents is even more difficult. It must deal with contrasting demands and values, especially in family therapy. The psychiatrist must refrain from labeling authoritarian Mediterranean parents as archaic. Ideally, the psychiatrist dealing with migrant patients should be assisted by a cultural anthropologist (Van Mol 1977) or by a person who knows both cultures, a "bridging person," as suggested by Hsu and Tseng (1972).

Mediterranean Psychiatric Practice in Gent

My view on the diagnosis and treatment of psychiatric problems in Mediterranean patients who live in Belgium is based on 9 years of practice in the psychiatric department of the University Hospital of Gent, including the university emergency department, to which all medical and psychiatric emergencies of this Flemish city are referred. In this chapter, I give particular attention to Mediterranean patients who visited the medical-psychiatric emergency ward with a combined presentation of physical symptoms and mental distress and who, after medical and psychiatric assessment, were diagnosed as having a psychiatric problem and were consequently referred to our university psychiatric department for hospitalization or outpatient treatment.

Although many psychiatrists working in the university psychiatry department found that their Mediterranean patients often presented with a complex clinical picture of physical and psychological symptoms, the results of a standardized registration were striking: in an emergency psychiatric situation, more than two-thirds of the Mediterranean patients presented mainly somatic symptoms, whereas fewer than one-third of the Belgian patients somatized in an identical situation. The presence of somatization has led psychiatrists to an overuse of diagnostic labels, wherein the somatic symptom presentation has the dominant role and the diagnosis of hysteria, hypochondriasis, and somatization disorders is—in our view wrongly—too often attributed to these patients. On the other hand, their real mental problems—depression, anxiety disorder, or psychosis—were often not well recognized.

The purpose of our research is first to provide a transcultural critique on the way Belgian psychiatry misinterprets somatization by automatically diagnosing a somatoform disorder. Secondly, we analyze the specificity of the Mediterranean way of conveying psychological distress in somatic symptoms and the cultural causes of this somatization. Thirdly, we formulate therapeutic guidelines, particularly for biculturally educated youngsters.

A Field Survey of Psychiatric Admissions of Mediterraneans

The Mediterranean psychiatric patient group we investigated consisted entirely of migrant workers and their families, so-called guest workers—*Gastarbeiter* (German) or *gastarbeiders* (Dutch)—mostly from villages and rural areas in Turkey, Morocco, Algeria, Tunisia, Italy, Greece, Yugoslavia, Spain, and Portugal. We excluded those who had lived in Belgium for fewer than 5 years. We wanted to avoid blurring the data by psychiatric problems that had been caused by migration or by early adaptational problems in the host country (Almeida 1975; Berner 1967; Carpenter and Brockington 1980; Häfner 1980; Hitch and Rack 1980) and instead focus on the interaction of Mediterranean illness behavior and Belgian medical practice. Five years seemed a reasonable period to allow acculturation with our health care facilities. The city of Gent (220,000 inhabitants, including 16,000 foreigners) has six large psychiatric institutions. Because none of these has a 24-hour service for psychiatric consultation or emergency psychiatric hospitalization facilities, the university hospital psychiatric department (UHPD) provides the only access to acute psychiatric care. The UHPD thus assesses every area patient in need of immediate psychiatric advice.

In the university emergency department (UED), a complete medical history and physical examination (clinical, electrocardiogram, and blood and urine screenings) are the standard procedure for all admissions. The resident psychiatrist conducts an additional psychiatric examination when the general practitioner's (GP) referral note indicates a psychiatric problem; when the patient or his or her family mentions any psychological problem, a history of psychiatric illness, or the use of psychotropic drugs; and when psychiatric symptoms or behavioral disturbances are observed in the UED. Psychiatric evaluation is also mandatory when the medical examination fails to objectify the somatic complaints or when the subjective somatic complaints are discrepant with the clinical findings. If this combined medical and psychiatric screening remains inconclusive, the patient stays in observation for 24 to 48 hours before being referred to either a medical ward or the psychiatric department. This screening process helps prevent erroneous admissions (e.g., a patient who is delirious because of hyperglycemia admitted to the psychiatric department or a patient with psychophysiological reactions to stress admitted to a medical ward).

After exclusion of patients whose incomplete medical psychiatric records made assessment of the predominant symptom pattern (somatic or psychological) impossible and of those without a proper DSM-III-R (American Psychiatric Association 1987) diagnosis, we compiled a group of 189 Mediterranean patients: 161 adults (82 females and 79 males, ages 19 to 53 years, with a mean age of 29) and 28 adolescents (21 boys and 7 girls, ages 15 to 18). Youngsters under 15 were excluded from the study, since they are admitted through the pediatric emergency service. Most of the 79 adult male patients were unskilled laborers (29 unemployed at the time of admission, 38 currently employed, and 12 running their own businesses). Of the 82 adult females, 79 were married and 24 were employed in housekeeping or factory jobs.

A reference group of 161 adult and adolescent Belgian psychiatric patients were selected, gender and age matched, from a comparable social class and admitted to the psychiatric department after similar recruiting and with identical medical and psychiatric screening procedures in the UED. In both the Mediterranean and the Belgian group, the dominance of either somatic or psychological complaints was recorded in the admission files. Definitive DSM-III-R diagnosis was not recorded until the psychiatric follow-up had been established.

In patients with predominant somatization, the somatic symptoms that constituted the most important reason for admission were subdivided into two categories.

1. Somatic symptoms that are not induced by the patient:
   a. Subjective bodily sensations for which no organic cause could be found: tiredness, fatigability, dizziness, fatigue, headache, low-back pain, abdominal pain, spasms of the digestive tract, and sexual dysfunction.
   b. Pseudoneurological symptoms: seizures, tremor, agitation, hypokinesis, pseudoparesis, pseudoparalysis, muscular spasms, burning sensation, glossodynia, and anesthesia.
   c. Psychophysiological disorders (psychosomatic syndromes in which psychological factors are widely accepted as one of the etiological factors): migraine, neurodermatitis, gastric ulcer, essential hypertension, ulcerative colitis, and hyperventilation.
2. Somatic symptoms that are self-induced, as the result of the patient's own action against his or her bodily integrity: attempted suicide, self-mutilation (wrist slashing and dermatitis artefacta), drug and alcohol abuse, anorexia, and bulimia.

On emergency psychiatric admission, 128 (68%) of 189 Mediterranean patients (161 adults and 28 adolescents) had predominantly somatic symptoms; only 61 (32%) in the same situation reported both somatic and psychological complaints, with an emphasis on the latter. In a gender-, age-, and socioprofessionally matched group of Belgian patients, only 46 (24%) were admitted with a clinical picture marked by a predominance of somatic symptoms, while the majority (i.e., 143 [76%]) reported psychic symptoms, often exclusively. The difference in somatization is not an artifact of recruitment or help seeking patterns, because both patient groups were recruited and screened in a similar manner.

Particularly striking, the frequent somatization of acute mental distress in these Mediterranean patients was not associated with an equally high proportion of somatoform disorders in their final psychiatric diagnoses. Indeed, somatoform disorders were present in equal numbers (68 Mediterranean and 66 Belgian patients). Of 161 Mediterranean adult patients, only 68 were diagnosed as having a somatoform disorder (19 with conversion disorder, 8 with hypochondriasis, 6 with psychogenic pain, and 21 with somatization disorder), whereas 128 had been admitted with predominantly somatic symptoms. Although only 24% of Belgian patients somatized on admission, the ultimate DSM-III-R diagnosis yielded a comparable number (66) with somatoform disorders (14 with conversion disorders, 13 with hypochondriasis, 10 with psychogenic pain, 18 with somatization disorder, and 11 with atypical somatization disorder). It should be noted that in both groups, a somatic mask often hides affective disorders, schizophrenia, or anxiety disorders.

Furthermore, the emotional excitability and the traumatic expression of mental distress that often characterize the psychiatric emergency admission of Mediterranean patients, did not correspond with a high proportion of histrionic personalities in this group (29 Mediterranean patients in comparison to 34 Belgian patients met criteria for histrionic personality disorders). This finding is remarkable, because more than 45% of the GPs' referral letters indicated diagnostic characteristics such as hysterical conversion symptoms or simulation. Of course, one can easily blame GPs, not only for missing a transcultural view in their psychiatric diagnosis but perhaps also of a racist bias. An attenuating circumstance is certainly that the psychiatric curriculum in Belgium up to recently did not include any teaching of the basics of transcultural psychiatry.

Belgian and Mediterranean psychiatric patients differ considerably in the frequency of substance use disorder, with frequent alcohol abuse (but also drug abuse) in Belgian patients. The low incidence of alcohol abuse in Mediterraneans is due to the prohibition of alcohol in Islam. This high occurrence of alcohol and drug abuse in Belgian patients is related to the high number of antisocial personality disorders found in the Belgian patient group.

The second important finding of our research is the striking difference in somatization patterns between adult and adolescent Mediterranean psychiatric patients. In Mediterranean adults, self-inflicted somatization (suicide attempt, self-mutilation, alcoholism, and drug abuse) constituted the main problem in only 38 patients, and 97 patients showed somatization that is not at all self-inflicted but that follows physiological pathways. In Mediterranean adolescents, the reverse seems to be true: only 5 adolescents somatized in a "physiological" way, whereas 15 adolescents resorted to self-inflicted somatization. Young Mediterranean psychiatric patients compared with a matched group of Belgian youngsters tended to present with different problems. Mediterranean adolescents are admitted mainly for self-inflicted symptoms (15), whereas among the Belgian youngsters, aggression toward others (7 cases of oppositional behavior, 3 of delinquency, and 4 of impulse control disorder) was characteristic.

Two Clinical Examples

Mamoun is a 47-year-old married Moroccan, originally from Marrakech, who has lived in Belgium for 18 years. He speaks fluent French, but his knowledge of Dutch is restricted to what he needs in the building industry, in which he worked until 6 months before his admission to the hospital. Communication with his Belgian doctors appears to be quite problematic, even though the latter are bilingual. He develops aches and pains, particularly in his head, neck, and shoulders. The physical investigations are negative, apart from mild cervical arthrosis. Mamoun is not satisfied with his medical treatment. The pains exacerbate, and he is admitted on the basis of repetitive complaints and prolonged sick leave. His GP writes a short note with a biased diagnosis of "mal-partout syndrome," commenting that he believes Mamoun is work shy. A 2-week observation with daily, personalized attention of a Moroccan-speaking male nurse reveals that Mamoun has serious family problems. His three sons and two daughters have good school results, but in his view they behave badly, particularly his daughters. He explains that they dress provocatively. In his trustful relationship with the nurse, Mamoun confides about his irritability, anger, work problems, conflicts with his wife (who is more tolerant of the children's behavior), and recent sexual dysfunctions, including low sexual desire and erection problems. With the diagnosis of major depression masked by somatic symptoms, Mamoun is treated effectively with a combination of psychotherapy and antidepressants. On discharge he has some residual pain, but he is able to resume work, although in a physically less demanding job.

Gönül is a 16-year-old Belgian-born girl, the eldest in a Turkish family with five children from the Cappadocia region. She is admitted after wrist slashing, consecutive to school problems and conflicts with both parents. Her parents are extremely shocked by her behavior. As the owners of two shops and a Turkish restaurant, they do well financially. The father understands Dutch, but the mother does not. Their other children perform satisfactorily in school, and Gönül had been a docile child until she transferred to a secretarial school, where she seems to be influenced negatively by her fellow students. She stays away after school, visits pubs (where she occasionally drinks excessively), and refuses to follow her parents' directives. The more firm the approach taken by her parents, the more rebellious her behavior becomes. Her psychiatrist works in close collaboration with a female GP who has spent some years in Turkey. The latter succeeds in convincing the parents that firm action will only lead to more rebellion and that finding a middle course between the traditional form of upbringing and the more progressive school rules and customs may be a better alternative.

Culture's Pathoplastic Influence on Mental Problems

Culture's influence on mental disorders and their epidemiology, incidence, clinical pattern, and even response to psychotropic drugs has been studied extensively (Bebbington 1978; Ellenberger 1965; Marsella 1978; Murphy 1965; Pfeiffer and Schoene 1980; Serpell 1976). The views on the pathoplastic influence on the presentation of psychiatric illness range from a universalistic position, which holds that psychiatric illness shows similar phenomenology in all cultures, to a culture determinist conviction that essential differences exist among various cultures. In the latter view, culture is decisive in shaping pathological behavior into culture-bound syndromes—that is, single and often exotic symptom patterns restricted to a specific culture or region. Research so far has shown that there are universally occurring psychiatric diseases whose psychobiological foundations seem to be the same in all human populations but that are transformed into culture-specific illnesses through the effects of cultural beliefs and norms (Kleinman 1980).

When psychiatrist and patient belong to different cultures, misinterpretation of symptoms and faulty diagnosis often occur. Psychiatrists' ethnocentric biases may lead them to infer pathology where there is none (Leff 1977), and it may prove difficult to distinguish between culturally specific belief systems and delusions (Westermeyer 1985). Adequate diagnosis may be hindered by the difference between the patient's explanatory model for illness and the doctor's concept of disease (Kleinman 1978). Moreover, because pathological behavior may mirror or overemphasize normal behavior, ignorance about a patient's culture hinders diagnosis (Littlewood and Lipsedge 1982). Finally, when linguistic differences impede psychiatrists' diagnosing, they are likely to be less influenced by verbal reports of symptoms than by nonverbal symptoms of mental illness (Hill 1974).

Somatization in the Expression of Psychiatric Disorder

Somatization—that is, the expression of personal and social problems in a code of bodily symptomatology, idioms of distress, and patterns of medical help seeking (Kleinman 1977, Lipowski 1988)—is a frequent characteristic of psychiatric disorder and is the main feature of the so-called somatoform disorders, a category of psychiatric diagnoses in which physical symptoms are the main presenting complaint. Considerable cross-cultural variations in somatization render the assessment of mental problems difficult. Worldwide studies of depression (Bebbington 1978; Katon et al. 1982; Matthew et al. 1981; Murphy 1965) have shown that depression in African and other non-Western cultures tends to be somatized in a symptom pattern of pain (stomach pain and abdominal cramps), constipation, and, in men, sexual dysfunction. The classical Western characteristics of depression as present in the DSM-III-R inclusion criteria (i.e., low mood, guilt, self-depreciation, anhedonia, and lack of initiative) are often absent. Specific for Mediterraneans, especially women, seems to be the expression of dysphoria into abundant somatization (Gaines and Farmer 1986).

Anxiety disorders have received less transcultural attention, but cross-cultural patterns in anxiety disorders were found through the comparison of Japanese *shinkeishitsu* (phobia of interpersonal relations) with North American agoraphobia (Good and Kleinman 1985). Phobic states are expressed in somatic complaints in African patients (Morakinyo 1985). Kleinman (1982), in reviewing the typical physical diagnosis of neurasthenia in Chinese patients, found that most of them met the DSM-III-R criteria of major depressive disorder. This finding demonstrates the interaction of somatization, depression, anxiety, and a range of psychosocial problems such as maladaptive coping and work problems.

Misdiagnosis in Psychiatry Through Somatization

The predominant manifestation of psychiatric illness through physical symptoms may lead to diagnostic failures in various ways. The psychiatric problem may remain undetected, or it may be wrongly diagnosed as one of the somatoform disorders, such as conversion disorder, Briquet's syndrome, somatization disorder, psychogenic pain, or hypochondriasis. The more overt or even dramatic somatization encountered in Mediterranean patients may lead falsely to the diagnosis of histrionic personality disorder. This false classification of somatic symptoms, the unfamiliarity with the pathoplastic effect of culture, and the bias toward the extroverted expression of mental distress have led northern European psychiatrists to mislabel their Mediterranean patients with diagnostic monstrosities such as the "Méditerranée syndrome" or the "Mamma-mia" syndrome (Ellenberger 1965). In our survey, comparison of the DSM-III-R diagnoses in the Mediterranean and Belgian psychiatric patients clearly showed that the overall incidence of somatization in the Mediterranean patients is not due to the prevalence of somatoform disorders but to a particular way of expressing mental distress.

The Causes of Somatization of Psychiatric Problems in Mediterraneans

In an in-depth analysis of the causes of this high incidence of somatization of psychiatric illness in Mediterranean migrants, different etiological factors were retained. First, the illness concept in Mediterranean culture makes less distinction between mind and body problems and is thus more holistic. Secondly, somatization is predominant in Mediterranean communities, because somatic symptoms constitute a direct message of distress. Thirdly—and this is specific for migrant workers—the body is the capital investment in the host country, the migrant's earning capacity being directly dependent on his or her health and fitness. Some authors claim that the basic tendency to express psychic distress somatically is linked to the lower social, economic, and educational status of the Mediterranean migrants (Barsky and Klerman 1983); however, this attribution was not valid for our patients, because our Belgian reference group was carefully matched to be comparable in terms of socioeconomic level and schooling.

Concept of Illness in Mediterranean Culture

In Mediterranean medicine, the body-mind dichotomy has been far less explicit than in the northwestern European illness model (Blacking 1977). A Mediterranean migrant patient's concept of illness is determined by features of Mediterranean medicine and by notions from the medical model of the host country. Hence, illness is not attributed to either the mental or physical sphere exclusively. Supernatural powers are included among the causes of both somatic and mental illness, and physical entities such as wind or water are accepted as causes of men-

tal illness. This holistic view leads to a psychosomatic model of both somatic and psychiatric diseases (Groen 1970; Pierloot 1961). The acceptance of physical and psychological—even supernatural—causes in
any disease is reflected in the therapeutic procedures of ethnomedicine. Some ethnomedical procedures resort to physical treatment for
psychiatric conditions. In Algiers, the use of medicinal plants is common for treating psychosomatic headaches. In Turkey, methods believed to restore the equilibrium between cold and warm body elements
(e.g., steambaths, dietary changes to "hot" or "cold" food, and bloodlet-
ting) are used in the treatment of psychiatric problems. The reverse
(i.e., the use of spiritual techniques for bodily ailments) is also part of
ethnomedicine. Religious healing, writing the name of the disease in
cabalist signs, reciting verses of the Koran, and wearing a blue-colored
eye are indicated in the treatment of various physical conditions. Naturally, ethnomedicine varies in different countries such as Turkey, Morocco, or Sicily. Also, within a country, the practice may vary among the
separate regions (Gailly 1982; Gailly et al. 1980). Still, the Mediterranean medical practice as a whole is characterized by an integration of
mental and somatic aspects of illness and by the use of psychosomatic
and somapsychic treatment strategies for all conditions.

Mediterranean patients may be inclined to somatization by the particular doctor-patient relationship and the customary diagnostic procedures in Mediterranean medicine (Foster and Anderson 1978). As a
rule, Mediterranean doctors require a passive attitude from their patients (Blacking 1977; Racy 1980), and diagnostic procedures applied
in rural health services rely on direct clinical examination and palpation
rather than on indirect technical procedures such as X rays and laboratory tests.

Somatic Symptoms Appeal
to Community Support

The migrant patients included in this study come from rural villages in
Tunisia, Turkey, Morocco, Algeria, and Sicily. Although these countries
vary culturally and structurally, there are basic similarities in the social

organization of these rural communities and in the way the community responds when one of its members needs support. In contrast to the health services in northwestern European communities, which are primarily state organized, the social support systems in rural Mediterranean villages depend principally on personal support from the other community members. Thus the somatization of mental distress in external mechanisms is preferred as an appeal for support, because mental illness is thought to be the sufferer's own responsibility (Gailly et al. 1980). Somatization in Mediterranean patients may be an acquired coping mechanism, an adaptive behavioral pattern that triggers the social support system. Somatization in Mediterraneans is structurally different from the negative concept of alexythymia (i.e., the inability to express personal feelings, emotions, and fantasy in verbal channels), as is the case in many psychosomatic patients (Marty et al. 1957). Somatization is seen as a positive and adaptive way of letting the body speak when in distress. Instead of psychologizing emotions, which is widespread among North American and northern European patients, somatization becomes a "metaphor for personal distress, and the personal feelings and thoughts are expressed through an external referent system" (Katon et al. 1982, p. 128). Furthermore, the linguistic barrier between physician and patient (many of the adult Mediterranean migrants have a poor vocabulary in Dutch or French) fortifies the use of concrete bodily denotations for psychological distress.

The nature of the symptoms and the anatomical localization of the somatization often convey a symbolic meaning. Because such meanings vary by the culture of the patient, a physician who does not possess a thorough knowledge of its symbolic connotations may have difficulty interpreting a complaint. The choice of an organ or organ system carries particular connotations. In Iran, heart discomfort is not limited to cardiac problems but comprises a complex collection of different stresses including those surrounding female sexuality (Good 1977); in Morocco, pain in the head or in the knee may symbolize an authority problem, often between a son and his father (Gailly et al. 1980). The meaning of different symptom localizations also varies with gender. In male Mediterranean patients, somatization in gastrointestinal symptoms often refers to sexual problems, particularly to impotence. Male patients often somatize professional problems through disturbance of the locomotoric apparatus or through muscular or articular pains. In female Mediterranean patients, feelings of anxiety or ambivalence toward pregnancy, contraception problems, and the like are mostly somatized through heart palpitations or complaints of a deficit of "clean blood" (Del Vecchio Good 1980; Nicholas 1972). The help of a physician or nurse, either of Mediterranean origin or with a thorough knowledge of Mediterranean cultures, is necessary to decode the symptoms presented by the patient's original culture (the emic aspect) into models that are useful for psychiatric diagnostic and therapeutic activity (the etic level) (Katz et al. 1969).

The Importance of Physical Integrity for a Migrant Worker

The migrant guest workers' situation is distinctive. Forced to migrate from rural communities to urban habitats in a foreign country to raise their standard of living through manual work (Binder and Simoes 1978), migrant workers have an earning capacity that depends on physical ability and integrity. Guest workers' bodies are their capital investment. Next to somatization as the expression of personal distress and social problems determined by a specific illness concept, health structures, patient-doctor relationship, and communicative patterns typical for Mediterranean rural communities, somatization is also related to the specific situation by guest workers or members of the migrant's family. Social survival by work and bodily integrity are so strongly intertwined for migrants that it is quite understandable that physical health is central to their concepts of health. Attaching personal, social, and financial well-being to the body as the main earning capacity will resonate in all of the migrants' distress situations of physical illness, mental problems, or social distress. As their capital investment, the migrant workers' bodies occupy the central position in their concept of health and are thus the obvious culprit for mental distress as well (Häfner et al. 1977).

Male Mediterranean guest workers often live under considerable pressure because they must provide financially for the "satellite extended" families in the homeland as well as their immediate families (Ozbek and Volkan 1979). This situation may lead to an anxiety of failure to fulfill these commitments. Because the reporting of physical symptoms is culturally regarded as neutral, it may be an acceptable excuse for failing to earn money. In contrast, psychological complaints and feelings of depression, anxiety, or guilt are less socially acceptable and involve higher degrees of personal responsibility.

Our emphasis on the importance of cultural factors in the frequency of somatization must not close our eyes to other, more material factors. Somatic symptoms may be induced by broader material conditions and health factors. Many guest workers have poor working environments and long working hours, and their housing conditions are often bad. These factors may produce chronic somatic symptoms, such as coughing, headaches, and low-back pain. Nutritional status and dietary habits may also be physically debilitating.

Self-Destructive Patterns of Somatization in Mediterranean Youngsters

Adult and adolescent Mediterranean patients differ in the extent to which somatic symptoms are self-inflicted. Conveying personal problems and mental distress in somatic symptoms is acceptable for adult and adolescent Mediterranean patients alike, but adolescents turn mainly to self-destructive symptoms and self-inflicted somatic lesions. The reasons Mediterranean youngsters appear to turn to self-inflicted pathology are unclear and may be a reflection of age rather than cultural factors. Adolescents in both northern European and Mediterranean countries often express psychiatric problems through aggressive symptoms (Schoolar 1973), such as suicide attempts, wrist slashing, and dermatitis artefacta, and indirect self-destruction, such as anorexia nervosa, bulimia, drug abuse, and alcoholism (Debout 1981; Gueye et al. 1981; Jacob 1981; Leblhuber et al. 1981; Pancic et al. 1981; Ross 1981; Sarro 1981; Wong and Matus 1981). The transition from a rural community to an urban setting may be partially responsible for a rise in suicidal and self-mutilative behaviors, as demonstrated by Kacha (1974) in rural Moroccan adolescents migrating to the city of Algiers.

Adolescents tend toward aggression, so the low incidence of outward aggression and the predominance of self-aggressive symptoms in

Mediterranean youngsters is striking. Only one 17-year-old Turkish boy was admitted for depression and delinquency. The boy had lost his father 1 year before in an industrial accident, and he claimed (rightly) that his mother and younger brothers and sisters had received insufficient insurance compensation.

Although our sample of adolescent patients is too small to reach an overall conclusion about the psychiatric morbidity of adolescent children of migrant Mediterranean workers, we hypothesize that Mediterranean adolescents in a mental crisis combine the somatizing tendencies from their parents' original culture with the age-related aggressive features in self-inflicted symptoms. In our therapeutic work with these adolescents, we encountered ambiguous life situations, with opposite demands from the parental standards on the one hand and the school and peer group on the other. The specific stresses of bicultural upbringing have been emphasized (Figueiredo and Lemkau 1978). These youngsters are disoriented by their lack of firsthand experience of their parents' culture. Their usually less-educated elders demand strict obedience (Kabela 1974; Verdonk 1979), whereas the Belgian cultural environment and the school emphasize self-assertiveness and the pursuit of personal goals (Guyot 1978). Finally, since these youngsters grow up in nuclear families, they lack the support of traditional extended or plurigenerational family structures (Ozbek and Volkan 1979).

Conclusions

Somatization of mental problems yields a risk for misdiagnosing the underlying psychiatric disorder, particularly when doctor and patient belong to different cultures. Belgian GPs tend to misinterpret the complex somatic and psychological symptom presentation of their Mediterranean migrant patients. Mediterranean migrants with acute psychiatric problems show a predominance of dramatic somatization in their symptom patterns when compared with Belgian patients with similar psychiatric problems and admitted after identical recruiting and referral procedures. Psychiatric diagnosis of these Mediterranean patients reveals neither a correspondingly high incidence of somatoform disorders nor histrionic personalities. Belgian physicians, GPs, and psychiatrists alike must integrate transcultural psychiatric principles into their work with Mediterranean patients.

Special care is needed in dealing with problems of biculturally educated Mediterranean youngsters. Adult and adolescent Mediterranean migrants convey psychological problems through contrasting forms of somatization: adults exhibit them in a more "natural" way—in subjective bodily sensations, psychophysiological symptoms, or psychosomatic syndromes—and youngsters display self-inflicted symptoms, such as wrist slashing, self-mutilation, and drug abuse. This combination of somatization and aggression in self-inflicted physical symptoms demands particular attention, and the psychiatric management of biculturally educated youngsters requires caregivers with an understanding of cultural differences.

Acknowledgments

I am greatly indebted to my husband, Dr. Marc De la Ruelle, for his comments and cultural critique in the writing of this chapter.

References

Almeida Z: Les perturbations mentales chez les migrants. Informations Psychiatriques 51:249–281, 1975

American Psychiatric Association: Diagnostic and Statistical Manual of Mental Disorders, 3rd Edition, Revised. Washington, DC, American Psychiatric Association, 1987

Barsky AJ, Klerman GL: Overview: hypochondriasis, bodily complaints, and somatic styles. Am J Psychiatry 140:273–283, 1983

Bebbington PE: The epidemiology of depressive disorder. Cult Med Psychiatry 2:297–341, 1978

Berner P: Psychopathologie des migrations. Encyclopédie Médico-Chirurgicale 5. Paris, Editions Techniques, 1967

Binder J, Simoes M: Sozialpsychiatrie der Gastarbeiter. Fortschr Neurologie Psychiatrie und ihre Grensgebiete 46:342–359, 1978

Blacking J: The Anthropology of the Body. London, Academic Press, 1977

Carpenter L, Brockington IF: A study of mental illness in Asians, West Indians, and Africans living in Manchester. Br J Psychiatry 137:201–205, 1980

Debout M: Passage, rite, et tentative de suicide chez l'adolescent, in Dépression et Suicide. Edited by Soubrier JP, Védrinne J. Paris, Pergamon, 1981

Del Vecchio Good MJ: Of blood and babies: the relationship of popular Islamic physiology to fertility. Soc Sci Med 14B:147–156, 1980

Ellenberger HE: Ethno-psychiatry. Encyclopédie Médico-Chirurgicale 5. Paris, Editions Techniques, 1965

Figueiredo JM, Lemkau PV: The prevalence of psychosomatic symptoms in a rapidly changing bilingual culture: an explanatory study. Soc Psychiatry 13:125–133, 1978

Foster GM, Anderson BG: Medical Anthropology. New York, Wiley, 1978

Gailly A: Etnogeneeskunde en psychiatrie bij Turken. Kultuurleven 1:67–80, 1982

Gailly A, Hermans P, Leman J: Mediterrane Dorpskulturen. Kultuurleven 9:820–840, 1980

Gaines AD, Farmer PE: Visible saints. Cult Med Psychiatry 4:295–331, 1986

Good B: The heart of what's the matter: the semantics of illness in Iran. Cult Med Psychiatry 1:25–58, 1977

Good B, Kleinman AM: Culture and anxiety: cross-cultural evidence for the patterning of anxiety disorders, in Anxiety and the Anxiety Disorders. Edited by Hussain Tuma A, Maser JD. Hillsdale, NJ, Lawrence Earlbaum Associates, 1985

Groen JJ: Influence of social and cultural patterns on psychosomatic diseases. Psychother Psychosom 18:189–215, 1970

Gueye MR, Collignon R, Boussou MM, et al: Evolution du suicide et de la dépression au Sénégal et en Afrique, in Dépression et Suicide. Edited by Soubrier JP, Védrinne J. Paris, Pergamon, 1981

Guyot J: Migrant Women Speak. London, Search Press, 1978

Häfner H: Psychiatrische Morbidität von Gastarbeitern in Mannheim. Nervenarzt 51:672–683, 1980

Häfner H, Moschel G, Ozek M: Psychiatrische Störungen bei Türkischen Gastarbeitern. Nervenarzt 48:268–275, 1977

Hill D: Non-verbal behaviour in mental illness. Br J Psychiatry 124:221–230, 1974

Hitch PJ, Rack PH: Mental illness among Polish and Russian refugees in Bradford. Br J Psychiatry 137:206–211, 1980

Hsu J, Tseng WS: Intercultural psychotherapy. Arch Gen Psychiatry 27:700–705, 1972

Jacob OP: Self-destructive behaviour: its importance for our culture. Some questions and consequences, in Dépression et Suicide. Edited by Soubrier JP, Védrinne J. Paris, Pergamon, 1981

Kabela M: Kinderen van Spaanse gastarbeiders. Maandblad voor Geestelijke Volksgezondheid 29:296–304, 1974

Kacha M: Le suicide en Algérie. Thèse. Université d'Alger, Département de Psychiatrie, 1974

Katon W, Kleinman A, Rosen G, et al: Depression and somatization: a review, parts I and II. Am J Med 72:127–135, 241–247, 1982

Katz MM, Cole JO, Lovery HA: Studies of the diagnostic process: the influence of symptom perception, past experience, and ethnic background on diagnostic decisions. Am J Psychiatry 125:109–119, 1969

Kleinman A: Depression, somatization, and the "new cross-cultural psychiatry." Soc Sci Med 11:3–10, 1977

Kleinman A: Clinical relevance of anthropological and cross-cultural research: concepts and strategies. Am J Psychiatry 135:427–431, 1978

Kleinman A: Major conceptual and research issues for cultural (anthropological) psychiatry (editorial). Cult Med Psychiatry 4:3–13, 1980

Kleinman A: Neurasthenia and depression: a study of somatization and culture in China. Cult Med Psychiatry 6:117–190, 1982

Leblhuber F, Schöny W, Fischer F, et al: Study of suicides committed by adolescents in upper Austria, covering a period of three years, in Dépression et Suicide. Edited by Soubrier JP, Védrinne J. Paris, Pergamon, 1981, pp 652–655

Leff JP: International variations in the diagnosis of psychiatric illness. Br J Psychiatry 131:229–238, 1977

Lipowski ZJ: Somatization: the concept and its clinical application. Am J Psychiatry 145:1358–1368, 1988

Littlewood R, Lipsedge M: Aliens and alienists: ethnic minorities and psychiatry. Harmondsworth, Penguin, 1982

Marsella AJ: Thoughts on cross-cultural studies on the epidemiology of depression. Cult Med Psychiatry 2:343–359, 1978

Marty P, de M'Uzan, David C: L'investigation Psychosomatique. Paris, Presses Universitaires, 1957

Matthew RJ, Weinman ML, Mirabi M, et al: Physical symptoms of depression. Br J Psychiatry 139: 293–296, 1981

Morakinyo O: Phobic states presenting as somatic complaint syndromes in Nigeria: sociocultural factors associated with diagnosis and psychotherapy. Acta Psychiatr Scand 71:356–365, 1985

Murphy HBM: Méthodologie de recherche en socio-psychiatrie et en ethnopsychiatrie. Encyclopédie Médico-Chirurgicale 5. Paris, Editions Techniques, 1965

Nicholas M: Croyances et Pratiques Populaires Turques Concernant les Naissances. Paris, Publications Orientalistes de France, 1972

Ozbek A, Volkan KD: Psychiatric problems within the satellited extended families of Turkey. Am J Psychother 30:574–582, 1979

Pancic I, Kenderovic FS, Ungar P, et al: Is the suicidal bringing up the social peculiarity of the most suicidal town of Yugoslavia? in Dépression et Suicide. Edited by Soubrier JP, Védrinne J. Paris, Pergamon, 1981, pp 183–188

Pfeiffer WM, Schoene W: Psychopathologie im Kulturvergleich. Klinische Psychologie und Psychopathologie 14. Stuttgart, Ferdinand Enke, 1980

Pierloot RA: Phénomènes psychosomatiques et signification du corps pour la personne. Acta Psychotherapeutica 9:295–303, 1961

Racy J: Somatization in Saudi women: a therapeutic challenge. Br J Psychiatry 137:212–216, 1980

Ross RR: Adolescent self-mutilators, in Dépression et Suicide. Edited by Soubrier JP, Védrinne J. Paris, Pergamon, 1981, pp 599–603

Sarro B: Annotations sur la conduite suicidaire en Espagne, in Dépression et Suicide. Edited by Soubrier JP, Védrinne J. Paris, Pergamon, 1981, pp 53–60

Schoolar JC (ed): Current Issues in Adolescent Psychiatry. New York, Brunner/ Mazel, 1973

Serpell R: Culture's Influence on Behaviour. London, Methuen, 1976

Van Mol M: Marokkaanse zieken tegenover Europese artsen. Streven 2:401–410, 1977

Verdonk A: Van gastarbeiders tot immigranten: de problemen van de tweede generatie. Maandblad Geestelijke Volksgezondheid 6/7:444–458, 1979

Westermeyer J: Psychiatric diagnosis across cultural boundaries. Am J Psychiatry 142:798–805, 1985

Wong R, Matus A: Concepts of child and adolescent suicide in two contrasting cultures, U.S.A. and China, in Dépression et Suicide. Edited by Soubrier JP, Védrinne J. Paris, Pergamon, 1981, pp 638–643

CHAPTER 16

Cohabiting With Magic and Religion in Italy

Cultural and Clinical Results

GOFFREDO BARTOCCI, M.D.

LUIGI FRIGHI, M.D.

GIANGIACOMO G. ROVERA, M.D.

NICOLA LALLI, M.D.

TERESA DI FONZO, M.D.

In beginning our analysis of the coexistence of magic and religion in Italy, we would like to outline a general psychopathological framework for magical, psychospiritual, and psychoreligious experiences (Lukoff et al. 1992). We aim to simplify the complex debate on these issues. The general tendency is to label magic as an archaism, a prelogical disruption of the normal flow of reason that, sooner or later, reflects a pathogenic potential.

Conversely, some consider religious belief systems as incapable of negatively influencing the development of the ego. The ego is believed to be fortified by values that underlie the sacred. Such is the position taken by Lukoff and others (1992), who, by relying on the concept of statistical norm, tend to consider the psychoreligious experience as an ontological element that favors prevention of mental disorders.

Such a simplistic approach to the function of the two forms of supernatural belief systems has not been attempted in the work of the many authors representing the Italian Schools of Anthropology and Psychiatry (Barcocci 1997; de Martino 1959/1993; Fagioli 1974/1985; Italian Institute of Transcultural Mental Health 1990, 1994). These authors prefer to consider a religious experience an undoubtedly frequent psychic event, although not necessarily a sure boost for the ego.

In this chapter, we explore how the cultural structures of magic and religious beliefs lend themselves to rationalizing a psychopathological experience common to all cultures, namely the loss of one's ego. Before opening our discussion of a few clinical cases that substantiate these subjects, we would like, for the sake of clarity, to give a phenomenological and psychodynamic definition of magic and sacred belief systems and establish crucial distinctions between them.

Belief in magic is here used to mean a given ideoaffective state, historically determined and culture bound, that tends to interpret the development of the external world and of one's own relationship with that world as being strongly conditioned by immaterial forces, characterized by human features. In traditional magic, it is humans and the intentions of humans that drive the intangible forces that transversely influence the actions of humanity.

Sacred belief, on the other hand, refers to a conception of the world, historically and culturally determined, that defers the power of human intentions to a superior power that is unmoving in time and transcends human action. Humans and the intentions of humans are practically powerless before the inscrutable power of God.

We have chosen investigative strategies of transcultural psychiatry in analyzing the meaning and function of systems of belief involving the supernatural. In our view, the perspective of transcultural psychiatry offers the best method of objectively outlining the great ethnographic variety of these experiences and subsequently making a comparative analysis of the links that exist among psychopathology, culture, and the supernatural in a given situation. It is surely not by chance that many of the studies on this subject have been conducted by transcultural psychiatrists. It would be difficult, for example, to imagine the following statement being made by a biology-oriented psychiatrist: "Delusions must be carefully evaluated with reference to cultural and religious belief systems" (Karno and Jenkins 1997, p. 902).

Those who have done field work and undertaken ethnographic studies have surely been able to see how striking the representation of magic and religion actually can be. In some cases the supernatural experiences are judged as "normal" existential elements; in other cases they are seen as involving pathological states of mind. These experiences have found an outlet in increasingly complex conceptions such as folkloric magic, which has revealed itself as an effective solution to crisis in some traditional cultures, or as occult magic, which combines features borrowed from sacred rituals and ideologies and is particularly widespread in modern societies.

Some of the highest supernatural experiences such as ecstasy, mysticism, and the communion with the Absolute can attract special social consensus and take on the structure of prevailing cultural institutions, as in the case of religions in the Western world. On the other hand, the supernatural experience, with the concurrence of certain other pathogenic elements, may take the form of atypical and disruptive individual expression that dooms the subject to isolation. It is this realm of psychopathology that we shall further explore.

The Coexistence of Magic and Religion With Rational Thought

In a previous article (Bartocci et al. 1995), we reported the results of a study that found in a few regions of Italy a cultural conglomeration, the coexistence of the rather contradictory components of magic and religion, with religion ultimately prevailing. The forms of cohabitation that we described as predominant in fifth-century Italy did not contain the dichotomy between magic and traditional religion that would later develop in the Middle Ages and persist to our day, to the point of their becoming irremediably antithetical. In witnessing the antinomy between magic and religion in our modern world, we can easily affirm that a cultural conflict corresponds to an individual psychological difficulty in integrating these two dimensions, to which we must add a third well-structured form of reasoning: positivistic thinking.

The clinical cases reported in this chapter and observed in the regions of Umbria and Latium exemplify a situation characteristic of many Italian regions: the fragmentation of a cultural axis mundi that is no longer sufficiently consistent to be an effective existential point of reference, a fragmentation that can be reflected in the individual ego. The Italian people, and with them most of the Western world, have been forced into a tenuous position, atop a very shaky tripod: religious weltanschauung, positivistic thinking, and the still-existing rubble of magic belief. This weakness in Western humanity's ontological foothold is exacerbated and reiterated by the unwise demarcation of prevailing religious belief from religion-based pathological delusions.

Even if it were possible to find well-grounded criteria for a comparative analysis of the norm in religious pathology (Simoes 1994), there is no clear-cut approach to the study of the psychodynamics of religious experience capable of loosening the cultural stronghold of the sacred in its topmost position on the Gaussian cultural norm curve. The "puzzling relationship between the individual delusions of psychotics and the false or highly improbable beliefs held by large numbers of people" (Prince 1971, p. 18) is certainly one of the most vague areas of modern psychiatry.

The definition of that group of shared beliefs relating to the supernatural that Prince refers to as "integranal beliefs" in fact still remains uncertain. Despite the fact that some beliefs are classified as "false or highly improbable," there is still no consensus on what constitutes, in Prince's words, "acceptable expression" that might clearly define the limits, the nosographic classification, or the psychodynamic function of these undoubtedly universal phenomena, notwithstanding their diverse expression (Rovera 1990).

Clinical Cases

We now present some clinical cases from the traditional dimension of magic and others imbued with religious elements.

The case of the Rossi sisters. This first set of cases is rooted in the disappearing peasant world in a place located only 100 km from modern Rome but far distant in its archaic appearance.

The Rossi sisters present a very similar premorbid personal history. They were raised in a typical Umbrian peasant family whose economic situation prevented them from receiving adequate schooling. They, like the men they married, dropped out of elementary school to work in the fields. At the time of our investigation, all of the Rossi sisters were middle-aged, married, and mothers.

The Rossi sisters went to the mental health center of the nearest town (25 km away) independently of one another. The patients were evaluated by several different physicians, who did not know of the familial relationship. Each was diagnosed with depression.

Tullia, the oldest, went to the mental health center at age 50, complaining of a light form of existential depression that had affected her for many years and that was characterized by traditional symptoms: apathy, lack of interest in her family and the future, and fear of being crazy. She was hospitalized once, briefly, at age 16 for hysteria.

The second sister, Rosalba, shared many of Tullia's complaints, yet she presented to the mental health center only once each spring, requesting a tonic treatment. She never received an antidepressant or was hospitalized.

The physician who first treated Orsola, the third sister, diagnosed her as neurasthenic with depressive traits. She was hospitalized in 1953, at age 29, for an ongoing condition of neurotic excitement.

Pia, the fourth-born sister, first came to the mental health center a few months after Orsola. She was initially hospitalized in 1967, at age 37, for neurotic depressive syndrome. She was subsequently hospitalized several times following either reported pregnancies or actual medical abortions. She suffered from panic anxiety, stemming from the fear that her children might be born "as ill as I am." She was administered antidepressants and subjected to an electroconvulsive therapy cycle.

Unlike her sisters, Orsola manifested manic attacks preceded by panic-driven states of anxiety in addition to depression. Orsola's elderly mother and invalid stepfather showed no concern until Orsola seemed a threat to her family and was subsequently hospitalized by force.

The physicians at the mental health center considered the possibility of a biologically inherited depressive syndrome affecting the Rossi sisters. However, no trace of hereditary dysthymia could be found in their numerous offspring or in the preceding generation. The disorder seemed to transversely affect only one generation, leading us to formulate a theory involving "micro-culture-bound" factors. Rumors circulating in town seemed to validate this theory; the townspeople agreed that the Rossi sisters were cursed as a result of their mother's witchcraft. Their mother always dressed in black and was believed to possess magical powers, enabling her to predict the future, detect the presence of spells, and heal those under the spell of the evil eye. It seemed that the mother had at some point in the past given up her practice of magic. The Rossi sisters never told doctors that their mother was considered a sorcerer.

In treating the Rossi sisters, their doctors concluded that the women were somehow trapped in the past, in a time when evil forces directed through the powers of their mother and the devil and witch-craft belonged to the world picture. They believed that the devil had robbed them of their souls and strength. Thus they did not make the transition into the modern world and were essentially robbed of form-ing egos congruent with those of the new world. The Rossi sisters spent their childhood and adolescence in the prewar and war periods. The postwar era signaled the change of the homogeneous peasant world by the encroachment of different cultures and a modern world. They had passively witnessed the events and had not taken part in the transcul-turalization process; they had been incapable of moving into the new world. They were caught between the old world of their mother and the new world of their offspring, unable to fit into either. They had been raised in the world of witchcraft and were then flung into the transient world of modernity. The modern medicine they turned to for help was ineffective. No source, including the church, was able to help the sis-ters. They were overcome by despair and ultimately found refuge in their illness.

The peasant and worker's world of the Roman suburbs: Maria. In the following clinical case, magic is inherent in psychopathological ele-ments. Maria, a housewife from the suburbs of Rome and mother of three girls, presented to the psychiatric outpatient department of the University of Rome after a 20-day stay in the hospital for a bout of delu-sions, which was successfully treated with neuroleptic drugs.

Maria recounted her history. She had become bored with her hus-band and family and, at a friend's suggestion, began reading the maga-zine *Cronaca Vera (Real Stories)*, containing a correspondence column for "kindred spirits." Maria found a mate in the person of a convict, with whom she corresponded regularly. The convict began enclosing four-leaf clovers in his letters to Maria, with the word *love* and their names written on the leaves.

Maria's infatuation with the convict developed into an obsession; she was so preoccupied with thoughts of him that she considered herself to be under a spell he had cast through the clovers. Consequently, she turned back to the magazine and responded to another column, that by the "Wizard of Milan," whom she believed could reverse the spell. The wizard replied, promising he would help her but also advising her to see a psychiatrist. In a later letter he confirmed her belief about being under a spell, which resulted in a heightened state of anxiety accompanied by her hearing voices.

Early one morning, she ran into a church screaming and caused a commotion at the beckoning of the voices she had heard. Maria confessed her sins to a priest and received communion. Immediately afterward, she became verbally and physically violent and was thus hospitalized. Her state upon admission was described as a severe case of psychomotor agitation accompanied by obscene language. She was successfully treated but attributes her improvement not to medicine alone but to the power of the Milan wizard in freeing her of the spell.

In both of these cases, if the psychiatrists had merely examined the patients according to nosographic classifications and ignored the cultural impact of belief in magic and the supernatural, they would not have fully understood the patients' conditions. Both the psychodynamic aspects and cultural background of the patient must be taken into account in arriving at a differential diagnosis and treatment plan.

An urban case: Anna. The approach just mentioned is also valid in examining an urban Roman case that synthesizes religion and magic. Anna first presented at the mental health center when she was 18 years old. She was accompanied by her mother, who was concerned about her daughter's increasing isolation and antisocial behavior. Additionally, Anna had begun hearing disturbing voices.

The patient claimed she heard comforting voices before she fell asleep at night. The voices often occurred in the daytime as well. Because her physicians were unsure whether these hallucinations were hypnagogic or straightforward, they did not prescribe medication so that they could observe the symptoms untreated.

During her second interview with doctors, Anna and her mother reported another relevant point: the girl had been receiving messages from the world of the afterlife through telekinetic writing.

Anna's father abandoned her mother before Anna's birth. Her maternal grandfather became a father figure to Anna, who lived with him during the summers in a farming village. Anna's grandfather died when she was 11 years old, and she had difficulty understanding death and her grandfather's disappearance. Anna initially sought help from her maternal aunt, a fortune-teller, but instead received solace in her neighborhood parish church. When she turned 14, she began spending all of her time in an evangelical community, well-known for the rigidity of its views and zealousness. At 16 she left this community because of its pressure for her to join a convent and become a nun. As a result of her leaving, she felt tremendous guilt, believing she had turned her back on God.

The telekinetic writing first began when Anna concentrated in silence for hours, focusing on receiving messages from angels and blessed souls, including her grandfather. During her reports to doctors, Anna expressed a strange combination of ecstasy and satisfaction about her mediumistic ability but showed that it also provoked fear in her. The therapist decided to undertake an active therapy that might slowly lead the patient to talk about reality. After a short time, Anna started placing less emphasis on her paranormal powers and began talking about her real world. Soon she began wearing feminine clothing and cosmetics and started dating. Anna still reported telekinetic phenomena and hearing voices, but she did so less convincingly and complained that the episodes occurred against her will.

The Roman upper class: Marco. The magical element does not appear in Marco's case; instead, the pathogenic power of atypical grafting of a religious belief is seen. At 25 years old, Marco was hospitalized under mandatory health care in the psychiatric ward of a Roman hospital for voice hallucinations, attempted suicide, and refusal to continue taking the neuroleptic therapy prescribed by his family doctor.

Marco was born in Rome of an Italian father and an English mother. He was enrolled in a private English school in Rome, where he was enormously successful. When he turned 18, following the dictates of the social standards of his wealthy family, he moved to New York to continue university studies in business administration. At the age of 24, he obtained his master's degree with honors and immediately enrolled in a highly professional postgraduate course in information technology. Professionally, Marco was accurate, punctual, and respectful, even though he tended to isolate himself. He could count on only a small number of friends made throughout his life, and none of these friendships was very close. The previous year, during his information technology course, he met a young Buddhist with whom he immediately became friends. This young man introduced Marco to a Buddhist community, where he began spending a lot of time. In the following 6 months, Marco presented symptoms of derealization and depersonalization. He felt completely extraneous to himself and to the surrounding environment and began having imperative and persecutory auditory hallucinations. He eventually returned to Italy, where he was admitted to a private clinic for approximately 1 month. During this period, he was subjected to neuroleptic and electroconvulsive therapy. When his symptoms abated, he returned to the United States and participated in psychoanalytic group therapy.

In October 1994 the symptoms that had accompanied his first crisis reappeared. His second return to Italy took on dramatic overtones, since it was interpreted as a sign of his nonrecoverability. This perception drove him to attempt suicide and to undergo forced hospitalization.

During his stay in the hospital ward, Marco managed to report to the interviewer, in lucid, precise, and totally nonaffective terms, that he had been upset by the meditation techniques he had learned and carried out with the Buddhist group. "They teach you to close your eyes and wipe out the world," he said, "and then to open them up again and project a different, ideal reality." "By closing your eyes," he added, "you can make yourself and others disappear. Imagination is the vehicle that leads to nothing, to inner peace." He continued to speak profusely about reaching a different dimension, of a "parallel world" in which time is canceled and reality disappears, and of an inner sensation of emptiness; "then came the voices," which were insulting and provocative. "They taught me to day-dream and since then, I have been seeing a beautiful and alien girl whom I cannot touch."

While in the hospital, Marco revealed his concern for his mental efficiency: "I'm not working," he repeated constantly. While in the ward, he became immersed in the reading of sacred texts (the Gospel and Old and New Testaments), which he explained by stating: "I need some points of reference. I need to confine and set boundaries to my mind." He again obsessively continued to repeat: "Buddhism is not for me. The Christian faith is my new spiritual guide; it can explain the mysteries. It is necessary to have a dogma, even if it makes you feel stupid; it doesn't matter." Later, he pressured the doctors on the ward with requests: "Please, program me. How can I program my dreams? Tell me what to do!" He acted like a robot, asking to be told when and how to eat and what to do during the day. He kept repeating, "I don't work anymore. I don't work anymore." After a week's stay in the hospital, Marco agreed to continue the therapy on an outpatient basis and was therefore discharged from forced hospitalization.

Conclusions

The clinical cases reported in this chapter highlight the interconnection that exists among magic, religious beliefs, and psychopathological disorders. Magic and sacred belief systems can, in some way, explain mental disorders in antiquity and within traditional contexts. In psychodynamic terms, we have observed that the cultural structures of magic and sacred belief systems lend themselves well to rationalizing, in cognitive terms, a very deep-rooted psychopathological experience common in all cultures: the loss of one's ego (Dodds 1951).

The etiopathogenic element constant in the cases reported here is the robbing of the ego (Frighi 1984). It can appear in a form that is acted out blindly (the four Rossi sisters), in the form of a fascination for powerful persons (Maria), in the form of existential damage associated with real affective deprivation subsequently exasperated by an attempt to make compensation for it by transcendent means (Anna), or in the form of active religious conditioning that induces detachment from external reality (Marco).

Any attempt aimed at resolving the shortcomings of one's presence in our modern world may take a wide range of approaches that, nonetheless, develop along two main frames of reference: our patient may either turn to the healing hand of humanity or appeal for the help from the omnipotence of God. The former approach entails the hope and trust we have in the existence of fellow humans being endowed with therapeutic skills, as well as awareness of the limitations of human effort. The attempt to recover by relying on the power of religious salvation or, more generally, on healing techniques that transcend a scientifically grounded therapeutic approach opens the way to a metaphysics that gives the illusion of providing a faster solution to the crisis.

Both paths are characterized by stops, crossroads, and wayside hostels that are consistent with each individual's ideological strategy. We find there well-organized cultural institutions and therapeutic systems: the presence of an inquiring human being, outpatient clinics, medical instrumentation, and hospital wards. Along the other path we find fortune-tellers, astrologists, wizards, charismatic figures, prie-dieu, sacred shrines, tabernacles, miraculous places of worship, and the epiphany of the sacred.

Each one of these paths deserves a detailed analysis. The question is, how does the interaction between magical and religious culture and psychopathology change within a society in which great inconsistency exists between very advanced technical and scientific achievements and the persistence of strong beliefs in the supernatural? Furthermore, considering the folds of each religious faith, we are led to ask ourselves: what is the influence of a religious creed as specific as the one put forward by orthodox monotheistic religions, and how are religions "humanized" by the copresence of redeeming messianic figures?

If we are to accept the existence of "[b]ehavioral patterns found in the United States that have been argued to be psychodynamically and structurally analogous to what are labelled in the literature the 'Culture-bound Syndromes'" (and among these Hughes et al. [1997, p. 998] also mention anorexia nervosa and type A personality), why can we not consider the existence of subtype X or Y personalities that are structured around different religious ideograms that can prove to be highly invasive and conditioning?

Islamic religious fundamentalism, besides corresponding to materialistic types of interpretations, can also be reported as the straightforward example of personality traits deriving from specific contents of the Islamic religion.

The cultural product of religious ideology drawn from biblical monotheism seems to be a powerful resonance chamber for the emotions and the dynamics pertaining to more than one sociocultural setup. If the Rossi sisters and Maria still belong to the folkloristic world of peasants and assembly-line workers to the extent that it is willing to bear, with religious resignation, the shame inflicted by the world of magic as well as the very sufferings of Christ; and if Anna, who belongs to the lower middle class, appears to be influenced by "banal" forms of the supernatural, we have still to consider the existence of cases like Marco's. The Roman upper middle class is a privileged social category that, despite its lay values, proves to be rather inclined to fall prey to the charms of the more sophisticated forms of the supernatural (that is to say, to the fine interweaving of a polymorphous plurality of religious forms).

It seems to be of particular interest to refer back to the case of Marco, because it clearly shows a psychodynamic situation induced by transcendence techniques borrowed from a religious ideology, such as Buddhism, that is renowned worldwide. The introduction of such sacred-related techniques in a personality structure that developed according to parameters that are specific to the Western culture in fact produced dramatic results that, even if they could be referred to possible premorbid personality disorders and thereby be stripped of their power of causation, nonetheless prove to be liable to produce an altered state of consciousness that has taken on clearly psychopathological hues.

The ritual of making the external reality actively and rationally disappear (to a lesser extent, these are the procedures used in autogenous training) was capable of triggering a process of derealization that became patently pathological but that, in minor forms, can be found in more than one religious technique (Bartocci and Rullo 1994).

On further analysis of Marco's case, we see that it does not present the clash between reason and the supernatural that we discussed in the introduction as much as an exacerbation of the rationalization, aiming to make the external world disappear through the apotheosis of the rational technique of abstraction. The performance of these extreme forms of transcendence turn out to be very difficult to handle if we consider that the specificity of the active annulment technique performed by Marco is exceptionally similar to the mental performances typical of autistic types of pathologies.

The symptomatology of clinical cases, the new atypical figures of healers, and the new therapeutic techniques stuffed with catechism all represent the outcome of a *current* situation that determines the appearance of figures that synchronize with the cultural, historical, and individual needs of the moment.

According to this view, the supernatural can no longer be described by the forms that are traditionally handed down, nor can it be exclusively attributed to the patent representatives of sacred or magical belief systems; rather, it is to be looked for in the concealed forms existing in apparently lay structures.

If it is true that magic is to sacred belief what an abacus is to a computer (de Martino 1959), by paraphrasing de Martino, we can affirm that, within the context of healing attempts, the canonical miracle of St. Gennaro in Naples is to transcendence techniques used in some healing procedures mixed with lay, scientific, magic, and religious elements what fireworks is to the atom bomb (Bartocci and Prince 1998).

Transcendence techniques are a fundamental point, because the territory conquered by sacred belief in the culture of the twentieth century is no longer as easily recognizable as religious institutions might suggest. Rather, the invisible space behind the camouflages can be found in many forms of healing activities that would like to be defined as scientific (Bartocci and Gigli 1992; Lalli 1979). In this perspective, it becomes increasingly evident that psychiatrists need expertise in drawing comparisons among the patient's history, culture, and psychopathology (i.e., have a training in transcultural psychiatry); however, it is also necessary for every psychiatrist to know the workings of religious techniques, whatever form they take, to suggest a diagnosis that might be differentiated according to varying forms of supernatural belief, just as any psychiatrist can differentiate between illusions and hallucinations and pseudologia phantastica and delusions.

We cannot forget that the responsibility of the psychiatrist is considerable (Bartocci 1997). It is, in fact, the therapist's task to accept patients who, although they manifest a range of forthright psychopathological mental productions, regardless of whether they are of a religious nature, are nonetheless the most liable to undergo a therapeutic program insofar as these individuals still require a lay scientific treatment and not an esoteric performance. To propose a therapy stuffed with catechizing elements to anyone turning to a psychiatrist seems to oppose the request for medical treatment. Great responsibility lies in trying to provide answers to anyone turning to a psychiatrist for help because the success of the attempt depends on the individual responsibility and expertise of the therapist.

References

Bartocci G: Trance spiritualità e cultura: tecniche psicobiologiche induttrici di Stati Alterati di Coscienza (ASC). Attualità in Psicologia 2:231–239, 1997

Bartocci G: Review of: World Mental Health: Problems and Priorities in Low-Income Countries by Desjarlais R, Eisenberg L, Good B, and Kleinman A. Transcultural Psychiatry 34:123–125, 1997

Bartocci G, Gigli M: Il Mondo delle Intenzioni. Napoli, Liguori, 1992

Bartocci G, Prince R: Pioneers in transcultural psychiatry: Ernesto de Martino (1908–1965). Transcultural Psychiatry 35:111–123, 1998

Bartocci G, Rullo S: Le apocalissi culturali ed individuali: reazioni psichiche di fronte alla morte. Attualità in Psicologia 9:77–86, 1994

Bartocci G, Frighi L, Lalli N, et al: La coabitazione del magico e del sacro in Umbria. Attualità in Psicologia (in press) 1995

de Martino E: Sud e Magia (1959). Milano, Feltrinelli, 1993

Dodds E: The Greek and the Irrational. Berkeley and Los Angeles, CA, University of California Press, 1951

Fagioli M: Istinto di Morte e Conoscenza (1974). Roma, Nuove Edizioni Romane, 1985

Frighi L: Tematiche di influenzamento nella cultura popolare e nella patologia psichiatrica. Rivista Sperimentale di Freniatria 5:1599–1620, 1984

Hughes CC, Simons RC, Wintrob RM: The "culture-bound syndromes" and DSM-IV, in DSM-IV Sourcebook, Vol 3. Edited by Widiger TA, Frances AJ, Pincus HA, et al. Washington, DC, American Psychiatric Association, 1997, pp 991–1000

Italian Institute of Transcultural Mental Health: Psicopatologia Cultura e Pensiero Magico. Edited by Bartocci G. Napoli, Liguori, 1990

Italian Institute of Transcultural Mental Health: Psicopatologia Cultura e Dimensione del Sacro. Edited by Bartocci G. Roma, Edizioni Universitarie Romane, 1994

Karno M, Jenkins JH: Cultural considerations in the diagnosis of schizophrenia and related disorders and psychotic disorders not otherwise classified, in DSM-IV Sourcebook, Vol 3. Edited by Widiger TA, Frances AJ, Pincus HA, et al. Washington, DC, American Psychiatric Association, 1997, pp 901–908

Lalli N: A Proposito di Victor Tausk. Rivista di Psichiatria 2:88–98, 1979

Lukoff D, Lu F, Turner R: Toward a more culturally sensitive DSM-IV: psychoreligious and psychospiritual problems. J Nerv Ment Dis 180:673–681, 1992

Prince R: General and theoretical issues. Transcultural Psychiatry Research Review 8:18–22, 1971

Rovera GG: Problemi transculturali in psicopatologia, in Psicopatologia Cultura e Pensiero Magico. Edited by Bartocci G. Napoli, Liguori, 1990, pp 27–44

Simoes M: L'irrompere del sovrannaturale: tra crisi spirituale e crisi psicotica, in Psicopatologia Cultura e Dimensione del Sacro, Vol 1. Edited by Bartocci G. Roma, Edizioni Universitarie Romane, 1994, pp 33–48

Education and Training

CHAPTER 17

Developing Curricula for Transcultural Mental Health for Trainees and Trainers

EDWARD FOULKS, M.D., PH.D.
JOSEPH WESTERMEYER, M.D., PH.D.
KAREN TA, M.D.

In this chapter, we focus on the place of cultural psychiatry in any mental health training curricula and outline recommendations for content and curriculum based on this rationale. The practice of psychiatry is being shaped by the same global and national forces bringing change in virtually all major institutions, including medicine. These forces include the rise of multiculturalism, world migration and pluralism, health care reform and managed care, and cultural considerations and formulation in psychiatric diagnosis (American Psychiatric Association 1994).

The principle of *cultural relativism* has evolved over the past several decades and has entered the public's political consciousness as *multiculturalism*. Major ethnic minority groups in the United States are now requesting that their respective histories, arts, sciences, values, and politics be given equal voice in higher education and in the greater society (Coughlin 1993). The proportions of ethnic minority students now in universities range as high as 30%–40% in California, New Mexico, Texas, and Louisiana (Chronicle of Higher Education 1997). Health care reform seeks to increase the proportion of minorities in medical schools over the next decade.

As a result of these socioeconomic trends, it is likely that medical and psychiatric education of the next decade will involve the following:

1. Training an increasing proportion of ethnic minority medical students and residents.

2. Training all students to render culturally sensitive health care to an increasing number of ethnic minority patients.
3. Training all students to work in liaison and cooperation with ethnic-specific alternative medical systems that show enhanced outcomes.

Categories are complicated when race and ethnicity mix. "Ethnic-identities are often constructed by their bearers in response to particular circumstances as, for example, in the way Trinidadians and Jamaicans became 'West-Indians' when they settled in New York" (Coughlin 1993, p. A-7). Panethnic identification as a Black or African-American entails yet another level of solidarity and allegiance to a broader political coalition. Pluralism in health and mental health care will require that the education of the next decade involve

1. Training in utilizing and referring to therapeutic approaches and systems across cultures that improve disease states or quality of life (e.g., Tai-Chi and dietary and lifestyle regimens).
2. Training for practice in a pluralistic work environment.
3. A need to reevaluate previous research and to reconceptualize future research related to sociocultural matters.

Health Care Reform in the United States

Current market forces are increasingly transforming the way medical care is being provided in the United States. This reshaping of American medicine has profound implications for undergraduate and graduate medical education. During the 1990s health insurance companies and health maintenance organizations (HMOs) have required patients to enroll in primary care clinics and to be examined by primary care practitioners before proceeding to obtain care from any non–primary care specialists. Hospital stays have become briefer because more diagnostic procedures are now conducted in community ambulatory settings and because payers are limiting allowable hospital costs.

The locus of medical education has accordingly followed these shifts of patient care from the inpatient specialty wards to outpatient primary care clinics, where continuity, preventive medicine, and holistic approaches to the patient are important values. Educating medical students and residents in clinics where continuity of responsibility for health maintenance is the principal mission has major implications for the development of relationships with patients and colleagues. The student-doctor working and learning on one team, in one community, with one cohort of patients *must* learn how to work well with others in a respectful, committed, culturally sensitive manner in order to be successful. Such enduring structures of educational experience contrast with traditional rotational models. Rotating on a monthly basis from one service to another involves leaving behind one set of patients and treatment team members and moving on to a new set. In such a process the student-doctor never really becomes committed and involved with patients or staff. The student-doctor is always a visitor rather than a true "resident" to the ward or clinic and has no opportunity to develop committed, long-lasting ties.

The rotational structure of traditional medical education creates a cultural environment that fosters certain values and personality characterisitcs that some students have described as dehumanizing. Such a culture has functioned well to promote the learning of disease processes and the technical aspects of treatments but has failed to emphasize the highest standards of a biopsychosocial perspective of medical care, which incorporates the essentials of cultural sensitivity.

These developments have already resulted in several rather ironic trends in the practice patterns of general internists and psychiatrists. While psychiatrists are finding it more parsimonious to provide medication evaluations for psychopharmacological treatments and leave the psychosocial interventions to psychologists and counselors, internists are becoming increasingly more holistic in their practices. Ballard and Brown (1990) have provided a chapter entitled "Culture, Ethnicity, and the Practice of Medicine" in a general introductory text on human behavior for medical students. *Through the Patient's Eyes: Understanding and Promoting Patient-Centered Care* (Gertens et al. 1993) has recently been reviewed in the *Journal of the American Medical Association (JAMA)*. Other recent articles in *JAMA* have also included research studies on "the effect of ethnicity on physician's estimates of pain" (Todd et al. 1994, p. 925) and "race, class, and the quality of medical care" (Ayanian 1994, p. 1207). Internists are already treating large numbers of patients with anxiety disorders and nonpsychotic affective disorders using tricyclics, selective serotonin reuptake inhibitors (SSRIs), anxiolytics, and psychotherapy via their counselor extenders.

These trends in health care reform will result in the following:

1. An increased presence of ethnic minority patients in general medicine and psychiatric practice.
2. A greater need for general training in cultural sensitivity for medical students and general medicine, family practice, and psychiatric residents.
3. A reduction in the numbers of psychiatric residents nationally.
4. An increased need for training the psychiatrist to function as a psychocultural expert.

The DSM-IV Cultural Formulations

The recently published *Diagnostic and Statistical Manual of Mental Disorders, 4th Edition* (DSM-IV), of the American Psychiatric Association (1994) now reflects an awareness that valid psychiatric diagnosis must be predicated on considerations of the cultural factors in each patient's life. This perspective is explicitly acknowledged in the introduction to the manual, which states that "A clinician who is unfamiliar with the nuances of an individual's cultural frame of reference may incorrectly judge as psychopathology those normal variations in behavior, belief, or experience that are particular to the individual's culture" (p. xxiv). It can lead the clinician to judge variations in normal behavior, belief, and experience as psychopathology, when such is not the case.

The biopsychosocial model has offered the conceptual framework by which trainees in psychiatry learn to diagnose, understand, and treat their patients. This framework has by now become the standard, determining the spectrum of courses basic to any psychiatric training curriculum. The multiaxial system of diagnosis in DSM-III-R (American Psychiatric Association 1987) previously allowed formal diagnosis according to severity of psychosocial stressors within a year before the psychiatric evaluation (Axis IV) and according to a global assessment of functioning of societal roles both at the time of evaluation and during the past year. No formal methodology was suggested or required for rating other cultural factors that might have critically influenced a patient's behavior and beliefs or the diagnostic process itself.

In contrast, the DSM-IV now includes a formal guideline for cultural formulation, Appendix I, and a glossary of culture-bound syndromes and idioms of distress. This cultural formulation highlights the effect of culture and the expression of symptoms on definition of illness and treatment consideration and effectively broadens the scope of the biopsychosocial model (Lu et al. 1995). Specifically, the clinician should provide a narrative summary on each of the following cultural factors:

A. *Cultural identity of the individual.* Specify the individual's cultural preference group(s). Attend particularly to language abilities, use, and preferences (including multilingualism). For immigrants and ethnic minorities, note separately the degree of involvement with both the culture of origin and with the host or majority culture.

B. *Cultural explanations of the individual's illness.* Identify 1) the predominant idioms of distress through which symptoms are communicated (e.g., "nerves," possessing spirits, somatic complaints, or inexplicable misfortune), 2) the meaning and perceived severity of the individual's symptoms in relation to norms of the cultural reference group, 3) any local illness category used by the individual's family and community to identify the condition, 4) the perceived causes or explanatory models that the individual and the reference group employ to explain the illness, and 5) current preferences and past experience with professional and popular sources of care.

344 · **Education and Training**

C. *Cultural factors related to psychosocial environment and functioning.* Note culturally relevant interpretations of social stressors, available social support, and levels of functioning and disability. Special attention should be given to stresses in the local social environment and to the role of religion and kin networks in providing emotional, instrumental, and informational support.

D. *Cultural elements of the relationship between the individual and the clinician.* Indicate differences in culture and social status between the individual and the clinician and problems that these differences may cause in diagnosis and treatment (e.g., difficulty in communicating in the individual's first language, in eliciting symptoms or understanding their cultural significance, in negotiating an appropriate relationship or level of intimacy, and in determining whether a behavior is normative or pathological).

E. *Overall cultural assessment for diagnosis and care.* Conclude the formulation with a discussion of how these cultural considerations specifically influence comprehensive diagnosis and care.

These and other cultural additions that have been incorporated into DSM-IV will serve to shape psychiatry residency education for the next decade in the following ways:

1. Quality assurance mechanisms will require that complete diagnosis include a cultural formulation.
2. Cultural caveats now included under each diagnostic category will become required basic knowledge in psychiatry.
3. Seminars and case-focused conferences will be developed to ensure that all residents have the opportunity to acquire this knowledge.
4. Competence in rendering a cultural formulation will be a standard required by board examinations in psychiatry.
5. Quality assurance and board requirements for inclusion of a cultural formulation will increase interest and motivation in trainees in a cultural curriculum.

Setting Goals: Career Opportunities and the Curriculum

The curricular goals for education and training in cultural psychiatry depend on several factors, including the nature of patients whom the trainee is likely to encounter during the residency and thereafter and the emerging roles required of the psychiatrist in an evolving health care system. Most multiethnic societies (with a common government, educational system, language, and mass media) require clinicians who can provide cross-ethnic and cross-cultural services. Even in a largely monolingual and monocultural society such as Japan, where a student is likely to encounter few patients from unfamiliar cultural settings, exceptions are likely to occur. For example, there are large numbers of a Korean minority and foreign business and embassy staff members from foreign countries in Japan.

Generalists in medicine and psychiatry should appreciate the methods of cross-ethnic and cross-cultural diagnosis and treatment of psychiatric disorders, as well as the theories and principles underlying these methods (Westermeyer 1987). Certain trainees require more specialized education and training to prepare them for work in special settings. For example, a Euro-American psychiatrist working for the Indian Health Service or a foreign-born psychiatrist providing services for native-born Americans will need enhanced training in specific cultural issues to function comfortably, sensitively, and successfully. Special consultation and academic roles, such as those performed by some psychiatrists in Washington, D.C., who serve the special needs of the foreign embassies there, include many foreign-born officials and their families. Psychiatrist trainees may wish to be prepared for academic careers. Most of the larger and more cutting-edge academic departments of psychiatry have at least one cultural psychiatrist on their staffs who can teach and research in cultural psychiatry. Another career pathway might be in psychiatric administration, where one must be able to conceive and manage cross-ethnic or cross-cultural services. In multiethnic societies, the public mental health specialist must be able to identify cultural, societal, and politicoeconomic factors that ameliorate or exacerbate psychiatric disorder (Casimir 1993). The education and training of clinicians must also take into account the opportunity for consultation by experts in cultural psychiatry.

Curricular Objectives and Planning

1. The Medical Student

Knowledge: Medical student clinicians require knowledge of fundamental principles regarding the concepts employed in studies of language, culture, and medical anthropology. Such concepts should be applied to the clinical context (Pachter 1994). Fundamental principles include understanding the following:

- Cultural concepts: worldview, emic or etic, values, norms (ideal and behavioral), identity, and ethnicity.
- Linguistic concepts: denotation or connotation, translation interpretation, idioms, and local jargon and referents.
- Medical anthropology concepts: cultural idioms of distress and conceptions of illness and illness presentation.

Medical students should have some idea about how culture and ethnicity can modify the importance of work, family, illness, and death in the lives of their patients. They should appreciate the ideal cultural norms with regard to family organization and loyalty (e.g., patriarchal-matriarchal authority, patrilineal-matrilineal inheritance, and patrilocal-matrilocal-neolocal residence). Does illness represent a personal failure or moral lapse in the sufferer? Or does it suggest the action of a malevolent spirit that has been offended by the patient or a family member? Or does illness raise the question of a curse by an enemy? Does the patient fear death from the malady? In the patient's culture, what follows after death?

Medical students should also appreciate the existence of certain culture-bound or culture-related disorders (Westermeyer 1988; Westermeyer et al. 1989). They should understand the concept of pathoplasticity and the role played by culture in certain psychiatric conditions (e.g., eating disorders, substance-related disorders, and various somato-form, hysterical, or crisis states).

Skill: During medical school, student clinicians should undertake diagnostic evaluations with patients from a variety of ethnic backgrounds. Some foreign-born patients should be assessed. At least one case requiring the services of a translator should be assigned. These tasks will require demonstration of skills in the following areas:

- Diagnostic interviewing across ethnicities and cultures: methods of establishing rapport, the importance of facilitation and clarification, potential problems associated with confrontation, language interpretation and education, ethnic differences in eye contact and interpersonal space (or body envelope), and nonverbal communication.
- Patient versus family interviewing, cultural differences regarding confidentiality and privacy, and presence of a family member during assessment.
- When to use an interpreter, preparation for becoming an interpreter, conceptual models regarding interpreters, differences between translators (who are trained to transcribe materials, usually written, from one language to another) and interpreters (who are trained to convey meaning, emotional coloration, and symbolism from one language to another, usually in a face-to-face interaction), problems in being an interpreter, and how to facilitate the work of a translator (Westermeyer 1990).

Attitude: Students must be helped in appreciating their own ethnicity and their ethnocentricity, as well as the ethnicity of their patients, and remaining sensitive to the worldviews of others (Waters 1990). In particular, they must be assisted in recognizing how their own ethnocentricity may interfere with medical care. Such opportunities abound around problems related to alcoholism and drug abuse, trauma, and venereal disease. For example, one student whose religion forbade the drinking of any alcohol suggested that a patient go through delirium tremens to "teach the patient a lesson." He was instructed that his attitude was problematic because it would risk the life of the patient and not lessen the risk of future drinking and his role as a physician was to help—not judge—people who had become ill as a result of any cause, including human foibles; as a physician in the United States, such an action would put him at risk for ethical and legal sanctions by his professional peers and by the courts.

2. The Psychiatry Resident

Knowledge: The general psychiatrist should have sufficient knowledge to conduct at least a screening evaluation and emergency treatment with patients from unfamiliar ethnic and cultural groups (Foulks 1980). This task requires knowledge of the following:

- The effects of education and acculturation on orientation to time and space, addition and subtraction, and pencil-and-paper tasks.
- The utility and limitations of cross-lingual and cross-cultural assessment using psychological tests, especially those requiring language or familiarity with mathematical symbols and paper-and-pencil tasks.
- The dosage levels of psychoactive medications that are affected by race or ethnicity because of pharmacokinetics (e.g., tricyclics and neuroleptics) and pharmacodynamics (e.g., lithium).
- The cultural factors that influence transference and counter-transference.

Skill: Psychiatric physicians at the residency level should be able to conduct a cross-ethnic or cross-cultural psychiatric assessment (Westermeyer 1985). This requirement sometimes includes the ability to work with a translator in undertaking such an assessment. They should also demonstrate competence in the biopsychosocial treatment and management of such patients. They should learn to recognize when value, ethnic, or linguistic differences may preclude proper treatment and how to establish liaison or referral strategies to appropriate cultural experts (Guerra et al. 1994).

Attitude: Psychiatric residents must be able to recognize that all un-familiar traits, behaviors, thoughts, or emotions in a patient are not necessarily the result of psychopathology (Lu et al. 1995). Likewise, they must consider that unfamiliar dimensions of a patient may not be simply cultural in origin. Perhaps most important, the clinician must recognize and deal with cultural countertransference, negative or positive, such as actually occurred in one training program when a Jewish-American resident encountered a Palestinian-immigrant pa-tient. The resident conducted a competent evaluation but stated that his negative feelings about the patient's ethnic group prevented his working with the patient. His supervisor made arrangements for an-other therapist. In this particular case the resident might have prof-ited through supervision if he had been able to begin work with such a patient.

A Model Curriculum for Psychiatry Residents

1. Seminar Series

A yearlong seminar series on sociocultural psychiatry, including topics relative to social psychiatry (Moffic et al. 1987), public psychiatry, and administrative psychiatry, would permit the previously mentioned ob-jectives to be met. Choice of topics should reflect several considera-tions in addition to those objectives listed, including the background and experience of the residency class. Foreign-born residents with ex-tensive cross-cultural experience but little formal education in medical anthropology will require a different curriculum than native-born local residents with in-depth medical anthropology knowledge but little cross-cultural or cross-ethnic experience. A mix of both types of resi-dents provides opportunities for mutual teaching-learning experiences within the residency group.

Seminar participants should be actively involved in each presenta-tion, which can be accomplished in one or two ways. First, participants may present the formal results of their readings and other preparations for the first one-third or one-half of the session, followed by comment and discussion. Or a specified participant might lead off the discussion with a prepared comment, following the presentation by an outside seminar leader.

Establishing cultural sensitivity in the seminar setting. Cultural biases and ethnocentricities are universal human traits observed in psychiatry residents as well as their supervisors (Lefley and Pedersen 1986; Spiegel 1976). Many of these traits are based in implicit assumptions regarding values, such as what is right and good (e.g., equalitarianism) versus wrong and bad (e.g., dominance) and what is healthy psychologically (e.g., mature individuation) versus pernicious (e.g., family or group symbiotic dependency). Some are also based on more premature, often unconscious, symbolic equations of race, color, seductiveness, potency, mystery, and evil (e.g., "pure white" versus "the darker side" or "black magic"). Conscious attitudes, often ignored or denied, regarding biases inherent and learned within the context of the dominant-majority society can interfere with the resident's ability to obtain appropriate diagnosis and conduct appropriate treatments. Establishing the desired cultural awareness and sensitivity, therefore, requires more than didactic courses or a list of readings. A valuable experience early on in such a seminar consists of the ethnic self-disclosure described by Moffic (Moffic et al. 1987, 1988; Spiegel 1976). He recommends that the seminar leader begin the exercise, modeling the activity. The steps in such an exercise follow.

- Describe one's own national origin(s), first language, family religion(s), family rituals and celebrations, and identity.
- State cross-ethnic and cross-cultural experiences, acquisition of second languages, changes in religious or ethnic identity over time, and similarities and differences in ethnic affiliation of spouse(s) or friends vis-à-vis one's own ethnicity.
- Indicate ways in which one's early acculturation was accepted or noted and later acculturation to foreign culture(s).

Pinderhughes (1984) has found certain group exercises in ethnic introspection regarding reference groups of origin to be particularly valuable in this regard. These cultural sensitivity groups are best arranged for residents in their second postgraduate year. Each resident is asked to prepare and present responses to the following questions regarding ethnic and social identity to the group:

1. What are your ethnic backgrounds?
2. Which one is your primary reference group?
3. Where did you grow up, and what other ethnic groups resided there?
4. What are the values of your ethnic group?
5. How did your family see itself—as similar to or different from other ethnic and racial social class groups?
6. What was your first experience of feeling different?
7. What are your earliest images of race or color?
8. What are your feelings about being white or a person of color? What are your advantages and disadvantages?
9. Discuss your experiences as a person *having* or *lacking* power or opportunity in relation to the following: ethnic identity (including religion), racial identity, class identity, gender role, professional identity, and family role.

Helping residents develop sensitivity toward specific ethnic minorities may require inviting representatives to join in this group process. In this case, it might be especially important to include several men and women representing the minority group(s) most frequently encountered in the daily clinical experiences of the residents.

Field experiences within minority communities served by residents' clinics have also been found to be useful in developing cultural awareness. In this regard, meetings with community boards, counsels, religious groups, and the like to discuss their concerns with mental health issues and services can be especially enlightening. Such meetings may have additional benefits in facilitating policy and procedural changes in the clinic, leading to better liaison and more congenial access to services for the minority community. We have found that such field experiences for residents quickly dispel cynical biases regarding the initiative and capabilities often found in disadvantaged minority communities. This change frequently results in the resident developing a more positive, proactive attitude toward working with members of the minority community (Foulks et al. 1995; Westermeyer and Hausman 1974).

2. Readings

A number of textbooks on one or another aspect of cultural psychiatry are available (Gaw 1982; Hall 1959; Holtzman and Borneman 1990; Lin et al. 1993; Tseng and McDermott 1981; Wilkins 1986). None of them is the ideal text for such a seminar series, although several would be useful either in whole or in part. Perhaps most useful is the seminar leader being aware of available texts in order to select core readings or to list references for residents who are leading particular seminars. Given available time in the seminar, some key articles can aid residents in understanding the history of the field and research methodology. Residents should be urged to begin their own regular journal readings. Of the four monthly psychiatry journals, the *Journal of Nervous and Mental Disease* and the *American Journal of Psychiatry* are most apt to have articles relevant to cultural psychiatry. Such articles appear infrequently in the *Archives of General Psychiatry* and the *Journal of Clinical Psychiatry*.

3. Conferences

Before completing their residency, psychiatrists should establish a habit of attending conferences, at which up-to-date information can be acquired. The annual meetings of the American Psychiatric Association and Hospital and Community Psychiatry regularly cover topics relevant to cultural psychiatry. General psychiatrists can keep abreast of the field by attending lectures, courses, plenary sessions, case conferences, and symposia on sociocultural psychiatry.

4. Acquiring Skill

It is difficult to imagine a psychiatry residency in the United States in which access to cross-ethnic and cross-cultural patients is not available. In fact, in a recent survey of psychiatry residency training programs in the United States, Samuel and Silberman (1994) found that 83% of programs reported that their residents' clinical caseload consisted of between 20% and 100% ethnic-minority patients. The important consideration is providing for the development of skill, which can be initiated by case conferences or interviews conducted by skilled cultural psychiatrists. Then residents should begin cross-ethnic or cross-cultural assessment and treatment of a few to several patients, with supervision by a cultural psychiatrist.

Special issues in teaching psychotherapy. The multicultural nature of the United States renders the teaching of therapies specific to each and every identifiable ethnic group a daunting and impractical goal. However, questions remain regarding the extent to which a standardized psychotherapy is possible and applicable across cultural groups. Recent research indicates that members of many major ethnic minority groups in the United States are as receptive to psychotherapy as the majority. Sanchez and Mohl (1992) found no difference between a sample of Mexican-Americans and Anglo-Americans in terms of referral, compliance, and resistance to psychotherapy.

Flaskerud and Hu (1992) found that neither race nor ethnicity had any effect on the number of treatment sessions, treatment modality, or treatment setting in a large sample of white, African-American, Latino, and Asian-American patients in Los Angeles. Rumbaut (1985), Kinzie and Fleck (1987), Mollica et al. (1985), and others have demonstrated the efficacy of culturally sensitive psychotherapy with Asian-American patients, refuting the cultural stereotype of Asians as being unable to express themselves in emotional terms.

The therapist's ability to listen openly in an empathetic, noncritical manner to what the patient is saying and to mutually decide on the goals of the treatment is fundamental to any treatment, no matter what ethnic group is concerned (Adebimpe 1981; Bell et al. 1983; Brantley 1983; Spurlock 1982). Previous studies indicate that these skills do not come naturally; cross-ethnic psychotherapy must be self-consciously examined and learned (Ward et al. 1974).

Although some authors have argued that patients prefer to be treated by a therapist from their own racial or ethnic group (Vontress 1976), no studies have demonstrated that African-American patients do substantially better in treatment when seen by racially matched therapists (Pena and Koss-Chioino 1992). The confusion with competence regarding this issue has been suggested by Sue (1988). The ideal in this regard is that, regardless of race, gender, or other difference between patient and therapist, all are superseded by the education, training, and skill (particularly the awareness, understanding, and effective management of countertransference) of the therapist to effectively bridge this gap.

On the other hand, clinical experience and the teaching and supervision of trainees demonstrates that empathy develops more naturally, and negative countertransference is lessened, when a sense of commonality (whether real or imagined) exists between patient and therapist. Racially matched or cross-matched, each configuration of patient and therapist has its own unique ways of catalyzing, facilitating, or potentially encumbering the psychotherapeutic process (Foulks et al. 1995).

Cultural differences may so fascinate the resident therapist that the treatment is distracted from the reality of the patient's core conflict to inquiries of a more anthropological nature. Comas-Diaz and Jacobsen's (1991) vignette of the psychotherapy of a Brazilian-American patient is particularly illustrative in this regard. In this case, substantial time was spent in therapy discussing the cultural meanings of interactions with friends during carnival, while the patient's biological proclivities toward and defensive use of hypomania were overlooked. Conversely, the majority therapist may deny that cultural differences have any relevance to psychotherapy and believe that all patients are or should be just like the therapist (Comas-Diaz and Jacobsen 1991; Westermeyer 1989). The exuberance of this revelation may often pave the way to unwarranted assumptions regarding social values, which may interfere with an insightful-empathetic enactment of mutual goal setting. In addition, the therapist may overlook and underemphasize the special needs associated with specific minority membership to the point of cultural insensitivity. On the other hand, overemphasizing the generally perceived needs of special populations leads toward negative (or even positive) cultural stereotyping.

Race or ethnicity, gender, religion, and socioeconomic status are potent factors that often set the patient at a perceived distance from the therapist (Yager et al. 1989). When the patient is a person of color and the therapist is white, the issue of racism is an inevitable factor interwoven with multiple other concerns. How these concerns, perceptions, and previous experiences of racism are manifested is dependent on many complex variables. The potential for countertransference enactments is great, however, especially if the therapist fails to promptly understand and effectively deal with these issues. By doing so, the therapist conveys a sensitivity to the patient's contextual history and experiences (Jones and Seagull 1977) that is self-affirming and facilitates an empathic engagement. Only then does the therapist establish a sense of credibility with the patient that provides opportunity for an effective, working therapeutic alliance (Sue and Zane 1987).

Issues of supervising residents in the treatment of such cases are equally complex. On the one hand, each resident should have individualized case supervision with a faculty member who can best represent and understand the special requirements of their ethnic minority patient(s). On the other hand, Cheng and Lo (1991) have argued that differences in culture between the patient and the therapist (and the supervisor) may offer unique insights while preventing overidentification and cultural myopic blind spots in the treatment. They argue that, with proper sensitivity, an outsider can provide a different set of values and alternatives to help the patient cope with the stresses taken for granted in living in American society. Cheng and Lo's argument applies to both majority therapist–minority patient and minority therapist–majority patient situations.

3. The Cultural Psychiatrist

Some residents may wish to pursue training beyond the 4 years required in general psychiatry to gain special expertise in cultural psychiatry. Although this field is unlikely to acquire the status of a boarded subspecialty in psychiatry, unique career pathways may be realized.

Knowledge: The expert in cultural psychiatry should acquire advanced knowledge in the following areas:

- Psychiatric epidemiology: similarities and differences in rates across cultures and ethnicities, differences in rates across time within the same culture (in association with diverse environmental influences), methods of sampling and data collection and their effects on the data, and history of psychiatric epidemiology.
- Sociocultural factors that can increase or decrease the rates of psychiatric disorder (e.g., rapid change, religious strictures and practices, and voluntary and involuntary migration).
- Psychopathology and culture: themes in culture-bound or culture-related syndromes, pathoplasticity in psychopathology across cultures, modes of cultural influence in various psychi-

atric disorders, special symptoms apt to be observed in those outside their own culture (e.g., somatization, suspiciousness, and paranoid symptoms), and various Axis III conditions that can produce or mimic Axis I disorders (e.g., sickle-cell disease, cerebral malaria, avitaminosis, various dementias, and heavy metal poisoning from folk nostrums).

- Methods of psychiatric assessment across cultures: interviewing techniques, mental status examination, use of rating scales, psychological testing, physical-neurological examination, and laboratory tests across cultures.
- Pharmacotherapy across cultures: compliance and culture, potential effects of concurrent folk nostrums, and pharmacokinetic and pharmacodynamic differences among races and ethnicities.
- Psychotherapy across cultures: models for working with interpreters; cultural transference and countertransference; and special cultural issues concerning couples, family, or group psychotherapy.
- Public health aspects: designing and implementing treatment systems for special populations and prevention using sociocultural knowledge and principles.
- Principles of teaching: the expert should be able to teach cultural psychiatry in diverse situations (e.g., consultation and liaison, lecture, and case conference).
- Principles of research: experts should have sufficient familiarity with research to interpret and apply up-to-date research findings, be able to conduct research procedures and teach and publish in their chosen field (e.g., review the literature and write a chapter or prepare and publish case reports), and have the opportunity during training to learn more advanced research techniques or work with other experts (e.g., psychiatric epidemiology, descriptive psychopathology, and treatment outcome).

Skills. The core skill in cultural psychiatry is the ability to assess and treat patients from ethnicities and cultures different from one's own ethnicity and culture. This skill includes the ability to plan and implement assessment and treatment, even with a patient whose ethnicity, culture, or language is unfamiliar to the expert. Second, the expert should be able to teach others the knowledge and skill that they require, whether at the generalist, specialist, or expert level. Third, he or she should be able to read and understand the research literature and to conduct research in selected areas. Fourth, the expert should be able to participate in the design of sensitive and effective psychiatric services for special populations. All of these core skills require experience under supervision. Since it may not be feasible to design a new project during a fellowship, fellows in cultural psychiatry should be able to play a responsible role in such a program. The latter experience can be supplemented by readings. In the postresidency phase of one's career, it may be necessary to seek further mentoring in the process of developing such programs (Collins et al. 1984; Westermeyer and Hausman 1974).

Attitudes. Cultural psychiatrists must have a willingness to explore their ethnocentric ideas and values, as well as their feelings toward their own ethnicity and culture. That is, they must be willing to discover their own unknown thoughts or feelings as these reflect their backgrounds. They must be able to recognize and cope with ethnocentricity in their students and trainees, without being upset or angered by it. (As a Zen master has phrased it, it requires "a very calm mind" to accept in others those foibles that we have had to struggle with in ourselves.) Since no cultural psychiatrist can learn all cultures and ethnicities, even in a lifetime, the cultural psychiatrist must anticipate a lifelong learning process.

A Model Curriculum for Fellows in Cultural Psychiatry

1. Seminar Series

A psychiatric fellowship in sociocultural psychiatry should include a seminar that would provide trainees with a broad knowledge about cultural issues in psychiatry. Topics should include epidemiological concepts, worldviews, and psychopathology across cultures. Other important topics include psychotherapy across culture and language, psychopharmacology across ethnicities and races, and psychological testing across cultures. The fields of medical anthropology, public health, and epidemiology can offer differing and valuable perspectives on transcultural aspects of mental health. Personal accounts or case reports may elicit interesting discussions among trainees.

The speakers invited to the seminar should depend heavily on seminar leaders who are mental health professionals experienced in transcultural mental health. They may be involved in research projects studying cultural issues in psychiatry or they may be in practice (e.g., community mental health or a refugee program). These experts may come from various disciplines, such as psychiatry, psychology, public health, and anthropology. People with cross-disciplinary training or experience can be especially valuable as seminar leaders.

Ideally, the coordinator for the seminar should be a faculty member assisted by an advanced fellow in the program. The faculty member should be responsible for planning the seminar series, assisted by the fellow. Either the faculty member or the fellow may invite the seminar leaders, although this can be excellent experience for the fellow to develop skills as an educational leader. The seminar should be well publicized by posted flyers and mailed invitations and schedules. The target audiences are psychiatry residents, attending psychiatrists from academic settings, mental health professionals in practice (especially those treating special patient populations), and anthropologists with mental health interests. Anthropologists and public health officials who have interest in serving ethnic groups may be invited to participate in the seminar. Following 30–45 minutes of formal presentation, the following 30- to 45-minute discussion period should be informal. Open discussion among the various disciplines should be facilitated.

2. Clinical Skills, Including Management, Administration, and Consultation

After acquiring knowledge about transcultural mental health issues and development of skills in treating patients across cultures, fellows should have an opportunity to apply their knowledge and skills in working with patients from diverse cultural backgrounds, as well as programs and teams providing such services. Supervisors should include cultural psychiatrists, some of whom may come from different cultural backgrounds themselves. Clinical options may include community mental health centers serving special populations and minority groups (African American,

Native American, Asian, and Hispanic) and clinics serving refugees, American-Indian reservations (under Indian Health Service), or poor rural patients. Trainees should be exposed to different social values among staff and patients. They should learn to recognize transcultural transference and to deal with countertransference issues in themselves, other trainees, and staff. They should be able to perform cross-cultural consultations referred by other psychiatrists or primary care physicians.

Cultural psychiatrists must be able to distinguish hallucinations from spiritual or preternatural experiences and delusions from cultural or religious beliefs. They should be comfortable with interviewing patients who are not fluent in English through translators. They must be able to obtain a relevant psychological consultation of patients whose assessment is limited by cultural and language barriers.

3. Teaching Skills

Fellows in such a program should have the opportunity to teach medical students about cultural issues raised in psychiatry practice, which can stimulate the students' interest in transcultural psychiatry. They should also take opportunities to present cases or subjects related to cultural psychiatry at case conferences and grand rounds.

4. Research Skills

Cultural psychiatry fellows should have opportunities to do clinically relevant research under supervision. They can review literature for specific topics. The trainees should have the opportunity to learn statistical and research principles before embarking on a project. With supervision and statistical consultation, they should be able to conduct a data analysis on a clinical topic (e.g., outcome study or descriptive study). Cultural psychiatry fellows should learn about the process of writing and publishing a paper.

References

Adebimpe VR: Overview: white norms and psychiatric diagnosis of black patients. Am J Psychiatry 138:279–285, 1981

American Psychiatric Association: Diagnostic and Statistical Manual of Mental Disorders, 3rd Edition, Revised. Washington, DC, American Psychiatric Association, 1987

American Psychiatric Association: Diagnostic and Statistical Manual of Mental Disorders, 4th Edition. Washington, DC, American Psychiatric Association, 1994

Ayanian J: Race, class, and quality of medical care. JAMA 271:1207–1208, 1994

Ballard B, Brown P: Culture, ethnicity, and behavior and the practice of medicine, in Human Behavior: An Introduction for Medical Students. Edited by Studemire A. New York, JB Lippincott, 1990

Bell C, Bland IJ, Houston E, et al: Enhancement of knowledge and skills for the psychiatric treatment of black populations, in Mental Health and People of Color. Edited by Chunn J, Dunston PJ, Ross-Sheriff F. Washington, DC, Howard University Press, 1983

Brantley T: Racism and its impact on psychotherapy. Am J Psychiatry 140:1605–1608, 1983

Casimir G: Rethinking work with multi-cultural populations. Community Ment Health J 29:547–559, 1993

Cheng L, Lo H: On the advantages of cross-cultural psychotherapy: the minority therapist/mainstream patient dyad. Psychiatry 54:386–396, 1991

Chronicle of Higher Education Vol 44, 1997

Collins J, Mathura C, Risher D: Training psychiatric staff to meet a multicultural patient population. Hosp Community Psychiatry 35:372–376, 1984

Comas-Diaz L, Jacobsen FM: Ethno-cultural transference and countertransference in the therapeutic dyad. Am J Orthopsychiatry 61:392–402, 1991

Coughlin E: Sociologists examine the complexities of racial and ethnic identity in America. Chronicles of Higher Education, May 24, 1993, p A-7

Flaskerud J, Hu L: Racial/ethnic identity and amount and type of psychiatric treatment. Am J Psychiatry 149:379–389, 1992

Foulks E: The concept of culture in psychiatric residency education. Am J Psychiatry 137:811–816, 1980

Foulks E, Bland IJ, Shervington D: Cross-ethnic psychotherapy, in Annual Review of Psychiatry. Edited by Ruiz P. Washington, DC, American Psychiatric Press, 1995

Gaw A: Cross-Cultural Psychiatry. Boston, MA, Wright, 1982

Gertens M, Edgeman-Levitan S, Daley J, et al: Through the Patient's Eyes: Understanding and Promoting Patient-Centered Care. San Francisco, CA, Jossey-Bass, 1993

Guerra L, Meza A, Ho H, et al: Medicine residents' practices in cancer screening in a Hispanic population. South Med J 67:631–633, 1994

Hall ET: The Silent Language. Garden City, NY, Doubleday, 1959

Holtzman WH, Borneman TH (eds): Mental Health of Immigrants and Refugees. Austin, TX, University of Texas, 1990

Jones A, Seagull AA: Dimensions of the relationship between black clients and white therapist. Am Psychol 32:850–855, 1977

Kinzie D, Fleck J: Psychotherapy with severely traumatized refugees. Am J Psychother 41:82–94, 1987

Lefley HP, Pedersen PB (eds): Cross-Cultural Training for Mental Health Professionals. Springfield, IL, Charles C Thomas, 1986

Lin KM, Poland RE, Nakasaki G (eds): Psychopharmacology and Psychobiology of Ethnicity. Washington, DC, American Psychiatric Press, 1993

Lu F, Lim R, Mezzich J: Issues in the assessment and diagnosis of culturally diverse individuals, in Annual Review of Psychiatry. Edited by Ruiz P. Washington, DC, American Psychiatric Press, 1995

Moffic MS, Kendrick EA, Lomax JW, et al: Education in cultural psychiatry in the United States. Transcultural Psychiatric Research Review 24:167–187, 1987

Moffic MS, Kendrick EP, Reid K, et al: Cultural psychiatry education during psychiatric residency. Journal of Psychiatric Education 12:90–101, 1988

Mollica R, Wyshak G, Coelho R, et al: The Southeast Asian Psychiatry Patient: A Treatment Outcome Study. Washington, DC, U.S. Office of Refugee Resettlement, 1985

Pachter L: Culture and clinical care. JAMA 271:690–694, 1994

Pena JM, Koss-Chioino JD: Cultural sensitivity in drug treatment research with African American males. Drugs and Society 12:157–179, 1992

Pinderhughes E: Teaching empathy: ethnicity, race, and power at the cross-cultural treatment interface. American Journal of Social Psychiatry 4:5–12, 1984

Rumbaut R: Mental health and the refugee experience: a comparative study of Southeast Asian refugees, in Southeast Asia Mental Health: Treatment, Prevention, Services, Training, and Research. Edited by Owan TC. Washington, DC, National Institute of Mental Health, 1985, pp 433–486

Samuel S, Silberman E: Training in cross-cultural and ethnic related issues for residents in psychiatry. Presented at the Annual Meeting of Directors of Psychiatry Residency Training. New Orleans, LA, 1994

Sanchez E, Mohl P: Psychotherapy with Mexican American patients. Am J Psychiatry 149:626–630, 1992

Spiegel JP: Cultural aspects of transference and countertransference revisited. J Am Acad Psychoanal 4:447–467, 1976

Spurlock J: Black Americans, in Cross-Cultural Psychiatry. Edited by Gaw A. New York, Wiley, 1982

Sue S: Psychotherapeutic services for ethnic minorities. Am Psychol 43:301–308, 1988

Sue S, Zane N: The role of culture and cultural techniques in psychotherapy: a critique and reformulation. Am Psychol 42:37–45, 1987

Todd K, Lee T, Hoffman J: The effect of ethnicity on physician estimates of pain severity in patients with isolated extremity trauma. JAMA 271:925–928, 1994

Tseng WS, McDermott JF: Culture, Mind, and Therapy: An Introduction to Cultural Psychiatry. New York, Brunner/Mazel, 1981

Vontress C: Racial and ethnic barriers in counseling, in Counseling Across Cultures. Edited by Pedersen PB, Lonner WJ, Draguns WJ. Honolulu, HI, University Press of Hawaii, 1976

Ward DC, Zanna MP, Cooper J: The non-verbal mediation of self-fulfilling prophesies in interracial interaction. Journal of Experimental Social Psychology 10:109–120, 1974

Waters M: Ethnic Options: Choosing Identities in America. San Francisco, CA, University of California Press, 1990

Westermeyer J: Psychiatric diagnosis across cultural boundaries. Am J Psychiatry 142:798–805, 1985

Westermeyer J: Cultural factors in clinical assessment. J Consult Clin Psychol 55:471–478, 1987

Westermeyer J: Some cross cultural aspects of delusions, in Delusional Beliefs. Edited by Oltmanns TF, Maher BA. New York, Wiley, 1988, pp 212–229

Westermeyer J: The Psychiatric Care of Migrants: A Clinical Guide. Washington, DC, American Psychiatric Press, 1989

Westermeyer J: Working with an interpreter in psychiatric assessment and treatment. J Nerv Ment Dis 178:745–749, 1990

Westermeyer J, Hausman W: Cross-cultural consultation for mental health planning. International Journal of Social Psychiatry 20:34–38, 1974

Westermeyer J, Bouafuely M, Neider J: Somatization among refugees: an epidemiological study. Psychosomatics 30:34–43, 1989

Wilkins CB (ed): Ethnic Psychiatry. New York, Plenum, 1986

Yager J, Chaug C, Karno M: Teaching transcultural psychiatry. Academic Psychiatry 13:164–171, 1989

Women and Children

CHAPTER 18

Children and Families
in Cultural Transition

Vincenzo F. DiNicola, M.Phil., M.D., Dip.Psych., F.R.C.P.C.

Children and their families who are in cultural transition present a complex but rewarding task for clinicians in mental health (Nann 1982). The task is made complex by the simultaneous flux and interplay of several variables (Bullrich 1989; Rakoff 1981; Westermeyer 1991):

1. The family's transcultural move from one society to another.
2. The growth and development of individual children.
3. The differential rates of adaptation of individual family members.
4. The different cultural definitions of interpersonal and mental problems and of culturally sanctioned solutions that shape help seeking behavior.

The task is rewarding because it provides the opportunity to work with people who are usually motivated to open and enter new doors of experience and willing to instruct their providers about their cultures of origin and to explore together newly adaptive approaches to living. This optimistic view may seem odd if one reviews the available transcultural literature, since much of it concentrates on the potentially disorienting effects of migration (Beiser 1989; Nann 1982; Pfister-Ammende 1973), the problems of getting immigrants to utilize mainstream health care services, or the underrepresentation of certain cultural communities in mental health services (Beiser 1989; Murphy 1973). There are both pragmatic and epistemological objections to this negative view of cultural transition.

Pragmatically, this literature deals with migration under the most difficult circumstances: waves of mass migration in earlier eras (e.g., the Irish in nineteenth-century United States), mass economic migration (e.g., *Gastarbeiter,* or guest workers, in postwar Germany), and war refugees and torture victims (e.g., Argentinians and Chileans [Allodi 1989]). Such accounts are as revealing about the limitations of health care delivery systems in host countries as about the cultural communities they hope to serve (Westermeyer 1991). A Canadian study of Soviet Jewish immigrants and their children (Barankin et al. 1989) found that children are doubly exposed to the direct impact of migration on themselves and to the adaptational difficulties of their parents. Nonetheless, the study highlighted the adaptive capacities of these families and outlined protective factors that make many immigrant children resilient and that can be used therapeutically. Furthermore, clinicians tend to mainly report problems. Few systematic studies have been undertaken on the experience of migration and cultural change among people without identified medical or psychiatric problems.

Epistemologically, transcultural research on migration has been shaped by *negative conceptions* of the transcultural encounter (Kracke 1987). According to the anthropologist Waud Kracke (1987), such negative conceptions include

1. "Culture shock" as a "self-limiting crisis" or "dysadaptation syndrome."
2. Immersion in another culture as "mourning."
3. "Anxiety" resulting from the overt expression of themes in another culture that are customarily repressed in one's own.

Kracke (1987) also outlines some more positive conceptions of the transcultural experience:

1. In the "regression-resocialization" model, initial problems in a culture induce a childlike regression followed by "growing up in the culture," or resocialization.
2. "Key relationships" with individuals in the culture lead to a construction of the larger society (modeled on the psychoanalytic notion of transference).

Transcultural psychiatry with children offers an opportunity to explore the transcultural encounter to construct new metaphors for child development (Valsiner 1989) and family experience and new tools for working with children and their families (DiNicola 1992). Constructing new metaphors requires a reworking of our notions of culture, child development, and family.

Looking Across at Growing Up: Two Immigrant Adolescents and Their Families

I would like to illustrate the aforementioned issues by examining the psychiatric problems of two adolescents and their families from cultural communities outside of the Canadian mainstream—an exercise that anthropologist Charles Super (1980) calls "looking across at growing up." These stories are about two teenagers whose families moved across cultures as immigrants. Despite numerous other differences, the teenagers have much in common: they are from cultures that support patriarchal family structures, their fathers are dominant and narcissistic, and their families as a whole tried to maintain the culture of their old homes while they were acculturating to their new homes.

Furthermore, their psychiatric problems emerged during adolescence, when violence or abuse triggered encounters with police, child welfare authorities, and psychiatric officials. The transcultural experience extended into and became a part of their therapeutic encounters with me. At times this experience was helpful and healing; at other times, the transcultural differences were a barrier. Lastly, these cases are representative of clinical work with adolescents in immigrant families, confirming the clinical lore that family moves are hardest for adolescents.

Parallel stories could be told about children and adolescents who experience cultural dislocation without moving. This situation is occurring among some native groups in Canada whose subcultures are rapidly changing. Observers hypothesize that the change is so great that the cultural continuity of families and communities is at stake. The devastating results for identity have created an epidemic of suicides among young native people in some northern Canadian communities (Gotowiec and Beiser 1993–1994). Similar intergenerational problems have been described in the rapidly changing societies in the Middle East (El-Islam 1983; El-Islam et al. 1986).

Alicia

Presenting problem. Alicia was a 15-year-old black Jamaican adolescent brought to my attention by the Children's Aid Society because of the violence she had directed toward her sister. The family also identified serious parent-child, marital, and family problems.

The violent incident occurred when Alicia and her 16-year-old sister, Marcia, were at home alone. During an argument, Alicia grabbed a knife and threatened her sister with it, lightly grazing Marcia's face. The police were called in, and the parents were contacted. The parents came home to face this situation with the police at their home and Alicia charged with attacking Marcia. The Children's Aid Society became involved because of protection issues, and Alicia was referred by the agency for a psychiatric assessment. Questioning revealed that over the preceding several months, Alicia had become increasingly withdrawn and sullen, angry at home, and failing at school. The violent exchange with her sister seemed to be the culmination of her family and social frustrations rather than a pattern of conduct disturbance.

Presenting family culture. The father, Gregory, was a well-educated, older black man from Kingston, Jamaica, where he had held a high-level government position. Marion, the mother, was a much younger, uneducated black woman from a rural Jamaican mountain town. In Jamaica, the parents had a *morganatic* marriage, that is, a socially sanctioned arrangement between two people of different "castes" without a conventional marriage. This arrangement gave Gregory the children he had always wanted and an attractive, constantly available younger partner. Marion received financial and practical support to maintain a house for herself and her children, where Gregory visited regularly and sometimes lived. They both agreed that she had free reign over the house and children and that he was a financially generous but busy and uninvolved father.

When political changes in Jamaica made Gregory's social position untenable, the couple opted to marry in order to immigrate to Canada.

In Jamaica, Marion had free reign over her daughters and her house, where the father was essentially a visitor. In Canada, they suddenly had to accommodate to a new arrangement: living together as married partners and sharing the parenting of their daughters. The patriarchal style of the father impacted jarringly against the matrifocal home of the three females. In Jamaica, Gregory's lifestyle of seeing numerous women was socially accepted (or so he said) and made possible by having two different homes. This arrangement gave him the narcissistic gratification he sought, but living together under one roof made it impossible. Confined to one relationship and now parenting his daughters for the first time, Gregory chafed at the restrictions in his marriage and demanded loyalty and obedience from his daughters. After a few years, because of the age difference and rigidly hierarchical relationship he demanded from his wife, Marion became more and more like a third daughter.

Transcultural family therapy.   During our first session, the two sisters, Alicia and Marcia, and their mother, Marion, sat quietly while Gregory explained why they had been sent to see me. The father told the story in great detail, patiently and deliberately. Attempting to include all of the family members, I posed questions or comments to them, asked for confirmation of details, and tried to get parts of the story from the perspectives of the mother and the sisters.

The father would listen attentively to my questions, then plow doggedly on, adding more details to his account or embellishing what others said. Within minutes, a pattern was set: Alicia and Marcia were sometimes successful in making some statements, but Marion was effectively silenced by her husband. I could not be sure about the feelings of the women in the family, but the father was clearly angry about the problems within the family and ashamed by the involvement of outsiders—police, the children's agency, and psychiatrists.

Noting this situation, I decided to move away from the presenting problem and work with the presenting culture. Because of Gregory's evident pain and shame and his dominant presence in the interview so far, I sensed that he would place me as an "outsider" to his world. My first transcultural intervention, therefore, was to adopt an outsider position. I expressed curiosity about Jamaica, noting that with my roots in

Europe and North America, I had never had the opportunity to live or work there.

Gregory launched into an informative and lively discussion of Jamaica, drawing a map of the island, describing his hometown of Kingston and the mountains where Marion had lived, and touching on the changing politics of the country. Again, I gently tried to draw Marion and the sisters into this exchange, with moderate success. So far, my approach had worked: there were more family interactions, less tension, and even some smiles and laughter as they described Jamaica and their home there. I now felt closer to Gregory, whom I perceived as working hard to be agreeable and helpful. I was genuinely fascinated by his culture, but I could also sense the pain of dislocation he must be feeling in shifting from a political mandarin in Jamaica to a midlevel civil servant in Canada.

The clinical issues I faced in this first session included the following: How could I help Alicia tell her own story with her family present? Given an unbalanced family, how could I join the family as a whole? Should I align with the father, who asserted himself, or side with the others, whose voices were not being heard? *Joining* is one of the first process issues in conducting family sessions. It was a problem from the outset with Alicia's family, because her father took charge and wanted me to fall in line with the rule of obedience that he obviously imposed on his family.

I decided to join the family *through the father*. I thought it useless to create a space for Alicia if this would heighten tensions in the family. After their experience with the police and the Children's Aid Society, I wanted to establish my therapeutic credibility by joining with the family as an ally rather than as an authority. Practically, I continued obtaining the history from the father, taking notes of his account, and occasionally checking details with other family members. The others looked as if they were pinned to their seats, helpless and hopeless. In a sense, I never succeeded at joining with the whole family. What I did note was a series of shifting alliances with different members of the family. I was able to engage Gregory as a person and, later, to join with Marion and the girls. However, the members never worked together as a family.

The parental couple. As therapy progressed, Marion's voice strengthened. I supported her in subtle ways, and gradually her daughters validated her right to tell her own story. Gregory's response was angry and dramatic.

He arrived at what was to be his last session stating with great ceremony that he had something to say. Ignoring the issues that had brought them into therapy, he complained that I had "questioned" whether he understood a word, treating him "like a boy in second form" (junior high school). In the previous session, when Gregory was discussing relationships with different women in his life, Marion asked him about a letter she had found from a woman that mentioned "eating a mango." From the looks they exchanged, I understood that this phrase had a sexual meaning. Gregory launched into a pedantic explanation about mangoes and then added, "I am dissembling." I suppose it was a kind of wink from one man to another, but it caught me off guard. Surprised, I asked him, "I do not understand. Do you mean you are not telling the truth?" Initially, Gregory may have been annoyed at my ignorance, but after the session, he apparently experienced my question as a narcissistic injury, which he resolved by rejecting me as a therapist.

But there is a greater systemic truth to his distress: the more damaging injury was coming from his wife, who was questioning their life together. My construction that he externalized the threat from the family system to the therapeutic system is supported by the words he used to end the session: "I must admit you have done one thing, which is to make this family 'circle the wagons.' You have made me realize that I must take things into my own hands as I should have done all along." He never returned. Marion responded to the offer of help for a time, and her relationships with her daughters greatly improved after her separation from her husband.

Alicia.   A reader of this chapter commented that Alicia gets lost in the description of the mother and father. This observation is astute: Alicia was lost in the fog of confused family relationships. If I had tried to engage the couple more overtly in marital therapy, Alicia's own dilemmas might have become clearer as the parental issues were acknowledged. The real issue is that Alicia got lost in the family move from Jamaica to Canada when the parental relationship was redefined. It is often true in troubled families that children are either ignored or recruited into dysfunctional roles. Children can be neglected when they are caught in triangles among other family members with stronger voices. Children can also develop psychiatric symptoms in an effort to resolve marital, family, or social problems and when they take on developmentally (e.g., adult) or structurally (e.g., parental) inappropriate roles.

Alicia's personal experience is complex. Although she was the identified patient, having threatened her sister with a knife, she felt that more often she was herself the victim of emotional and physical abuse within the family. Alicia felt she had been her father's favorite and was puzzled and distressed by his anger toward her. After her father's exit from therapy, when the family problems were explored in marital, family, and cultural terms, Alicia quickly experienced relief. Her relationships with her mother and sister improved dramatically with her father's emotional withdrawal from therapy and became stabilized when he left the home.

The family.   Experience with family therapy teaches that changing family alliances can create family tragedies. In this family, the changes were brought on by the combination of transcultural change from Jamaica to Canada, by the changing needs for self-definition that adolescence brought to the daughters, and by the mother's increasing realization that her morganatic marriage had given her too little. The mother's acculturation to Canada meant that she wanted more within her marriage, but, to her husband, this desire became an unbearable lien against the limited sources of his self-esteem. In structural family therapy terms, the family system regained the stable structure that had worked in Jamaica with a return to a matrifocal family.

In cultural terms, the parents could not adapt their marriage and family structure in ways that are culturally viable in mainstream Canadian society. Some family therapists suggest an acculturation model for migrants, using the notion of two homes, where the task is a constant integration of the old home into the new home (Turner 1991). The individuals in this Jamaican family were attempting this integration in different ways and at different rates, resulting in the family as a whole being unable to achieve a workable balance between the old and new homes. When the family reverted to its previous Jamaican structure, the therapy had to be renegotiated with them to deal with individual issues (especially the mother's and Alicia's) and with dyadic relationships (mother-daughter and sibling).

Samya

Presenting problem.   Samya was a 13-year-old girl who accused her father, Khaled, of physical and sexual abuse. In the course of an investigation of physical abuse discovered at school, Samya made an allegation of sexual abuse by her father when she was 12 years old. She was removed from her home. During her stay at a group home, Samya alleged she was raped. Her parents were distraught and angry, accusing the Children's Aid Society and the group home of unreasonably removing Samya from the parental home and then neglecting her. They blamed the society for Samya's behavior and for the alleged rape, pointing out that the social worker had supported "Samya's right to sexual expression."

    The Children's Aid Society and the Family Court Clinic were unable to establish a working relationship with the family. I was asked by the court to consult with the family as a transcultural psychiatrist and family therapist. I agreed to take on a clinical role with the child and her family if the court and the Children's Aid Society considered the investigation and legal issues resolved. In fact, they were stymied by the family but were happy to negotiate a therapeutic rather than a legal solution. My own goal was clear: to pursue therapeutic change rather than to clarify the charges and countercharges. What follows, then, is a psychological and therapeutic account of experiences rather than a journalistic rendering of actual events, which was outside of my agreement.

Presenting family culture.   Samya and her family are from the Middle East. The family members variously identified themselves as "Arabic" (a racial, ethnic, and political affiliation), "Palestinian" (a historical, geographic, and political affiliation), "Syrian" and "Lebanese" (where the father and mother grew up), and "Muslim" (a religious and political affiliation). Khaled, who was most vocal in his affiliations, ambiguously defined himself as Christian or Muslim due to his mixed parentage; he and his siblings attended French Catholic schools. After several other childless marriages, Khaled married a Lebanese cousin, Halifa. The birth of their first daughter inspired Khaled to leave the Middle East to live a new, more peaceful life. This man, who was passionately political and religious, declared that he held Samya "above my heart, above my God."

A transcultural reconstruction.   As a young child, Samya had enjoyed her special status with her father ("above God"), who treated her throughout her childhood as a princess. However, when she entered puberty, she started looking beyond the family and her father for affection. Samya had suggested (inconsistently and vaguely) that she had been sexually active before anything sexual occurred with her father (which was similarly vague and contradictory at different tellings). In my reconstruction, Samya's sexual awareness (and possible activity) set off a power struggle with her father, who experienced her as a changeling (changed, transformed, by Western culture and damaged by the perceived loss of her virginity) and as unavailable to him. In terms of Western family therapy, observers had felt quite uncomfortable with the father's lack of boundaries with his maturing daughter, his sense of ownership of Samya, and his instrusiveness into her emotional experiences.

Using the metaphors of his culture, Khaled labeled her as "betraying" him and as "promiscuous" and "ruined" when she (appeared to have) acted out her proscribed sexuality. Although no one could ascertain exactly what had happened, it is possible that since she was "spoiled" in his eyes, Khaled acted out his distress and culturally sanctioned disgust toward her by violating her trust and making sexual advances to her. Alternatively, to Samya, her father was a kind of mirror reflecting back to her a crucial source of her self-esteem. It is possible that in seeing herself "damaged" in his eyes she may have offered herself to him to prove her "loyalty" and "innocence" (virginity). In a more complex alternative, from an object relations perspective, father and daughter may have experienced fears and fantasies that could not be contained within the boundaries of the incest taboo. The spillover may have been partly projective fantasy and partly acted out facts on either or both their parts. The girl's charge of sexual abuse may represent any combination of fact and fantasy, guilt and fear. Certainly, the father-daughter interactions in the family sessions were filled with many highly charged, ambivalent, and anxious exchanges. The mother tended to side with her husband and appeared to be angry with Samya. Perhaps her anger was about the privileged relationship between her daughter and her husband; perhaps it was because Samya brought shame on the family. Observers of the sessions commented on what seemed, from a Western perspective, to be the mother's lack of sympathy for her daughter's distress.

Transcultural family therapy.   A portal of entry into this family's culture opened for me at the outset. After hearing of the father's complaints about the Children's Aid Society, the court, the lawyers, and Canadian society in general, I asked a few simple questions about their view of the problem and what solutions would be acceptable to them. Pursuing questions about how such problems are experienced in Lebanon or Syria was unhelpful because they denied that such things happen there, although this denial seemed unrealistic (see El-Islam 1983; El-Islam et al. 1986). The question for me was: How could I enter a family culture marked by pride and mutual support, whose solidarity was amplified through its involvement with the individualistic culture of North America, and whose wounded pride had made them rigid and defensive?

My approach to breaching this family's wall of solidarity was to join the members in their cultural style in order to understand their cultural assumptions. I should mention that I have a very special interest in the Middle East, having briefly lived and studied in Israel. Unlike my work with the Jamaican family, I could play with the option of adopting an insider role with this family or take a stronger outsider role as a Jew working with Arabs.

Needless to say, one can only consider such options if these personal identifications are sincere and genuine. Furthermore, the beneficial use of one's personal, family, and cultural background as therapeutic resources requires both personal growth and clinical experience. Useful tips for this approach include working with a cotherapist and a clinical supervisor and attending experiential workshops on personal, family, and transcultural matters.

So I posed this question in a session: If a family problem occurs, to whom do you turn for help? The answer was unequivocal: To the elders of the family. Accordingly, they were invited to bring one of the child's grandparents to a session, whom I called the "head of the family" and their "moral leader." It was a request they could not refuse, because they had suggested it and it was culturally sanctioned. We also progressed in defining their dilemma not as a psychiatric problem or a protection issue but as a "cultural question," which the father further redefined as a "human question."

When Samya's maternal grandfather arrived at the next session, I received him as the head of the family and placed him prominently as the guest of honor. Although I worked through a family member translating Arabic to English, my actions and my words conveyed a simple message: as head of his family, he could advise me about how to help his "children." He glanced at his grandchildren. "No," I said, "those children—Samya's parents." Ah! he nodded with understanding. The grandfather, who was visiting Canada for the first time from Beirut and spoke only Arabic, had a clear-headed view of *that* child's problem. Khaled, he said, was trying to raise his family in Canada the way people live in Beirut or Damascus. From what he could see about Canada, "this was a different place with different rules."

Khaled, who was very quick-witted, laughed self-consciously at this comment. He realized that his father-in-law had made an observation that no one else could have stated with any authority to him. Most Canadian therapists would not know enough to make such a statement, nor would Khaled have accepted it from them. This beginning set the stage for a very different kind of family interaction than was possible by the sanctions of Canadian courts or Western family therapists. Although what followed was an eventful, stormy course of family therapy, Samya was eventually returned home. The family and our team were able to work together with mutual respect, despite the eruption of the Gulf War between Iraq and the United Nations forces. Khaled was constantly on the verge of leaving the country to join the struggle. My own feelings were also high at this time. At the end of one session, I put a hand gently on his shoulder and suggested that we should both stay to take care of our families in Canada. Khaled did stay and take care of his family. By the family's own cultural measures of healthy child development and family life, the outcome was very successful indeed.

Case Discussion: Transcultural Processes

Many transcultural issues can be identified in these two cases. We can examine the reasons for migration and how the host country and new culture are imagined. Alicia's father was ousted by a change of government in Jamaica and Samya's family was seeking a peaceful haven from the political and military unrest of the Middle East. We can also examine each family's attitudes toward their starting points in how the native country and culture of origin are defined and redefined. Samya's family had idealized their origins, a process amplified by their problems in their new culture. Alicia's father sought political asylum in Canada but did not bargain on changing his family life.

Just as important to the construction of a therapeutic system is the cultural "fit" between the family and its therapist. Although I am different in many ways from both families—in terms of culture, religion, race, class, and ethnicity—it was possible to find points of joining. This connection was attempted by a combination of insider and outsider positions with each family.

Differential rates of acculturation. Looking at the differential rates of acculturation among family members is instructive. In both families, the children were adopting mainstream Canadian cultural values at a pace and in a way that threatened the internal cohesion of their families. In Alicia's family, this situation was doubly threatening in that both the children and the mother challenged the father's dominant role. Not surprisingly, Alicia's family could not withstand this double challenge, and a breakup ensued.

In each case, culture was explicitly brought to therapy by the families themselves, and their experiences reveal the dominant metaphors for culture, for migrants, and for diversity in their cultures of origin and in the host culture. Treatment of these families was not an academic exercise. Attending to these parameters allows one to map out the boundaries between the immigrant family and the host culture. I have suggested that the perspectives of insiders and outsiders (DiNicola 1986) usefully capture much information and help to predict how the encounter of different cultural values is resolved.

Insiders and outsiders. The language of insiders and outsiders helps to place where both the family and the host culture position each other and, in turn, where the therapist is placed in his or her transcultural encounter with the family. To Alicia's and Samya's fathers, I was potentially an intruder from an alien culture. In each case, this alien role was given to me by the father, but I was able to negotiate a more positive role for at least some of the members in each family. For some members of each family, I was a welcome outsider, a teacher about a world they wanted to enter. I had such a role for Alicia's mother and secretly throughout for Samya herself. While remaining different, I became a useful transcultural interpreter for Samya's family members, to the point that they relaxed the boundaries separating cultures. They began to share their political struggles and their home experiences (we conducted a session in their home as part of Samya's first supervised home visit).

Culture-bound developmental myths. The transcultural issues that arise from the family crises of the two adolescents, Alicia and Samya, include whether adolescent turmoil is a universal developmental stage or limited to certain cultures. In Canada, as in most Western societies, adolescent turmoil has become enshrined in folklore and in developmental psychology and child psychiatry (Rutter et al. 1976). Is adolescent turmoil inevitable for Alicia, who was raised in Jamaica, or for Samya, whose Arabic-Muslim family culture strongly values family loyalty and obedience? An anthropological review of 186 societies outside of the industrial West (Schlegel and Barry 1991, p. 198) confirmed the view of "adolescence as a social stage in all human societies." This thorough review of available research, however, failed to find the turmoil that is supposed to characterize adolescence in Western society in traditional societies, nor does it seem to characterize adolescence in modernizing societies outside of the West. Adolescent turmoil seems to be a Western European myth about adolescent development. Like culture-bound syndromes that occur only in limited sociocultural circumstances (e.g., amok in Southeast Asia and anorexia nervosa in Western societies [Simons and Hughes 1985]), adolescent turmoil is a culture-bound Western myth about life's stages. Only when they are challenged do these beliefs become obvious as myths, as the following outdated pedagogical myths attest: "children should be seen and not heard" and "spare the rod, spoil the child." Families also have their own private myths about their members, like the family therapy notion of the "scapegoat." Seltzer (1988) has written about how to edit and change the impact of such "destructive myths" in transcultural family therapy.

Clinical work in transcultural family therapy nonetheless reveals that generational problems exist in rapidly modernizing cultures. Japan is a very interesting example because of its advanced technological development and its relative openness to Western notions of child psychiatry and family therapy (for a Japanese perspective, see Shibusawa 1992; for a dialogue about the differences between British and Japanese families, see Tamura and Lau 1992). Rapid cultural change within a society can lead to differential rates of adaptation among family members (El-Islam 1983; El-Islam et al. 1986) and differential rates of acculturation when families move across cultures.

Cultural clash. Both cases reveal how difficult and how powerful the clash of values can be when one cultural tradition encounters another. For Alicia's mother, Marion, the clash was in the therapeutic encounter, because she was herself rejecting some aspects of her culture of origin. The clash occurred among members of the family, and only when Marion sought an ally outside of her family did it hamper the therapeutic alliance: to take the sting out of his wife's complaints, Gregory tried to disqualify me as a therapist. Samya first went outside of the family with her complaint but then retreated into the solidarity of the family, perjuring her own testimony. Confronted with legal sanctions, all of the family members preferred their own culturally sanctioned solutions to anything that an alien Western culture could offer.

As I read it, the stalemate between Samya's family and Canadian authorities was due to a cultural clash of values. The authorities responding to Samya's allegations adopted a rigid stance toward her family, leaving no room for discussion of different cultural and family perspectives. This situation was amplified by statements made to Samya's family about her right to express herself in a variety of ways, including dating and sexual activities. When the family members were forced to comply with the Children's Aid Society plan of care for Samya, and she then made a further allegation of rape while in the society's care, Canadian society lost all credibility in their eyes. The investigation was profoundly misguided: there was a confusion between the society's definition of child abuse and the family's culturally sanctioned rules for individual behavior (Samya and Khaled) and family interactions (father-daughter). Since the parents felt that their entire family and cultural value system was under assault, they avoided discussion of particular issues (Samya's allegation against her father). My therapeutic success with Samya's family was in positioning myself as someone who could resolve the differences between Canadian society and their own culture by negotiating goals that were acceptable in Canadian society achieved by means that were generated by their own culture.

Cultural adaptation. Conducting cultural family therapy raises the issue of the family's adaptive strategies (DiNicola 1992). These strategies can be examined in various ways, modeled on Kracke's (1987) analysis of negative and positive conceptions of the transcultural encounter. Mapping out boundaries of insiders and outsiders (DiNicola 1986), as discussed, can be revealing.

Another approach is to examine how families negotiate cultural change, which depends on how they bear their culture of origin, how they experience the host culture, and what models each of those cultures makes available to that particular family. If cultures provide a smorgasbord of choices, the subculture of the family and its class, caste, religion, and attitudes will determine the members' adaptive styles. One adaptive style is to develop a "creole culture" (DiNicola 1992)—a local blend of two or more cultures created through the layer-by-layer buildup of cultural elements, much like the syncretic religions of Brazil and the Caribbean. When this strategy is not possible in the face of cultural differences, family members sometimes employ "double description" (White 1986). Within the family culture, members endorse one set of cultural values, while outside of the family they experiment with and learn another. This is more workable as a family strategy than as an individual one, since it exposes the individual to loyalty conflicts within the family (DiNicola 1986).

We can call the overall process of adaptation *acculturation*, which spans the spectrum from *assimilation*, or total immersion into the host culture (such as the older United States image of the melting pot), to *estrangement,* or total separation (such as the former South African policy of apartheid). In the two families presented here, Samya underwent acculturation (adapting to the culture but retaining her cultural identity), while Alicia's father felt estranged or alienated from Canadian culture and from his own family as they assimilated Canadian cultural values.

Culture and identity. The working assumption of child psychiatrists and social scientists has been that when the cultural background is in flux, the child's core identity is less grounded, as expressed in Erikson's (1960) notion of "transitory identity" in children who are uprooted. In postmodern society, however, such transitoriness may be more normative, and the child as a cultural changeling may have more positive connotations. For example, bicultural children may develop a personal synthesis of worldviews reflecting the different cultures they have lived in to form a third culture: "This is an international population that has loosened its ties to a home country but does not become totally integrated into the host country" (Werkman 1978). Such children develop a sense of who rather than where they are.

A Model for Transcultural Family Therapy

The clinical approach taken with these patient cases was to understand and treat the adolescents using transcultural family therapy. Detailed arguments can be made for family therapy as a natural context for child psychiatry (DiNicola 1990) and for a synthesis of family therapy and transcultural psychiatry (DiNicola 1985a, 1985b).

At the heart of *transcultural family therapy (TFT)* is a transcultural encounter between the family and the therapist. This encounter is a special instance of the family's transcultural experience in a new and potentially alienating society. It can also be a provocative and demanding experience for the clinician. In my construction of this special relationship (DiNicola, 1985c, 1986, 1993, 1994), everything can be negotiated between the family and the therapist. The therapist must be attentive to the family system's definitions of self and family, as well as to what constitutes problems and solutions in the family's worldview. What demands even greater flexibility and therapeutic resources is that the therapist must be prepared to examine, adapt, or even discard the usual assumptions, methods, and goals of therapy.

The fundamental attitude and the most basic tool in TFT is *transcultural translation*. It is a much more workable attitude than cultural relativism or tolerance. Relativism and tolerance do not invite an encounter but rather mutual indifference. Conducting therapy requires a more active involvement motivated by curiosity about differences or the desire to build bridges across differences. The effort to translate and work across differences (rather than tolerating them) encourages both parties—families and therapists—to relinquish clichés, myths, and stereotypes and together to explore new perceptions, explanations, and ways of being. Working with diversity across age, culture, gender, and religious differences, I confirm my belief that "[a]ll therapy is a form of translation—of language, of culture, and of family process" (DiNicola 1986, p. 189).

Key Features of Transcultural Family Therapy

We can identify some general features of TFT with reference to the two cases presented here (adapted from DiNicola 1994):

1. TFT Deals With Culture Change

TFT sees families across cultures or in cultural transition. Having worked with several cultural communities in their home cultures and also as immigrants, I regard these as two very different experiences. The therapist should not underestimate the impact of a family's experience of strangeness in another culture, often under less than ideal circumstances and not of their own choice. Alicia's family felt forced to move and obliged to change the marital arrangement, whereas Samya's family was financially quite well off and had a sense of having other options if living in Canada did not work out.

2. TFT Is a Transcultural Encounter

Constructing a therapeutic system across cultural differences is a transcultural encounter. Contracting with each family to do therapy necessarily involves culture at the outset, because culture has shaped the members' most basic assumptions and premises about what a family is (the apparently fluid but orderly household arrangements that Alicia's family followed in Jamaica) and how they define problems and solutions (Samya's family denied the problems that were identified but was even more strenuous in rejecting the solutions offered by Canadian society).

3. TFT Adds Cultural Complexity to Family Therapy

In TFT, the encounter is as different from family therapy as family therapy is from individual psychotherapy. Viewing therapy through the perspective of system theory, we can see the individual as the first unit of observation and therapy. By expanding the field of observation to the family system, we gain a broader perspective with a correspondingly larger set of therapeutic possibilities. TFT is a further expansion of the systems observed to the levels of society and culture, bringing even more therapeutic variables into play. For example, TFT uses translation within sessions and analyzes different models and rates of acculturation among family members.

4. TFT Is a Cultural Product

TFT recognizes that all therapeutics are cultural products. Since family therapy was developed for Western mainstream populations (DiNicola 1985a, 1985b; Kaslow 1982), its techniques need to be adapted when applied in different cultures (Shibusawa 1992) and for immigrants (DiNicola 1985c). TFT may also be valuable in helping therapists step outside of their normative assumptions when dealing with newly accepted social circumstances (e.g., family therapy for interracial families or gay couples and their children).

5. TFT Examines the Family's Presenting Culture

TFT examines the family's presenting culture much as a physician examines the patient's presenting complaint. The families of the two adolescents described presented their own private versions of their cultures for my understanding, validation, and (in part) healing. Even the most resistant members—the father in each family—understood that some part of their old world was at odds with their new one and that change was inevitable. Their resistance was rooted in the fact that they wanted change, but on their own terms.

6. TFT Generates an Emic Perspective

By directly observing the family's presenting culture, one is enabled by TFT to examine culturally sanctioned definitions of the self and the family, what constitutes a problem, and what constitutes a solution. The therapist seeks insider, or *emic,* definitions. My therapeutic maxim for working with families across cultures is to go with the culture. In Alicia's family, where her parents' marriage was breaking down, this meant trying to understand the rules that governed her parents' relationship in Jamaica and tracking it through their move to Canada. In Samya's family, which found itself at odds with Canadian authorities, going with the culture meant finding some authority within the family's culture with whom I could negotiate.

Tools for Transcultural Family Therapy

Different approaches call for special tools, so it is useful to identify the particular tools that were employed with the two families presented here (adapted from DiNicola 1994):

1. Transcultural Translation

TFT works on the translation of culture as well as language, making family therapy a process of transcultural translation. The "hook" that worked with Samya's family was inviting the Lebanese grandfather as a kind of consultant. The tool making the invitation work in the session was translation. Transcultural translation enabled us to communicate across cultures very effectively. On the other hand, with Alicia's father, who spoke English in nuanced and artful terms, we seemed to be divided by a common language. The apparent ease of speaking in the same language made the transcultural barriers harder to perceive.

2. Multiple Codes

TFT is attentive to many languages or "codes," including communication by gesture and body language and the symbolic language of fables, myths, and folktales (see Greenbaum and Holmes 1983). TFT explores cultural metaphors to convey diverse experiences rather than only cognitive or theoretical explanations. The anthropologist and psychiatrist Arthur Kleinman's (1988) notion of elucidating the patient's "explanatory models" is a way to get clinicians to stop thinking in their way and to start thinking in the patient's way.

Although this approach is widely considered empowering by North American clinicians, many individuals and families are at a loss or feel threatened when asked about their explanatory models or theories. One transcultural problem is that in some cultures, people expect their doctors to be authoritative and directive and experience such questions as a demand to come up with their own answers. Western psychotherapies give priority to psychological mindedness, with an emphasis on the *individual* as the focus of therapy, using the *introspective* method to explore *intrapsychic* dynamics, with personal *independence* as a therapeutic goal (adapted from the work of transcultural psychiatrist Raymond Prince; see DiNicola 1985c). TFT acknowledges that human experience is vastly broader than cognitive schemata or mental mechanisms, taking place in a social context based on interpersonal interactions that create culture.

Paradoxically, by attending to the unique aspects of a particular family's culture and experience, the clinician can help its members build their own bridges across cultural differences to find common points of contact. Samya's father made a fascinating qualification when I reframed his family predicament as a cultural problem. By insisting that these were "human problems," I think he felt validated enough as an Arab by me that he wanted me to grasp something fundamental, perhaps universal, in their plight.

3. Insiders and Outsiders

TFT maps out the family's boundaries, using the perspectives of insiders and outsiders. It is important to understand where the family wants to place the therapist—as an insider ("one of us"—Samya's family soon accepted me with all of the generosity of Arabic hospitality) or an outsider ("one of them"—Alicia's father felt the need to draw a sharp boundary between his family and others by "circling the wagons"). Two further points are crucial. First, neither the insider nor the outsider role is in itself superior. Each can be beneficial or a trap; each role must be assumed consciously by the therapist. Second, one can occupy either or both positions within the same family (if this is done with genuineness) as a way to model adaptive cultural strategies.

4. Cultural Strategies

TFT explores the family culture's adaptive strategies. An attitude of curiosity in the therapist allows families to share in an intimate way their strategies of acculturation (e.g., Samya) and even estrangement (e.g., Alicia's father, Gregory). Stories of other families known to the participants or from history, literature, or movies can be helpful as models. I try to learn at least one new cultural family story from each transcultural family I see.

5. Cultural Family Life Cycle

TFT attempts to understand the individual child in a family life cycle framework generated by the family's culture. This approach allows the therapist to normalize even potentially explosive issues such as adolescent turmoil, differential rates of adaptation, and generational differences as normative family events in the face of change. In both Alicia and Samya, adolescent development was easily lost among the cultural and family issues. One had to attend to these broader issues before the individual voices of the girls could be heard.

Conclusions

Eric Erikson said that mental health is a condition of being "at home with one's family and with the future" (Nann 1982, p. 142).

There are several conceptual and experiential barriers to the use of TFT for children with mental disorders. These troubled children may seem strangers to us, because they are from different places (culture), have disturbing and alienating experiences (mental disorder), or the world of their childhood (development) has become unfathomable to their families or their therapists.

Nonetheless, transcultural therapy with children can be a rich opportunity to construct new metaphors for child development and family experience and new tools for working with children and their families (DiNicola 1985a, 1985b, 1985c, 1986, 1992, 1993). Its use may require a reassessment of our notions of culture, child development, and family. The three key propositions for transcultural child psychiatry include the following (DiNicola 1992):

1. Culture Is Integral to Self-Identity

Culture is one of the integral sources of the self. One examines the presenting culture of the child and his or her family much as one examines the presenting complaint in medicine. Culture should not be construed as a dirty window obscuring supposedly more fundamental biological variables, nor as an icebreaker in therapeutic work used as a prelude for diagnosis and treatment. Cultural variables should be relevant throughout all of the traditional phases of clinical work.

2. Child Development Is Contingent and Contextual

That child development is contingent and contextual means that childhood and adolescence are social, cultural, and historical constructs. Each society's experience of young people is deeply informed by prevailing beliefs. The cultural embedding of developmental beliefs is often more evident when looking at other societies. Westerners seem to find reports of suicides over academic achievement among Japanese schoolchildren tragic but absurd, whereas only comparative studies and the more recent efforts of specialists can disabuse Westerners of the notion of adolescent turmoil, which has the effect of denying or even normalizing the social epidemic of suicidal behavior among Western youth. The developmental psychologist Jaan Valsiner's (1989) culture-inclusive developmental psychology offers a powerful new paradigm to integrate culture and child development.

3. Familism Is Normative

The family is the significant living context for examining the definitions and experiences of stages of life. Family is the key context for therapeutic interventions aimed at redefining ages and stages and for adapting to new social and cultural realities. Transcultural family therapy is a model for doing family work with children across cultures.

Taken together, culture-inclusive developmental psychology and transcultural family therapy can provide powerful tools for understanding and treating children in transcultural flux whose identities can be complex, confusing, and transitory. The defining image for the twentieth century may come to be the endless exiles created by countless revolutions and wars. The worldwide conditions of exile and migration in this century continue to create problems but also a heretofore unimagined degree of cultural interpenetration. In future decades, children and their families may feel more enriched than isolated by such transcultural encounters. Our cultural future may be in the hands of the creative individual adaptations of "third-culture kids" and their family and communal evolutions into "creole cultures." Helping children in transcultural transition become at home with their families may aid them in developing the mental health that Erikson envisioned to enjoy a future that is culturally enriched (rather than merely complex), offering many choices (not just confusion), and syncretic (rather than transitory) identities, with each cultural encounter building upon the last.

References

Allodi F: The children of victims of political persecution and torture: a psychological study of a Latin American refugee community. International Journal of Mental Health 18:3–15, 1989

Barankin T, Konstantareas MM, de Bosset F: Adaptation of recent Soviet Jewish immigrants and their children to Toronto. Can J Psychiatry 34:512–518, 1989

Beiser M: Migration and mental health. Annals of the Royal College of Physicians and Surgeons of Canada 22:21–25, 1989

Bullrich S: The process of immigration, in Children in Family Contexts: Perspectives on Treatment. Edited by Combrinck-Graham L. New York, Guilford, 1989, pp 482–501

DiNicola VF: Family therapy and transcultural psychiatry: an emerging synthesis, I: the conceptual basis. Transcultural Psychiatric Research Review 22:81–113, 1985a

DiNicola VF: Family therapy and transcultural psychiatry: an emerging synthesis, II: portability and culture change. Transcultural Psychiatric Research Review 22:151–180, 1985b

DiNicola VF: Le tiers-monde à notre porte: les immigrants et la thérapie familiale [The third world in our own backyard: family therapy with immigrants]. Systèmes Humains 1:39–54, 1985c

DiNicola VF: Beyond Babel: family therapy as cultural translation. International Journal of Family Psychiatry 7:179–191, 1986

DiNicola VF: Family therapy: a context for child psychiatry, in Treatment Strategies in Child and Adolescent Psychiatry. Edited by Simeon JG, Ferguson HB. New York, Plenum, 1990, pp 199–219

DiNicola VF: De l'enfant sauvage à l'enfant fou: a prospectus for transcultural child psychiatry, in Transcultural Issues in Child Psychiatry. Edited by Grizenko N, Sayegh L, Migneault P. Montreal, PQ, Éditions Douglas, 1992, pp 7–53

DiNicola VF: The postmodern language of therapy: at the nexus of culture and family. Journal of Systemic Therapies 12:27–41, 1993

DiNicola VF: The strange and the familiar: cross-cultural encounters among families, therapists, and consultants, in Please Help Me With This Family: Consultation Resources in Family Therapy. Edited by Andolfi M, Haber R. New York, Brunner/Mazel, 1994, pp 33–52

El-Islam MF: Cultural change and intergenerational relationships in Arabian families. International Journal of Family Therapy 4:321–329, 1983

El-Islam MF, Abu-Dagga SI, Malasi TH, et al: Intergenerational conflict and psychiatric symptoms. Br J Psychiatry 149:300–306, 1986

Erikson EH: Identity and uprootedness in our time, in World Federation for Mental Health: Uprooting and Resettlement. Geneva, World Federation for Mental Health, 1960

Gotowiec A, Beiser M: Aboriginal children's mental health: unique challenges. Canada's Mental Health 41:7–11, 1993–1994

Greenbaum L, Holmes IH: The use of folktales in social work practice. Social Casework 64:414–418, 1983

Kaslow FW: The history of family therapy in the United States: a kaleidoscopic overview, in The International Book of Family Therapy. Edited by Kaslow FW. New York, Brunner/Mazel, 1982, pp 5–37

Kleinman A: Rethinking Psychiatry: From Cultural Category to Personal Experience. New York, Free Press, 1988

Kracke W: Encounter with other cultures: psychological and epistemological aspects. Ethos 15:58–81, 1987

Murphy HBM: The low rate of mental hospitalization shown by immigrants to Canada, in Uprooting and After. . . . Edited by Zwingmann C, Pfister-Ammende M. New York, Springer-Verlag, 1973, pp 221–231, 340–341

Nann RC: Uprooting and Surviving: Adaptation and Resettlement of Migrant Families and Children. Dordrecht, Reidel, 1982

Pfister-Ammende M: The problem of uprooting, in Uprooting and After. . . . Edited by Zwingmann C, Pfister-Ammende M. New York, Springer-Verlag, 1973, pp 7–18, 323–330

Rakoff V: Children of immigrants, in Strangers in the World. Edited by Eitinger L, Schwarz D. Bern, Hans Huber, 1981, pp 33–146

Rutter M, Graham P, Chadwick O, et al: Adolescent turmoil: fact or fiction? J Child Psychol Psychiatry 17:35–56, 1976

Schlegel A, Barry H III: Adolescence: An Anthropological Inquiry. New York, Free Press, 1991

Seltzer WJ: Myths of destruction: a cultural approach to families in therapy. Journal of Psychotherapy and the Family 4:17–34, 1988

Shibusawa T: Post-partum psychosis in a father: Japanese cultural dynamics, in Transcultural Issues in Child Psychiatry. Edited by Grizenko N, Sayegh L, Migneault P. Montreal, PQ, Éditions Douglas, 1992, pp 119–130

Simons RC, Hughes CC: The Culture-Bound Syndromes: Folk Illnesses of Psychiatric and Anthropological Interest. Dordrecht, Reidel, 1985

Super CM: Cognitive development: looking across at growing up, in Anthropological Perspectives on Child Development. Edited by Super CM, Harkness S. San Francisco, CA, Jossey-Bass, 1980, pp 59–69

Tamura T, Lau A: Connectedness versus separateness: applicability of family therapy to Japanese families. Fam Process 31:319–340, 1992

Turner JE: Migrants and their therapists: a transcontextual approach. Fam Process 30:407–419, 1991

Valsiner J: Child Development in Cultural Context. Toronto, Hogrefe & Huber, 1989

Werkman S: A heritage of transience: psychological effects of growing up overseas, in The Child in His Family. Edited by Anthony EJ, Chiand C. New York, Wiley, 1978, pp 117–133

Westermeyer J: Psychiatric services for refugee children: an overview, in Refugee Children: Theory, Research, and Services. Edited by Ahearn FL, Athey JL. Baltimore, MD, Johns Hopkins University Press, 1991, pp 127–162

White M: Negative explanation, restraint, and double description: a template for family therapy. Fam Process 25:169–184, 1986

CHAPTER 19

Psychological Consequences of Torture
Clinical Needs of Refugee Women

MARTA YOUNG, PH.D., C.PSYCH.

The distinctive and traumatic experiences of refugee women result in mental health needs that require specialized and comprehensive approaches to treatment (Morris and Silove 1992; Silove et al. 1991). In this chapter I examine current assessment, diagnostic, and treatment approaches to the rehabilitation of women survivors of torture. Each year, a large number of refugees emigrate to Western countries, such as the United States and Canada. Statistics further reveal that more than 80% of the adult refugee population are women (Kuoch et al. 1992), many of whom have been detained or tortured (Fornazzari and Freire 1990; Laurence 1992).

Torture is typically defined as "state-induced pain and suffering, whether physical or mental, which constitutes an aggravated and deliberate form of cruel, inhuman, or degrading treatment or punishment" (Amnesty International 1984). More than 98 countries practice torture on their citizens, with over 30 of them doing so systematically. Leading offenders include Iran, Iraq, Cambodia, Chile, China, Libya, Pakistan, Turkey, El Salvador, Guatemala, and, most recently, Bosnia-Herzegovina.

Current estimates suggest that between 30% and 60% of the world's 15 million refugees have been tortured. Although the majority of torture victims were traditionally thought to be young men (Rasmussen and Lunde 1980), more recent studies indicate that women are detained and tortured just as frequently (Fornazzari 1989). Furthermore, widespread evidence suggests that women are frequently subjected to sexual torture (Amnesty International 1990; Cole et al. 1992;

Mollica and Son 1989). Goldfeld et al. (1988) documented incidents of extensive rape and sexual torture of Cambodian, Laotian, Vietnamese, Chilean, and Salvadoran women. Similarly, a survey of Latin American women survivors of torture revealed that 64% had experienced various forms of sexual torture, with 44% reporting violent rape (Allodi and Stiasny 1990). These findings have led the United Nations High Commissioner for Refugees to designate women as a particularly vulnerable segment of the refugee population (Refugee Women in Development 1990).

The first two sections comprise an overview of the current methods and aims of torture practices, thereby describing the sociopolitical context of torture. In the third section, I review the relevant literature on the characteristic physical and psychological sequelae seen in women survivors of torture. This part is followed by discussions on assessment and diagnostic issues. Next, current approaches to psychotherapy and treatment are provided. The final sections briefly address potential burnout and future directions for clinical and empirical research.

Methods of Torture

Methods of torture can be physical, psychological, pharmacological, or sexual in nature. However, these various types overlap considerably. Physical torture, for example, often has a psychological component to it, and sexual forms of torture typically encompass physical and psychological aspects. Physical methods include beatings (e.g., slapping, punching, and kicking); electrical torture; cold water torture (e.g., submarino, or being continually dunked in cold water, and being forced to take cold showers and then stand in front of an air conditioner); application of burning cigarettes, chemicals, or scalding water to the skin; broken bones; removal of nails; and misuse of medication (Goldfeld et al. 1988).

Psychological methods involve verbal abuse and humiliation, false accusations, threats of execution of the individual or family members, observation of mock executions, observation of the torture or execution of others, isolation, sense and sleep deprivation, and extensive and prolonged interrogation (Agger 1989; Allodi and Cowgill 1982; Allodi and Stiasny 1990). Pregnant women are subjected to unique forms of physical torture. Electricity is sometimes applied to the fetus, and severe beatings in the abdominal area are not uncommon. Women who deliver in prison often witness the torture and killing of their babies or the removal of their babies by the torturers, who illegally give them up for adoption (Argentina).

Although physical and psychological forms of torture are well documented, survivors and mental health professionals have only recently focused attention on sexual methods of torture (Agger 1988; Bustos 1988; Mollica and Lavelle 1988). Many women do not disclose incidents of sexual torture, most likely due to the taboo surrounding this topic in many cultures and to the intense shame and trauma felt by the women who survive such torture.

Sexual torture can be carried out in one of two ways. The first involves forcing the prisoner to take part in sexual relations that are traumatic and humiliating, and the second consists of inflicting physical pain to the genitals and breasts (Agger 1989). Primary methods of sexual torture include heterosexual and homosexual rape, rape of women by specially trained dogs, application of electrical currents to genitals, observation of "unnatural" sex acts, forced masturbation, fellatio (oral coitus), rape by sons and husbands in front of torturers, and witness to the sexual torture of others (Mollica and Son 1989). In addition to these methods, there is often a general atmosphere of sexual aggression whereby one is pawed, forced to be naked, threatened sexually, and constantly subjected to lewd comments (Lira and Weinstein 1986).

Aims of Torture

The major aim of "modern" torture is to destroy the psychic integrity of the individual (Becker et al. 1990; Reid and Strong 1988; Silove 1988; Silove et al. 1991). As stated by Genefke (1987, p. 44), "the primary purpose of torture is not primarily to extract information. . . . [I]t is to destroy the victim's personality to break down, to create guilt and shame, to assure that he [or she] will never again be a leader."

From a clinical viewpoint, the aims of torture can be likened to a "twisted, up-side-down version" of what is typically accomplished in psychotherapy (Ritterman 1987, p. 43). As stated by Silove et al. (1991, p. 482),

> the sophisticated techniques used are often perversions of the principles which underlie psychotherapy, namely the heightening of the person's level of arousal, altering his or her level of awareness, loosening previously held beliefs and assumptions, and fostering an emotionally charged relationship with the perpetrators. The wider goal of this process, which is too often aided and abetted by medical practitioners, is to render political leaders and social militants powerless, so as to prevent further political opposition to the ruling regime and to act as a strong deterrent to other political opponents in the community.

Thus the aim of torture not only encompasses the individual but is also family and community oriented in that it seeks to destroy families and to terrorize entire communities.

Psychological and Physical Sequelae of Torture

Recent reviews of the literature indicate that the observed sequelae of torture can be organized into three major themes: incomplete emotional and cognitive processing, depressive reactions and life events, and somatic or physical symptoms (Ramsay et al. 1993; Turner and Gorst-Unsworth 1990). Furthermore, women who have been sexually tortured often exhibit certain identifiable reactions. Symptoms related to the incomplete processing of emotions and cognitions include recurrent and intrusive recollections of the event, intense distress when exposed to internal or external cues that remind the individual of the torture, associated hyperarousal (sleep difficulties, angry outbursts, and memory and concentration difficulties), and persistent avoidance of stimuli associated with the traumatic torture experience (Allodi and Stiasny 1990; Fornazzari and Freire 1990; Larsen and Pagaduan-Lopez

1987; Mollica et al. 1987b; Ramsay et al. 1993). The symptoms described are essential elements of posttraumatic stress disorder (PTSD), as outlined in DSM-IV (American Psychiatric Association 1994).

The experience of torture is also linked with a number of significant losses. Many survivors have to deal with the loss of body parts (e.g., limbs and eyes) and loss of their general health. In addition, many survivors face a lowered status at work, within the family, and among friends. Women refugees also frequently have to deal with the effects of losing family members through disappearances and summary executions. Fornazzari and Freire (1990), in a sample of Latin American women survivors of torture living in Canada, found that 40% of the women had close family members who had been executed or were missing. Such occurrences present formidable challenges for family members, who often cannot adequately mourn the loss because they are not certain whether the person is dead or alive. Women who were tortured while pregnant often lose their babies through either miscarriage, lack of adequate medical attention, or removal at birth. These losses are further compounded in asylum seekers, who must also deal with loss of country and culture, downward mobility, and rejection from host nationals (Turner and Gorst-Unsworth 1990). Not surprisingly, women survivors often exhibit a constellation of depressive symptoms that are linked to the many losses they have experienced (Becker et al. 1990).

Common somatic and physical sequelae of torture include headaches, stomach pains, scarring from lacerations and burns, fractures, tuberculosis, deafness and blindness, weight loss, broken teeth, skin rashes, chronic pain syndromes, head injuries, and difficulty walking due to trauma from beatings on the soles of the feet (Agger 1986; Allodi and Cowgill 1982; Allodi and Stiasny 1990; Fornazzari and Freire 1990; Larsen and Pagaduan-Lopez 1987; Mollica et al. 1987a). Pregnant women often miscarry or give birth to babies who suffer from serious medical complications resulting from the torture or lack of medical attention. Women's reproductive organs frequently are severely damaged physically by untreated pregnancy-related complications (Amnesty International 1990). Fornazzari and Freire (1990) found in their study that 26% of the women who had been subjected to physical torture had demonstrable physical sequelae.

Sexual dysfunction (particularly anxiety, avoidance of sexual relations, vaginismus, and chronic pelvic pain) is not uncommon in women who were sexually tortured (Bustos 1988; Goldfeld et al. 1988; Lira and Weinstein 1986). It has been noted that women who have survived sexual torture often have symptoms similar to those seen in rape victims (e.g., flashbacks during sexual activity, seeing one's partner as the rapist during sexual intercourse, and intrusive thoughts). However, some important distinctions exist between these two forms of sexual violence: "In rape, the act is experienced as being without meaning, while sexual torture can be conceived of as being meaningful if viewed as a part of a systematic process of destruction. Therefore, sexual torture has cultural and political dimensions which are different from rape in Western society" (Agger 1989, p. 313).

The previously mentioned symptoms of sexual torture can be particularly distressing for women and have been found to be more intense than those experienced from other forms of torture (Lira and Weinstein 1986). In one study of 28 Latin American survivors of torture, including sexual torture, the women still showed considerable adjustment difficulties 3 years after their traumatic experiences (Allodi and Stiasny 1990). Women who have been raped have to deal with not only shame and humiliation but often traumatic social repercussions as well. In certain cultures, the social stigma attached to rape survivors is such that they are often rejected by family members and friends. Cambodian women, for example, sometimes attempt to recapture their honor by renaming their rapists as husbands. Women who become pregnant as a result of rape face particular emotional and cultural challenges.

Diagnosis

Research investigating the effects of torture suggests that the most common diagnosis given to women who present with histories of incarceration and torture is PTSD (Allodi and Stiasny 1990; Mollica and Caspi-Yavin 1991; Mollica et al. 1987a; Pope and Garcia-Peltoniemi 1991). It has been found to afflict more than 50% of refugees who come from countries where torture is prevalent (Mollica et al. 1987a) and 70% of survivors of torture (Garcia-Peltoniemi and Jaranson 1989). In cases in which it seems appropriate to diagnose PTSD, it may be useful to specify its relation to experiences of torture and detention to differentiate it from other subcategories of PTSD (e.g., rape trauma, childhood sexual abuse, and therapist-patient sex syndrome).

PTSD in such populations is often associated with at least one other psychiatric diagnosis, usually major affective disorder (Garcia-Peltoniemi and Jaranson 1989; Goldfeld et al. 1988; Kinzie et al. 1984; Mollica et al. 1987a; Ramsay et al. 1993). Several studies have found that 80% of those diagnosed with PTSD were also diagnosed as having a mood disorder (Mollica et al. 1992; van der Veer 1992). A comorbidity rate of 50% has also been found between PTSD and anxiety disorders, particularly panic disorder and generalized anxiety disorder (van der Veer 1992). Other common diagnoses include pain disorders, organic brain syndromes (Westermeyer 1989), and adjustment disorders (Mollica et al. 1990).

Survivors of torture can also manifest transient symptoms characteristic of personality disorders (Sack et al. 1986). Passive-dependent and passive-aggressive traits, for example, may signal "adaptive" personality styles, acquired to survive the torture experience and live in a repressive regime. Similarly, common symptoms of PTSD (e.g., avoidance of close personal relationships and emotional numbing) may also mimic features of personality disorders. Personality disorder diagnoses should therefore be made with extreme caution with this population to prevent misdiagnosis (van der Veer 1992). Suggestions include delaying such a diagnosis until the survivor has resettled or waiting until treatment has been instituted. Patients may also exhibit personality changes due to brain damage secondary to torture.

Unfamiliarity with the sequelae exhibited by survivors of torture can lead to misdiagnosis and to treatment of presenting problems without attention to the real etiology. An example of such a case involves a 30-year-old woman who emigrated from Chile. She complained to her physician of memory and concentration difficulties. In particular, she reported that she was having problems taking notes during university lectures, because her "mind often wandered," and that she often forgot appointments and deadlines. A complete neurological examination and the in-depth neuropsychological assessment that followed were inconclusive, at which point she was referred for psychotherapy. After several months in therapy, the woman revealed that she often had recurrent and distressing nightmares and recollections of the severe physical and sexual torture she had endured during 5 days of incarceration in Chile 6 years before.

Another example involves the case of a 35-year-old Cambodian woman who was referred by the Children's Aid Society for neglecting her two children, ages 4 and 6. She apparently had difficulty taking care of her children (i.e., feeding them and monitoring their whereabouts), was severely depressed and withdrawn, and tended to be irritable. She was required to attend parenting classes and was referred to a psychiatrist for her depression. She was given antidepressant medication and asked to return for a follow-up visit in 2 weeks. A few days later, she made a serious suicide attempt and was hospitalized. During an in-depth clinical interview, she shared that she had spent several years in a "reeducation" camp, that her husband had been tortured and killed, and that her youngest child had died of malnutrition and disease.

Clinical Assessment

Dealing with cultural and linguistic differences.   Women survivors of torture are not only severely traumatized individuals but also migrants who often come from different linguistic and cultural backgrounds. One of the first challenges confronting a clinician is overcoming cultural differences so that he or she can develop "cultural empathy" (Dahl 1989). Survivors may differ in their presentation of symptoms based on their cultural background. Some evidence suggests, for example, that there are important cross-cultural variations in somatization (see Chapters 12 and 15 of this text) that may affect the survivor's treatment expectations. Westermeyer (1989) has suggested a number of useful strategies to help deal with patients who focus mainly on somatic symptoms, including 1) allowing the patient to give a full description of his or her somatic symptoms with facilitation and clarification by the clinician; 2) reviewing symptoms of all physiological systems; 3) briefly explaining the role of psychological, familial, social, and cultural factors in health; and 4) exploring these sensitive areas with the patient.

Furthermore, there are important differences in the causes various cultures ascribe to illness and to traumatic events. In various cultures (e.g., India, Cambodia, and many African cultures), illness is seen as being a result of coming into contact with malevolent spirits, witchcraft, and sorcery (van der Veer 1992). Cambodian survivors of torture feel responsible for their suffering, blaming it on their bad karma (Mollica and Son 1989). Understanding the patient's cultural framework becomes a crucial task for the therapist. Important sources of culturally relevant information include the patient, cultural interpreters, and anthropologists familiar with the patient's particular country or region of the world (Westermeyer 1989).

Another important cultural difference that may impact the establishment of a trusting therapeutic alliance is the degree to which a patient feels comfortable disclosing personal and distressing information to a stranger. Women survivors of torture, particularly sexual torture, often have great difficulty opening up to therapists. Their reasons include fear, shame, and distress at having to retell their stories; difficulty in trusting (particularly if the therapist is male); and doubt regarding the success of a psychotherapeutic approach to their torture-related trauma (Drees 1989).

Linguistic obstacles are often present when providing clinical assistance to survivors of torture. At times, the therapist or patient may be using a second language, leading to possible misunderstandings or communication difficulties (Westermeyer 1989). In many situations, the use of an interpreter's services is required. Working through a third party can pose several challenges to the attending therapist. Choosing a male interpreter when working with women survivors of torture may affect their comfort in describing the sexual torture and resultant sexual problems. Although some patients may feel comfortable with an interpreter from their own country, others may be profoundly distrustful of such a choice for political reasons. In addition, interpreters may make important translation mistakes, may change open-ended questions into leading ones, and may add to the questions and answers. Another potential problem occurs when the interpreter has experienced traumas similar to the patient's. This circumstance may lead the interpreter to avoid the subject, state that the patient does not want to talk about the events, or make translation mistakes (Westermeyer 1989). Therefore, clinicians must choose qualified and trained interpreters and the patient-interpreter match must be evaluated (e.g., for gender, political affiliation, and family tribe). A more thorough discussion of issues related to the use of interpreters and bilingual psychiatric assistants can be found elsewhere (Westermeyer 1989).

Nature of the therapeutic alliance.   The importance of having a working alliance that is characterized by an "ethically non-neutral attitude" toward the patient's presenting problems has been underscored by clinicians working with survivors of torture (Becker et al. 1990). In particular, it is "necessary to make explicit the political, social, and psychological alliance established between patients and the therapists who choose to work with victims of the régime. . . . [I]t is taken for granted that the patient's disturbance is the result of a traumatic experience inflicted purposefully and criminally for political reasons" (Becker et al. 1990, p. 142). Implicit in this alliance is the view that survivors of torture are not "sick" in the psychiatric sense of the term; that is, they are not neurotic or psychotic. Rather, their symptoms can be seen as consequences of having experienced extremely painful and traumatizing events (Becker et al. 1990). Therefore, this "bond of commitment" seeks to depathologize and demedicalize the symptoms often seen in survivors of torture.

Clinical interview.   One of the most important sources of diagnostic and clinical information is the clinical interview (van der Veer 1992). A comprehensive assessment not only includes a standard evaluation of psychiatric and psychosocial functioning but also assesses trauma history, including torture, pre- and posttrauma stressors (e.g., deaths in the family and migration or acculturation stressors), family history, pretrauma functioning, and current problems in adjustment and functioning (e.g., occupational, financial, and housing difficulties). Many refugees also suffer from debilitating pain syndromes caused by the extreme physical torture they have experienced. It may therefore be productive to refer survivors to a physiatrist or rehabilitation psychologist for an in-depth chronic-pain assessment (Turk and Melzak 1992).

It is also essential that women survivors of torture undergo a complete medical examination by a physician familiar with the consequences of torture. Many women have suffered the effects of starvation and frequently have untreated physical illnesses. Given the extent of sexual violence experienced by refugee women, they need to be examined for possible venereal diseases, pregnancy, and damage to their sexual organs. In addition, although symptoms such as headaches and memory and concentration difficulties may be stress related, many survivors of torture have suffered severe blows to the head. As a consequence, neurological and neuropsychological assessments may be warranted to rule out organicity.

Semistructured interview schedules. Self-rating scales have been found to be useful in the diagnostic process (Cienfuegos and Monelli 1983; Mollica and Caspi-Yavin 1991; Mollica and Lavelle 1988; Westermeyer 1989). A number of currently used self-rating scales have been translated and restandardized in many languages. Examples include the General Health Questionnaire, the Zung Self-Rating Depression Scale (Zung 1965), the Symptom Checklist—90 (SCL—90) (Derogatis et al. 1974), the Cornell Medical Index (Brodman et al. 1949), and the Minnesota Multiphasic Personality Inventory (MMPI) (Hathaway and McKinley 1943). Readers interested in obtaining information and copies of these translated and restandardized tests can contact the Refugee Assistance Program at the National Institute of Mental Health, Rockville, Maryland (Westermeyer 1989).

In addition, several semistructured interview schedules have recently been developed to document specifically trauma-related events and symptomatology (Allodi Trauma Scale [Allodi 1985] and Harvard Trauma Questionnaire [HTQ] [Mollica et al. 1992]). Many of the self-report measures dealing with torture, however, have not been tested psychometrically (e.g., Allodi Trauma Scale). One exception is the HTQ, which has recently been found to be a reliable, valid, and sensitive instrument for measuring torture, trauma, and PTSD in Cambodian, Laotian, and Vietnamese samples (Mollica and Caspi-Yavin 1991; Mollica et al. 1992).

The HTQ is a cross-cultural self-report instrument that measures torture, trauma, and related symptoms. It is composed of three sections. The first section consists of 17 trauma events (e.g., lack of food or water, murder of family or friends, and torture). Respondents are asked to report whether they have experienced, witnessed, or heard about any of the listed events. The second section includes a series of open-ended questions that require respondents to describe the most terrifying or traumatic situations they encountered in their country of origin or during resettlement. The third part lists 30 symptoms related to trauma and torture. Of these symptoms, 16 are related to DSM-III-R (American Psychiatric Association 1987) criteria for PTSD and 14 are symptoms commonly seen by the authors in their clinical experience with survivors of trauma and torture (e.g., "feeling ashamed of the traumatic or hurtful things that have happened to you" and "feeling as if you are going crazy").

Clinical experience with the instrument demonstrates that survivors of torture respond more positively to trauma-related questions when they are presented in a neutral, impersonal form (i.e., in a questionnaire format) than when similar questions are posed during a traditional open-ended psychiatric interview. Indochinese patients reportedly stated that it helped to "put words around" the trauma events (Mollica and Caspi-Yavin 1991).

Pharmacotherapy.   Although a thorough discussion of the use of medication is beyond the scope of this chapter, pharmacotherapy and other biologically based interventions often play an important role in the rehabilitation of survivors of torture (Silove et al. 1991). Many survivors have psychiatric disorders, such as depression, anxiety, and PTSD, that require active pharmacological intervention. Interested readers are directed to Westermeyer's (1989) chapter on somatotherapies and Rivero's (1992) chapter on the use of psychotropic medication.

Treatment Issues

Although awareness of the need for specialized treatment services for survivors of torture has increased in the past decade (Chester 1990), treatment approaches for highly traumatized and tortured refugees remain in their infancy (Goldfeld et al. 1988; Mollica and Lavelle 1988). Current approaches to working with survivors of torture distinguish between time-limited techniques that aim at stabilizing the patient and longer-term treatment options that attempt to help the survivor emotionally integrate his or her traumatic experiences (van der Veer 1992).

Time-limited goals. Survivors of torture are often significantly distressed and overwhelmed when first seen in therapy. Primary goals therefore include helping patients regain adequate functioning with respect to everyday behavior and reducing symptoms (van der Veer 1992). One supportive technique is to give survivors the opportunity to tell their stories so that they can express the overwhelming and distressing feelings they may be experiencing. In addition, providing explanation and information regarding the cause of their symptomatology can decrease any fears that survivors may have about "going mad," thereby alleviating anxiety.

At times, concrete assistance may be most beneficial for patients' immediate well-being. Women in exile must deal with the trauma, but they also suffer from a "concatenation of subsequent stressors which disempower them in the social, cultural, and political spheres" (Silove et al. 1991, p. 482). In particular, women refugees have to overcome a number of obstacles including language, housing, employment, acculturation, and prejudice and discrimination. Many women are seriously underemployed or experience severe downward mobility given their previous education and work experience (Stein 1986; Westermeyer 1986; Wiseman 1985). For some, residency status may be unresolved for several years, during which time they live in constant fear of being deported to the repressive country of origin.

These obstacles can lead to the emergence of immediate and concrete needs (such as finding a home or a job or applying for welfare) that need to be resolved. Often, refugees expect those with whom they have current contact, including their therapists, to solve these problems. Although therapists may not be able to address all of their concerns because of time or resource constraints, it is essential that an appropriate referral be made as a means of meeting a wider array of refugees' needs and establishing trust in the therapeutic relationship.

Longer-term therapeutic techniques. Many survivors try to cope with their torture-related trauma by attempting to forget it and pretending it never happened. In many cases, however, the trauma continues to live in the form of psychological distress and psychosomatic symptoms. Recounting the trauma is often seen as cathartic and is an important component of therapy with women survivors of torture. Several authors, however, have suggested that simply recounting and reliving the trauma is not, in and of itself, therapeutic and can in fact lead to an increase in intrusive and painful thoughts, with a concomitant increase in distress and symptomatology (Mollica and Lavelle 1988). It is equally important that the trauma be seen in a new context. Therefore, the clinician's main goal is to help patients reframe what has happened to them. This reframing allows survivors to avoid getting stuck in the pain by experiencing it in a more meaningful way (Agger 1989; Lindy 1986).

One reframing method is the testimonio, or oral history, developed by Chilean psychologists Lira and Weinstein under the repressive regime of Pinochet and initially published under pseudonyms (Cienfuegos and Monelli 1983; Dominguez and Weinstein 1987). This method consists essentially in helping survivors record in detail the painful and traumatic experiences they have gone through. In essence, the therapist encourages them to bear witness to their abuse by encouraging them to express experiences that had been relegated to the private domain. While the patient provides a detailed account, the therapist should help the survivor express emotional reactions to the torture. The testimony thus moves continually between the cognitive and emotional levels, seeking to integrate the affect with the traumatic experiences. While doing this work, it is important to respect the women survivors' defenses by encouraging and allowing them to work at their own paces. If survivors are pressured to open up too quickly, they risk being overwhelmed and revictimized.

Another important function of the testimony method is to help survivors reframe their experiences. One way in which this reframing is achieved is by *normalizing* and *validating* the patients' reactions and experiences. Therapists can provide reassurance to survivors that their symptoms are not defects but are indeed common in women who have undergone similar experiences. Comments such as "these are normal reactions to abnormal situations" and "many women who have been tortured have symptoms similar to yours," as well as continually emphasizing their strength and survival skills, enhances the patients' self-esteem. Through normalization of the torture experience, its aftereffects, and the resulting coping skills, survivors come to understand that their reactions were appropriate to the situations and necessary to survival. Their symptoms are not "crazy," and the survivors have the option to change or to modify symptoms that are no longer adaptive in their current lives.

Furthermore, it is essential to help survivors deindividualize the blame and reattribute the responsibility for what happened to them to their torturers and to the repressive and violent tactics of the regime. In this way, each survivor can see his or her "private symptoms as part of an attempt at ideological destruction" (Agger 1989, p. 314). In other words, it is important to reconceptualize the abuse by countering the denial and stressing its reality. Survivors need to understand that they are not responsible for their torture, nor did they cause the torture to occur because of something inherent in their personalities or characters.

Once the testimony is completed, the therapist and survivor read through it, rework it, and edit it. Thus, by repeatedly working through the trauma, cognitions and feelings can be processed until the traumatic events are objectified, and the "evil is moved onto the white paper" (Agger 1989, p. 315). In essence, "the testimonio, by retracing the thread of a life course until it was broken by the repression, and the survival skills that promoted life after the traumatic events, facilitate a recovery of personal and social identity, a mending of the lifeline" (Aron 1992, p. 184).

The following case provides an illustration of this kind of work. Juana is a 38-year-old woman who had recently emigrated from El Salvador to the United States. She was a secondary school teacher in her homeland and was active in human rights issues. Two years previously, she and her 18-year-old son were arrested in the middle of the night in their home. Both were severely tortured, and her son died of torture-related injuries while detained. Juana presented as severely depressed. In addition, she described feeling guilty, because she believed she had caused her son's death by her political involvement. Juana, provided with a safe place and the opportunity to tell her story, was able to begin coming to terms with what had happened to her and her family. It was important, however, to continually validate and normalize Juana's reactions and feelings and to help her reframe the trauma. A turning point in therapy occurred when Juana was able to resolve the issue of responsibility by transferring the blame from herself to the torturers and the repressive political situation in El Salvador. The transfer of responsibility allowed her to face her extreme powerlessness and helplessness in protecting herself and her son, thereby leading to greater self-empathy and self-esteem. Reconceptualizing the traumatic experiences and connecting her feelings with the torture allowed her to then grieve and mourn in a healthy fashion over her son's death and her other losses.

Reactions of Therapists

Dealing with torture-related trauma is not difficult only for survivors but also for the professionals who witness their pain. This effect has been referred to as burnout, "vicarious trauma" (United Nations High Commissioner for Refugees 1993), and "secondary post traumatic stress disorder" (Dolan 1991). The symptoms of secondary posttraumatic stress in health care providers are similar to those seen in survivors of torture. Symptoms include insomnia; lack of interest in relationships and sex; sadness and depression; feeling overwhelmed and incompetent; recurrent, intrusive thoughts of the trauma; nightmares or dreams about torture; generalized anxiety; withdrawal; cynicism; and discouragement (Bustos 1990; Dolan 1991; United Nations High Commissioner for Refugees 1993). Although therapists may differ with respect to their vulnerability to secondary posttraumatic stress, these symptoms have been observed in many highly trained and experienced clinicians.

These symptoms can be prevented or alleviated by engaging in physical activity, taking time off, using relaxation techniques, joining a support group for professionals involved with survivors of torture, seeking individual or group supervision, and managing one's caseload by ensuring an adequate balance of presenting problems (Dolan 1991; United Nations High Commissioner for Refugees 1993). The recognition of physical and psychological limits ensures that all professionals working with this highly traumatized population will provide continued ethical interventions.

Conclusions

Given the current political and economic upheavals worldwide, there is little reason to believe that the influx of refugee women to North America and Europe will abate in the years to come. Women survivors of torture will therefore continue to require highly specialized medical, psychiatric, and psychological services to help them alleviate their pain and suffering. Despite the pressing demand for assessment and treatment services, there is a dearth of professionals trained to deal with torture-related trauma. Similarly, knowledge about the clinical rehabilitation of women survivors of political torture in general and of sexual torture in particular is limited.

These conclusions underscore the need for further development of culturally sensitive treatment models for this patient population. In addition, research on the psychological and clinical needs of women survivors of torture is urgently needed. Areas to be explored more fully include the effects of gender and age on adjustment following torture; the usefulness and limits of a PTSD diagnosis for women survivors, given that it was primarily derived from the experiences of male veterans; the effects of sexual violence on women's well-being; and the identification of variables that moderate the impact of torture. In addition, treatment outcome studies are sorely needed. Although these suggestions are far from exhaustive, they provide a starting point for a greater understanding of refugee women's experiences and needs. Hopefully, this understanding will lead to the development of more specific approaches to the treatment of women survivors of torture.

References

Agger I: Seksuel torture af kvindelige politiske fanger. Nordisk Sexologi 4:147–161, 1986

Agger I: Die politische Gefangene als Opfer sexueller Folter [Female political prisoners as victims of sexual torture]. Zeitshrift für Sexualforschung 1:231–241, 1988

Agger I: Sexual torture of political prisoners: an overview. J Trauma Stress 2:305–318, 1989

Allodi F: Physical and psychiatric effects of torture: a Canadian study, in The Breaking of Bodies and Minds: Torture, Psychiatric Abuses, and the

Health Professions. Edited by Stover E, Nightingale EO. New York, Freeman, 1985, pp 58–78

Allodi F, Cowgill G: Ethical and psychiatric aspects of torture: a Canadian study. Can J Psychiatry 27:98–102, 1982

Allodi F, Stiasny S: Women as torture victims. Can J Psychiatry 35:144–148, 1990

American Psychiatric Association: Diagnostic and Statistical Manual of Mental Disorders, 3rd Edition, Revised. Washington, DC, American Psychiatric Association, 1987

American Psychiatric Association: Diagnostic and Statistical Manual of Mental Disorders, 4th Edition. Washington, DC, American Psychiatric Association, 1994

Amnesty International: Torture in the Eighties. New York, Amnesty International, 1984

Amnesty International: Women in the Front Line. New York, Amnesty International, 1990

Aron A: Testimonio: a bridge between psychotherapy and sociotherapy, in Refugee Women and Their Mental Health: Shattered Societies, Shattered Lives. Edited by Cole E, Espin O, Rothblum E. Binghamton, NY, Harrington Park Press, 1992, pp 173–189

Becker D, Lira E, Castillo MI, et al: Therapy with victims of political repression: the challenge of social reparation. Journal of Social Issues 46:133–149, 1990

Brodman K, Erdmann AJ, Lorge I, et al: The Cornell Medical Index. JAMA 140:530, 1949

Bustos E: Sexuality and exile in traumatized refugees: a psychodynamic understanding. Nordisk Sexologi 6:25–30, 1988

Bustos E: Dealing with the unbearable: reactions of therapists and therapeutic institutions to survivors of torture, in Psychology and Torture. Edited by Suedfeld P. New York, Hemisphere, 1990, pp 143–163

Chester B: Because mercy has a human heart: centers for victims of torture, in Psychology and Torture. Edited by Suedfeld P. New York, Hemisphere, 1990, pp 165–184

Cienfuegos A, Monelli C: The testimony of political repression as a therapeutic instrument. Am J Orthopsychiatry 53:43–51, 1983

Cole E, Espin O, Rothblum E: Refugee Women and Their Mental Health: Shattered Societies, Shattered Lives. Binghamton, NY, Harrington Park Press, 1992

Dahl CI: Some problems of cross-cultural psychotherapy with refugees seeking treatment. Am J Psychoanal 49:19–32, 1989

Derogatis LR, Lipman RS, Rickels K, et al: The Hopkins Symptom Checklist (HSCL): a self-report symptom inventory. Behav Sci 19:1–15, 1974

Dolan Y: Resolving Sexual Abuse: Solution-Focused Therapy and Ericksonian Hypnosis for Adult Survivors. New York, WW Norton, 1991

Dominguez R, Weinstein E: Aiding victims of political repression in Chile: a psychological and psychotherapeutic approach. Tidsskrift for Norsk Psykologforening 24:75–81, 1987

Drees A: Guidelines for a short-term therapy of a torture depression. J Trauma Stress 2:549–554, 1989

Fornazzari X: Psychiatric care of Latin American immigrants and refugees: a comparative study. Paper presented at Health, Political Repression, and Human Rights Conference, Costa Rica, November 1989

Fornazzari X, Freire M: Women as victims of torture. Acta Psychiatr Scand 82:257–260, 1990

Garcia-Peltoniemi R, Jaranson J: A multidisciplinary approach to the treatment of torture victims. Paper presented at the Second International Conference of Centres, Institutions, and Individuals Concerned With the Care of Victims of Organized Violence, San Jose, Costa Rica, 1989

Genefke I: Cited in Ritterman M: Torture: the counter-therapy of the state. Networker 43–47, 1987

Goldfeld AE, Mollica R, Pesavento BH, et al: The physical and psychological sequelae of torture: symptomatology and diagnosis. JAMA 259:2725–2729, 1988

Hathaway SR, McKinley JC: Minnesota Multiphasic Personality Inventory. Minneapolis, MN, University of Minnesota, 1943

Kinzie J, Frederickson R, Ben R: Posttraumatic stress disorder among survivors of Cambodian concentration camps. Am J Psychiatry 141:640–649, 1984

Kuoch T, Wali S, Scully M: Forward, in Refugee Women and Their Mental Health: Shattered Societies, Shattered Lives. Edited by Cole E, Espin O, Rothblum E. Binghamton, NY, Harrington Park Press, 1992, pp xv–xvi

Larsen H, Pagaduan-Lopez J: Stress-tension reduction in the treatment of sexually tortured women: an exploratory study. J Sex Marital Ther 13:210–218, 1987

Laurence R: Part I: torture and mental health: a review. Issues in Mental Health Nursing 13:301–310, 1992

Lindy J: An outline for the psychoanalytic psychotherapy of post-traumatic stress disorder, in Trauma and Its Wake. Edited by Figley C. New York, Brunner/Mazel, 1986

Lira E, Weinstein E: La tortura sexual. Paper presented at the Seminario Internacional: Consecuencias de la Represion en el Cono Sur Sus Efectos Medicos, Psicologicos, y Sociales, Montevideo, Uruguay, May 1986

Mollica R, Caspi-Yavin Y: Measuring torture and torture-related symptoms. Psychological Assessment 3:581–587, 1991

Mollica R, Lavelle J: Southeast Asian refugees, in Clinical Guidelines in Cross-Cultural Mental Health. Edited by Comas-Diaz L, Griffith EH. Rexdale, Ontario, Wiley, 1988, pp 262–304

Mollica R, Son L: Cultural dimensions in the evaluation and treatment of sexual trauma. Psychiatr Clin North Am 12:363–379, 1989

Mollica R, Wyshak M, de Marneffe D, et al: Indochinese versions of the Hopkins Symptom Checklist—25: a screening instrument for the psychiatric care of refugees. Am J Psychiatry 144:497–500, 1987a

Mollica R, Wyshak M, Lavelle J: The psychosocial impact of war trauma and torture on Southeast Asian refugees. Am J Psychiatry 144:1567–1572, 1987b

Mollica R, Wyshak M, Lavelle J, et al: Assessing symptom change in Southeast Asian refugee survivors of mass violence and torture. Am J Psychiatry 147:83–88, 1990

Mollica R, Caspi-Yavin Y, Bollini P, et al: The Harvard Trauma Questionnaire: validating a cross-cultural instrument for measuring torture, trauma, and post-traumatic stress disorder in Indochinese refugees. J Nerv Ment Dis 180:111–116, 1992

Morris P, Silove D: Cultural influences in psychotherapy with refugee survivors of torture. Hosp Community Psychiatry 43:820–824, 1992

Pope K, Garcia-Peltoniemi R: Responding to victims of torture: clinical issues, professional responsibilities, and useful resources. Professional Psychology 22:269–276, 1991

Ramsay R, Gorst-Unsworth C, Turner S: Psychiatric morbidity in survivors of organized state violence including torture: a retrospective series. Br J Psychiatry 162:55–59, 1993

Rasmussen OV, Lunde J: Evaluation and investigation of 200 torture victims. Dan Med Bull 27:23–243, 1980

Refugee Women in Development: What Is a Refugee? Washington, DC, Refugee Women in Development, 1990

Reid J, Strong T: Rehabilitation of refugee victims of torture and trauma: principles and service provision in New South Wales. Med J Aust 148:340–346, 1988

Ritterman M: Torture: the counter-therapy of the state. Networker 43–47, 1987

Rivero W: The Use of Psychotropic Medication in Counseling and Therapy With Refugees: Psychological Problems of Victims of War, Torture, and Repression. New York, Wiley, 1992

Sack WH, Angell RH, Kinzie JD, et al: The psychiatric effects of massive trauma on Cambodian children, II: the family, the home, the school. Journal of the American Academy of Child Psychiatry 25:377–383, 1986

Silove D: Children of apartheid: a generation at risk. Med J Aust 148:346–353, 1988

Silove D, Tarn R, Bowles R, et al: Psychosocial needs of torture survivors. Aust N Z J Psychiatry 25:481–490, 1991

Stein B: The experience of being a refugee: insights from the research literature, in Refugee Mental Health in Resettlement Countries. Edited by Williams CL, Westermeyer J. Washington, DC, Hemisphere, 1986, pp 5–23

Turk DC, Melzak R: Handbook of Pain Assessment. New York, Guilford, 1992

Turner S, Gorst-Unsworth C: Psychological sequelae of torture: a descriptive model. Br J Psychiatry 157:475–480, 1990

United Nations High Commissioner for Refugees. Draft Guidelines: Evaluation and Care of Victims of Trauma and Violence. Geneva, United Nations High Commissioner for Refugees, 1993

van der Veer G: Counselling and Therapy With Refugees: Psychological Problems of Victims of War, Torture, and Repression. New York, Wiley, 1992

Westermeyer J: Migration and psychopathology, in Refugee Mental Health in Resettlement Countries. Edited by Williams CL, Westermeyer J. Washington, DC, Hemisphere, 1986, pp 5–23

Westermeyer J: Psychiatric Care of Migrants: A Clinical Guide. Washington, DC, American Psychiatric Press, 1989

Wiseman J: Individual adjustments and kin relationships in the "new migration": an approach to research. International Migration Review 23:349–367, 1985

Zung WWK: A self-rating depression scale. Arch Gen Psychiatry 12:371–379

CHAPTER 20

Culture and Psychiatry
An Indian Overview of Issues in Women and Children

Usha S. Naik, M.D.
M. Sharda Menon, M.D.
Sayed Ahmed, M.D., M.P.H., Dr.P.H.

The history of India can be traced back more than 5,000 years, when the Indian subcontinent was witness to one of the world's best-known civilizations, the Indus Valley civilization. Amazingly enough, despite the passing of millennia, evidence of the continuity of that culture is still discernible. Beginning with the Hindu religion, whose origins date from prehistory until the Vedic period in 1,500 B.C., Buddhism and Jainism in the fifth and sixth centuries B.C., the advent of Islam from the eleventh century, Sikhism in the fifteenth century, and finally Christianity centuries before British colonial rule, the country has evolved and assimilated much from the global transmogrifications. The most important aspect of this history is the assimilation of these changes into the fabric of "Indianness." India today is a country of diverse races, religions, sects, castes, languages, and dialects. These distinctions color every aspect of life in customs, rituals, selection of marriage partners, child rearing, education, family configurations, employment, and attitudes; India is still called a subcontinent because of this very diversity.

Paradoxes abound: while Bombay, India's largest city, provided both the Miss Universe and the Miss World titleholders in a single year, it also has the world's largest slum. Big business and corporate organizations are obvious, as are holy men, genuine and otherwise. India, perceived newly as a consumer market, is now the target of the satellite media, precipitating dramatic changes in dress, music, and other preferences and possibly values.

The current population of India is more than 850 million individuals: 440 million are male, and 410 million are female. It is estimated that there are 330 million children below the age of 16 (Census 1991; UNICEF 1994a). The 1995 "population clock" anticipates a population of more than 920 million. There are approximately three psychiatrists per one million people. From this disparity, it is obvious that treatment measures applicable in other parts of the world are not appropriate in India. The country has formulated a National Mental Health Plan whose main objectives are 1) to ensure minimal health care for all sections of the population, 2) to apply mental health knowledge in health and social development, and 3) to promote community participation (Srinivasa Murthy and Burns 1987).

Some anthropologists have tried to define an Indian ethnosociology that "could offer a second lens through which all could look, a second language in which all could speak" (Marriott 1989). However, the Indian response has been against a single formulation of this nature (A. Sharma 1992; R. Singh 1992). In India, a land of diverse languages, religions, and subgroups, the transcultural approach is so much a part of daily routine that it has been underinvestigated. Most therapists speak at least three languages and accept patients or their relatives' opinions regarding cultural practices. The maturation of the Indian psychiatrist can be anecdote ridden, because the psychiatrist and patient are often from very different backgrounds. During my own residency training, I diagnosed paranoid schizophrenia in a patient who expressed that magic was being performed on him. His wife, however, collaborated his story. "Magic" was being done. His neighbors were placing lemons and eggshells outside of his door to get him to leave the neighborhood.

Transcultural psychiatry is fraught with such dangers, and in the past social anthropologists have diagnosed entire populations as paranoid. To avoid overgeneralizations, it is more prudent to use cultural information as a backdrop against which the individual's personal and human qualities must be studied. If in this chapter we refuse to describe an Indian culture, it is because one could spend a lifetime understanding one subgroup, only to find a myriad of microcosms still requiring elucidation. In this chapter we focus on culture and development, issues in child psychiatry, women's issues in psychiatry, the Asian Indian immigrant, and future areas of research.

Culture and Development

Although the relationship between environment and health is more apparent in the study of physical health, many components of the environment influence the mental health of the individual. They include diverse elements such as climate, man-made physical components including human settlement, and societal factors (Nadkarni 1993). Jahoda and Lewis (1988) have outlined the influence of culture on development as 1) the physical and social settings of everyday life, 2) the culturally regulated methods of child care and rearing, 3) cognitive development, and 4) social change.

Physical and social settings.   Economic considerations result in a wide disparity in living conditions. Definitions of poverty used in other countries are not relevant in India (Garbarino 1992). Poverty, with all of its attendant physical and social ills, is defined in terms of the proportion of income spent on food and is estimated at 30% of the Indian population (UNICEF 1994b). Affluence and literacy are associated with higher-quality amenities, toys, milder discipline, and better education (Aphale 1976). Child-centered rituals are more common in traditional families. In personality studies, deprived children are found to be more reserved, conservative, and group dependent and less stable emotionally (Seth et al. 1982). Malnutrition is found in as many as 63% of children (UNICEF 1994b). Specific vitamin deficiencies compound the problem. Effects are seen in delayed development, lassitude, apathy, irritability, and depression (D. I. L. Agarwal et al. 1992; Carney 1990; UNICEF 1994b; Upadhyay et al. 1992).

The description of social values outlined in the following is also based on generalizations. All Indians do not take care of their elderly parents, nor are all girls subjected to deprivation. Described are social values that are "cherished," or preferred, values. Behavior does not necessarily conform to these values.

Families may consist of three generations living under one roof, called a joint family, although more than two related married couples cohabiting under one roof have also been described as joint. The family is organized by a hierarchy determined by gender bias. An "individual's obligations to those above him and his expectations of those below him are immutable" (Kakar 1990). The emphasis is on conformity to family goals at the sacrifice of personal autonomy and pursuits. The advantages of the joint family include additional caregivers for children, which is particularly useful to the working mother and for security in illness, unemployment, and old age. The disadvantages are lack of privacy, obligation to multiple authority figures, and some stifling of individual achievement.

In a review, J. B. P. Sinha (1990) has distinguished between cherished and operative values:

1. Embeddedness, or to remain a part of one's group, has as its most striking example familism, wherein the family is the prime concern, sometimes to the detriment of other responsibilities.
2. In striving to maintain harmony and tolerance, the coping methods used are necessarily nonconfrontational; third-party mediation is acceptable.
3. Duty in contrast to hedonism is strongly emphasized to children; sports and hobbies are often considered a waste of time.
4. Preference for personalized relationships means an increased expectation for caring and being cared for. This trait may be seen even in therapeutic relationships.
5. Preference for hierarchy is an important factor in all social relationships, familial and extrafamilial.
6. Devaluation of self is proper. An individual is expected to be modest and self-effacing. Self-effacement is considered a virtue but may be misunderstood as low self-esteem when the quality is detected in another culture (Fry and Ghosh 1992).

Religion and religiosity are important organizers of daily life; social and devotional aspects of religion are widely understood and practiced. By offering meaning and purpose in life, religion provides emotional buffers and enhances coping strategies. Devotion to religion also explains some of the tolerance toward deviance and an acceptance of adversity on the basis of a preordained fate.

Access to education is determined by economic and gender factors. Only 52% of girls enter fifth grade. In Indian studies, aggressive behavior and scholastic backwardness have been considered more serious than emotional problems. However, innovative programs have been developed for training teachers in handling problem behavior in schools (Kapur et al. 1980; Somen 1989).

Culturally regulated customs of child care and rearing. Levine describes child rearing to have three hierarchical goals, the achievement of the first being necessary to reach the second and third levels.

1. The physical health and survival of the child.
2. Development of the child's capacity for economic self-maintenance.
3. Development of the capacity for maximizing other cultural values such as morality and prestige.

Adaptive child rearing practices become incorporated into folk wisdom and later become custom. Traditionally, children are demand fed. They are also dressed by a caregiver for a longer period than in Western cultures. Children sleep with their parents, and infants are never kept in a different room, even if physical space permits. These activities are child initiated in many instances, and rigid schedules are not common. Changing some of the less-adaptive child rearing practices has been found to be possible using a community-based approach (Naik and Plumber 1992).

The indulgence adults show in their children's early childhood markedly contrasts the authoritarianism seen in later childhood. Milder forms of punishment are employed in upper socioeconomic strata, and physical punishment is used in lower socioeconomic groups (Aphale 1976). Traditionally, praise is not used to effect behavioral change. Shame is inculcated as opposed to guilt (Baig 1979). Overprotectiveness and increased authoritarianism have been found in families of children with behavioral problems (G. Agarwal et al. 1979; Nigam et al. 1978).

Described in detail later, the discrimination against the female child takes place before birth and persists throughout her life (Anandalaxmi 1991; Kartal 1991). Maternal attitudes change, possibly during the separation (individuation) period, with reduced attentiveness and reciprocity (Graves 1978). In practice, discrimination by the mother is likely material rather than emotional deprivation. The education of the female child is related to poverty, home responsibilities, religious factors, and coeducation (Chanana 1990). Certain universal factors are found in child rearing; fathers being less involved, preferential discrimination of fathers for girls, and mothers favoring boys are not particular to India (Isley and Langford 1991).

Cognitive development. Several assessment tools have been standardized, and Indian reference values are now available. These tools include the Weschler, Simon-Binet, Baley, Gessell, and Vineland Scales. Several scales have been produced to suit the Indian context, and some have been used across cultures, including the Temperament Scales (Malhotra 1988; Malhotra and Randhava 1983). Socioeconomic deprivation and concurrent malnutrition adversely affect performance. Schooling, urbanization, and other social advantages have contributed to improved performance by students on language and arithmetic tests. In cross-cultural studies, equal competence in verbal and pictorial learning in Indian and Western subjects has been noted (S. D. Sinha 1979). Using home-based programs, even in underprivileged sections of society, it has been found possible to enhance cognitive ability using infant stimulation measures (Gill et al. 1990; Naik and Plumber 1992). Study of race as a variable is not considered politically correct (Lamb 1992).

In studies of cognition, distinction between the form and the content of thought has not been adequate. Enough evidence exists to show that the way we think is the same across cultures, although beliefs and cosmologies may be different. There is less controversy regarding socialization, which refers to "the process by which children become effectively functioning members of a particular society" (Jahoda and Lewis 1988).

Language development is a special feature in the Indian child because of the multiplicity of languages acquired. Children may speak one language at home and require two or more other languages at school. By the time children are 3 or 4 years of age, they may have acquired the ability for imitation, analogy, formal instruction, and exploration in two languages. Children also learn contextual specificity, or when to use which language (Bhatia 1990).

Social change.   Urbanization, television, the inroads of satellite television, and rap music are exerting their influence in the globalization of culture. This phenomenon in urban areas has become a cause of major concern (Hoskote 1994). Programs with violent and aggressive themes are reported to make children more aggressive and disobedient. Prosocial themes induce self-control, cooperation, and friendliness. Children tend to view more adult programs than they did previously (Blair 1993; Mayuri and Monite 1992; Tonge 1990).

The number of mothers working to supplement family income has increased significantly. In the absence of proper alternative care, increased antisocial behavior has been seen in children (Saxena et al. 1986). In the West, the concept of family is changing, and the number of single-parent families is on the rise. However, the rates of divorce in India vary from state to state, with the highest in Kerala, 34 per 1,000, and the lowest in Haryana, 1.6 per 1,000 (Sareender et al. 1992).

Migration may be voluntary or forced and can cause many social and emotional changes (du Toit 1990). Rural-to-urban migration causes much disruption. Rural children have been found to exhibit better home adjustment, whereas urban children show better adjustment in school and college. In migration to different cultures, the minority status operates in preventing direct extrapolation of information from the culture of origin (Devos 1980).

Child abuse in India has not been studied adequately. Segal (1991) describes different forms of abuse:

1. Societal abuse refers to poverty, child labor, and prostitution.
2. Physical abuse includes physical and sexual abuse, benign neglect, and failure to provide.
3. Nonphysical abuse results from parental alcohol and drug use and emotional and educational neglect.

Some disorders seem to be transferred with culture. With new ideas of body shape and dieting ("the Barbie Doll image"), anorexia nervosa is making its appearance in India. This occurrence parallels reports of bulimia in Bradford and other parts of England in Asian populations.

Issues in Child Psychiatry

The Indian Association for Child and Adolescent Psychiatry was formed in 1991. Child psychiatry is a rapidly growing specialty in India but requires no separate board certification as a subspecialty. Some clinics in pediatric hospitals serve children exclusively, but most children's clinics are run in regular clinics, treating children only on allotted days.

Most clinics use the ICD-10 or DSM systems of classification. For lack of space, all individual child psychiatric disorders cannot be listed. However, Table 20–1 summarizes the annual statistics for the Depart-

Table 20–1. **Annual new case registration 1991: Department of Child Psychiatry, Niloufer Hospital, Hyderabad, India**

Case diagnosis	Number of cases	Percentage
Developmental delays and mental retardation	986	47
Specific developmental delays	249	12
Attention-deficit disorders	124	6
Emotional disorders	190	9
Conduct disorders	94	4.5
Special symptoms	134	6.4
Pervasive developmental disorders	45	2
Primary neurological disorders	272	13
Total number of cases registered	2,094	

SOURCE: Department Statistics, U.S. Naik, Gowri, M. Devi, M. Joshi, P. Das, and S. Joseph, unpublished data, 1991).

ment of Child Psychiatry, Niloufer Hospital. This clinic is located in a government hospital for women and children. It serves only children below the age of 12 and operates 6 days a week.

In most child guidance clinics in India, mental retardation and developmental disorders account for 40%–50% of clinic referrals, whereas in a Western setting, these problems may have a rank order of 5 or 6 following emotional, conduct, and personality disorders (Silver 1983). Under special symptoms are listed a variety of conditions including enuresis, stuttering, and breath-holding spells. Many children with epilepsy are referred for assessment and continue to be seen for follow-up treatment in psychiatric settings.

Different studies rank the prevalence of child psychiatric disorders as ranging from 5% to 20% of the child population. Emotional disorders are reported more commonly than conduct disorders in both clinic and community surveys. In one major two-stage study, 20% of children were detected to have problems. Of these, 5% had mental retardation, 2% had speech disorders, 8.8% had enuresis, 1.6% had emotional disorders, 1.6% had epilepsy, and 0.5% had conduct disorders (Jiloha and Murthy 1981; Varghese and Baig 1974). In Asian families in the United Kingdom, proportionally fewer children were referred for treatment. There were fewer broken homes, fewer conduct disorders, and more somatoform complaints. Fears were treated with more tolerance (Hackett and Hackett 1991; Stern et al. 1990; Wong 1990).

In their survey, Narang et al. (1991) found socioeconomic differences, with conduct disorders, truancy, and mental retardation predominating in lower socioeconomic groups, and food refusal, food fads, and temper tantrums predominating in the higher socioeconomic groups.

Treating the Indian Patient

Psychiatrists from other countries wishing to work in India would need to use empathy, sensitivity, and patience as their main skills. Language would be the first barrier, but in a country with 14 languages, patients usually bring their own interpreters to the clinic. If a Kannada-speaking patient came to Hyderabad, he or she would bring along a Hindi-, Telugu-, or English-speaking relative. However, the therapist's language skills do serve to keep patients in therapy (Flaskerud and Liu 1991; Westermeyer 1990).

Who presents the history? Seldom the patient. In the case of a child, the most important family member is usually the paternal grandparent. In the first visit, a large number of people may accompany the patient. Deference should be given to the spokesperson, who might be a relative or an important village functionary in the case of a rural patient. Ignoring the spokesperson and demanding that the parent or spouse alone speak would be embarrassing to the whole party. Confidentiality and privacy are not really required until later in the interview. Even some educated mothers may say the child's problem is due to *nazar* or *drishti,* translated as "evil eye" or, more correctly, "envious eyes." While accepting the medical explanation, families may simultaneously placate the gods and sort out planetary influences. Acceptance of disability or suffering is, at least at a superficial level, described as the hand of fate. However, these attitudes should not be allowed to interfere with the management plan. Counseling in child rearing practices should be discussed with senior members in a joint family, usually the paternal grandmother, if change is to be effected. Counseling the mother alone would be less useful.

The child with emotional problems almost always has difficulty in school. The three wishes test has the first response in reference to school performance, usually worded, "I want to come first." Conversion symptoms peak before annual examinations. A special area of inquiry is the tutoring teacher, a ubiquitous entity in the lives of urban children, who provides extra coaching after school hours. Children seldom have hobbies, and recreational activities are of low priority. Symptoms should be analyzed for their form and content; it may be difficult for the child to express his or her emotional problems.

When the patient's beliefs are not clear to the therapist, it is always better to check with other family members, as in the following instance. S, a 12-year-old boy, presented with a 3-day history of acute anxiety. His main preoccupation was with what would happen after death. When interviewed, S stated that he had been shown a knife and threatened with death by four boys on his way home from school; this threat stemmed from a previous squabble. The boy's father helped in patching up the quarrel. To answer S's question about death, it was more appropriate to check with the parents, since it is not the therapist's view but the family's that needs reiteration.

Tact is required in dealing with the family's beliefs and value systems. They should never be mocked or derided. A family's belief in religious rituals or charms should be accepted. Admitting ignorance about a ritual is preferable to suggesting that it will not work. Obviously, harmful practices such as the branding of children with epilepsy should be prevented. Behavior modification is an accepted method of treatment, condoned by parents for behavior problems and enuresis. Families drop out of therapy the moment the index case shows improvement. Family support is a positive outcome variable and can be expected in the majority of cases.

In spite of linguistic and cultural differences, empathy can be understood and appreciated by patients of different cultures. Patients do well with brief, supportive psychotherapy that is directive, goal oriented, and time limited. Long-term analytically oriented therapy with accompanying free association is often threatening for the patient used to medical authority. Longer-term therapy is possible in Westernized and urbanized middle-class patients, with whom the therapist may be able to identify more easily. Usually, however, unless the goals and duration of therapy are clearly spelled out, a high dropout rate is likely. Erna Hoch, a Swiss psychiatrist who has worked for more than 30 years in India, has identified factors operating against a Western psychotherapeutic approach—namely, traditional family organization, discouragement of egoistic and individualistic striving, and concepts regarding the "guru-chela" relationship, or the relationship between the teacher and the student—that alter the transference process (Neki 1973).

Not keeping appointments is unlikely to be due to negative transference but to more prosaic elements of daily life such as missing a bus or illness in the family. Excuses can seem feeble—a wedding, an engagement, or a distant relative's funeral—but these are important activities for women, and missing them would probably have more negative repercussions than missing a visit to a doctor.

Administration of medication or a prescription may be required; even vitamins complete the "medicalness" of the encounter. With the high prevalence of vitamin deficiencies, providing them, along with a statement about how they keep the body strong and that the patient should remember the discussions in the therapy session, is a useful practice. Pharmacotherapy in children follows this maxim: for the shortest period of time at the lowest dosage. Studies of drug metabolism have shown that both therapeutic and adverse effects have lower thresholds in the Asian patient.

Traditional healing practices have been divided into three categories by Kleinman: 1) the professional sector: biomedicine, 2) folk health care: alternative medicine, and 3) popular medicine: what patients and relatives do to deal with illness (U. Sharma 1993). In India and other Asian countries, traditional healing practices are seen as important. Both the Unani and the Ayurvedic schools are officially recognized. Their concurrent use may sometimes facilitate or improve response, especially in conversion and dissociation states. Tolerance of both kinds of medicine keeps the patient in therapy. Traditional practices should be discouraged only when they are known to be harmful. Some traditional practices, such as yoga, are returning to Indian schools, especially following their validation in the West (Someswarananda 1989).

Women's Issues in Psychiatry

The socioanthropological approach to the management of mental disorders states that environmental influences, particularly the social and man-made physical components, should no longer be viewed as either having only a pathoplastic effect on mental illness or contributing to the esoteric syndromes commonly referred to as the "culture-bound syndromes" (Littlewood 1990). The protagonists of this new transcultural psychiatry propose that culture is often the core determinant of the presentation of the various types of mental illness and also substantially influences the prognosis, even of illnesses that are now believed to have a biological basis (Birchwood et al. 1992). The social role performance of people with mental health problems, vis-à-vis the role expectations of significant others, is likely to play a major part in influencing the course and outcome of the illness. A sociological perspective is also likely to provide critical input for the clinician in developing appropriate management strategies, because it aids in the understanding of help seeking behavior and clarifies issues related to the appraisal of stress and the coping mechanisms undertaken by the afflicted individual.

Clinicians seeking to enhance their skills in the management of psychiatric problems of the female gender in the Indian subcontinent must understand the interplay of the ecological, political, social, psychological, and spiritual elements and their impact on both mental health and mental illness. In the following section, we thus present a very broad review of the key social systems that interface with the Indian woman and briefly discuss the impact of these issues on the management of psychiatric problems of women in India. Subsequent sections deal with issues of presentation and management of both psychoses and neuroses of the female gender in India.

Key demographic details. In a country of 850 million, the gender ratio is adverse to women (i.e., the number of women per 1,000 men has generally been less than 1,000 and is continuing to decline). Although firm empirical data to explain this phenomenon are lacking, Shiva (1992) has argued that this decline is a result of a conscious gender bias, which is translated into termination of female fetuses, predetermined and systematic malnutrition of the female child, pockets of female infanticide, and high maternal mortality due to poor health practices and repeated pregnancies. The picture in terms of literacy rates for women is equally depressing, with only 30% of India's female population being categorized as literate.

Subsistence agriculture is almost exclusively the domain of women in rural India, and it is estimated that women spend most of their time working—at survival tasks of maintaining the household and at income-generating tasks needed to keep the family and economy alive; 94% of women are engaged in the unorganized sector, 81.4% in agriculture, and the rest in occupations that are mostly unskilled and poorly paying. A small percentage of women in urban areas hold jobs in the organized sector but often have to work in conditions that are not conducive to physical or mental well-being. The mean age of marriage for Indian women is 16.3 years, although the age sanctioned under the prevailing law is 18 years.

Health services utilization studies show that women consistently underutilize the health services compared with men. Hospital records show more male than female admissions, and women are brought for treatment far later into their illnesses than are men. This situation is truly paradoxical in a country where 75% of health system workers are women, although assigned peripheral roles.

Wadley (1988) has drawn attention to the inherent contradictions that exist in defining the identity of the Indian woman. Mythology and traditional folklore have embodied women with the characteristics of the goddess Shakti, who is regarded as the destroyer of evil. On the other hand, society rewards and reinforces behaviors by women that place them in a nurturant and passive role. Mane (1993) has hypothesized that this constant shift from passivity to strength creates highly stressful situations for women. At a practical level, Venkoba (1987) has emphasized that the basic identity of the Indian woman is defined only in the content of her relationship with an adult male relative (i.e., she is the wife or mother or daughter of a male), and because she has to accept a submissive, docile, nonassertive role, she often finds it difficult to deal with negative emotions.

Family and community represent the biotic component of the ecosystem, and understanding the status of Indian women in the context of the family is important. The woman is regarded primarily as the homemaker, and personal independence or autonomy is not encouraged. Marriages are generally arranged by the families, and unmarried girls usually live in their parental homes until the time of their marriage. The hierarchy in the marital home is fairly rigid, with the women having to assume subservient roles in their relationships with both husband and mother-in-law. All major decisions are generally made by those who occupy the higher positions in the family hierarchy. In view of the pronounced gender bias in favor of male offspring, motherhood is accompanied by increased stress if the offspring are only female. Confidentiality and privacy are not core issues in India, and families participate in all decisions regarding a patient. In fact, it would be culturally incongruent not to involve families in major or minor decisions that concern adult patients, particularly women.

On balance, however, the Indian family has positive attributes that could contribute to the care and support of females with psychiatric problems. Among these attributes are the bonds of kinship and mutual interdependence, which are hallmarks of all sociocentric cultures, including India's. These bonds lead to a tacit understanding that the family has an obligation to care for the weaker members of the family. Although the traditional joint family system has gradually declined, a new concept of "functional jointedness" has taken root. This concept implies that although all of the family members do not live under the same roof or eat out of a common kitchen, they continue to honor their obligations to their kin. This situation creates a significant support system, and reports have shown that a majority of the mentally ill continue to live with their families (Thara and Rajkumar 1992).

The preceding section has briefly reviewed the sociocultural phenomena that influence the psychological well-being of the Indian women. A sensitivity to both gender and cultural issues is critical not only in arriving at the diagnosis but also in formulating treatment strategies.

Epidemiological studies have revealed a point prevalence rate of 2.6–17.2 per 1,000 population for schizophrenia in India, with no gender differences (Dube 1970; Varghese et al. 1973). Although most Western reports argue that women have a later age at onset, clinicians in India take a guarded view on this issue because women are traditionally taken for treatment much later than men. This circumstance has the potential to create an impression about a later onset of illness, and it is well established that the same is true in the case of physical illness. Mental health professionals also report other reasons for the prevalence that are presently speculative, but examining these reasons independently would be worthwhile. Many clinicians argue that the initial presentation of schizophrenia in women is more subtle as compared to that in men, who generally present with core psychotic features. Because both patients and families tend to report an array of nonspecific symptoms, clinicians often diagnose schizophrenia.

Added to these findings is the concern of families that a psychiatric diagnosis would stigmatize the family and harm the marriage prospects for the patient. Consequently, there is a tendency to underreport disturbing behaviors, at least in the initial assessments, which could further delay the diagnosis. Clinicians should thus very thoroughly examine younger female patients and exercise a vigilance about symptoms that appear vague and nonspecific, because they could be forerunners of psychotic breakdown.

Clinical reports from India indicate that women often exhibit marked behavioral problems. These difficulties could be linked to biological stressors in the form of menstruation and childbirth, although the role of social stressors cannot be ruled out. Intercurrent depression is another clinical challenge that has not been resolved satisfactorily. The special problems faced by mental health professionals in India include the negative attitudes of spouses toward their ill wives. Whereas female spouses are generally more tolerant toward their ill husbands, men tend to be very critical toward psychiatrically disabled wives who do not match their expectations of social role performance, particularly in the context of household tasks. The management of deserted and divorced women with schizophrenia is emerging as a major issue in urban areas, with the existing mental health infrastructure being increasingly strained to offer security and protection to these women.

Incidence studies on major depression have reported rates ranging from 5% to as high as 25% (Varghese et al. 1973; Wig et al. 1978). Although the discrepancy in these rates could be explained by differences in methodology, the most striking feature emerging from all of these studies is that Indian women present with a wide array of somatic symptoms. There is a consensus among psychiatrists in India that while depressed mood is rarely expressed subjectively by patients, reference is generally made to lowered vitality, generalized weakness, and a plethora of physical symptoms ranging from headaches to persistent gastric symptoms. The suicide rate from depression in India is about 1.2%, much lower than the statistics reported from the developing world (Venkoba and Nammalvar 1979). In a seminal work of 100 cases of suicide by Indian women (Venkoba 1987), the authors reported that 51% of suicides in Indian women were due to marital problems and 37% were due to other stressful circumstances and adverse life events. Only 23% of women who completed suicide attempts had a diagnosable history of mental illness. Therefore, all patients with depression or who have attempted suicide require a comprehensive assessment of their family circumstances. Involving the family in therapy is also important, but it should be done judiciously and after attempting to understand the polarizations and complexities that prevail in a typical Indian family.

Prevalence rates for neurotic and somatoform disorders have ranged from 25% to as high as 48%, depending on the population sampled. The preponderance of women in this category of psychiatric disorders is clearly established, as is the role of adverse environmental factors. The common precipitating factors have included marital maladjustment and physical illness. Clinicians also report that most Indian females present with an admixture of anxiety and depressive symptoms, and attempting to unravel the individual components does not enhance the efficacy of the therapy. In fact, most clinicians prefer to add antidepressants to the treatment regimen even when the patients report primarily symptoms of anxiety, since they believe that the component of depression has often been somatized. Subramaniam et al. (1980), in reporting on 267 cases of somatoform disorder, have indicated that 75% of their sample exhibited conversion symptoms, while only 20% had dissociative symptoms. Possession syndrome, in which the female reports that she has been possessed by some supernatural force, quite often a religious deity, is today regarded by clinicians as a culturally sanctioned presentation of depression. Treatment includes a judicious combination of antidepressants, anxiolytics, and supportive psychotherapy, because possession syndromes often occur in response to stress that has exceeded the individual's coping capacity.

In the Indian setting, supportive psychotherapy (which should be eclectic in its orientation) has a major role to play in the management of neuroses. This approach is in contrast to Western teachings that advocate insight-oriented therapies. Supportive psychotherapies are used more frequently, because insight-oriented therapies are often time consuming, and Indian female patients may not participate in therapy that requires regular visits to the mental health professional. Patients may also perceive insight-oriented therapies as threatening.

The Asian Indian Immigrant

The Asian Indian immigrant to the United States generally comes from a middle-class, professional background and enjoys that appropriate status in India. English is the language of instruction in all higher education, a result of our colonial past. Prospects of academic excellence, monetary advantages, and the intense competition for jobs in India prompt the move, and migration is voluntary. The first generation of immigrants includes highly motivated professionals with a determination to succeed. They need to prove themselves to their white counterparts, as well as to their families. They face real or imagined discrimination, and Indians have been said to take criticism poorly. This rapidly upwardly mobile group experiences more positive aspects of change, although assimilation may remain incomplete.

The second generation of immigrants, mostly born in the United States, face more problems regarding identity. A friend, now practicing pediatrics in the United States, remembers telling her children, "You're brown, not black," when they asked her their color. Parental values clash with those of adolescents regarding Western dating patterns, particularly so in the case of daughters. Acculturation takes place at different rates for different characteristics. Table 20–2 provides a simple generalization of psychosocial changes that occur in the same cultures with time and more rapidly when migration takes place from traditional cultures.

In observing social change, two dimensions—place and time—appear. When individuals emigrate from other continents to the United States, several changes take place regarding family roles and structures. These changes, however, have occurred before. Many of the qualities depicted in traditional cultures existed 50 years ago in Western societies. Some of these changes are related to economic independence of parents from children and vice versa. Some factors, such as religion, may not be fluid and require assimilation.

Conclusions

Transcultural psychiatry should search for the universals—going beyond the content of illness to the form. Although anthropological peculiarities are interesting, they serve mostly to perpetuate stereotypes. A therapist who has imbibed stereotypes during training may lose his or her sensitivity when confronted with a patient from another culture. All learning should eventually be to the patient's advantage.

Certain studies have compared, for example, urban middle-class American toddlers with toddlers from a tribal village in India. While the

Table 20–2. **A comparison of traditional Indian culture and United States/European culture**

	Traditional cultures	U.S. and North European cultures
Family	Hierarchical	Democratic
	Patriarchal	Mostly patriarchal
	Cohesive	Looser bonds
	Extended or nuclear	Nuclear, single parent
Women	Undervalued	Less obviously undervalued
	Homemakers primarily	Personal goals
	Restricted movements outside home	Unrestricted
Children and personality	Authoritarian upbringing	More freedom in upbringing
	Conformist	Creative
	Modesty, humility	Assertiveness
	Preference of clear hierarchies	Less formal hierarchies
	Guilt if family obligations are unfulfilled	Fewer familial expectations
	Self-effacing	Realistic appraisal
	Dependency	Autonomy
	View of self as interdependent	Independent

differences may be interesting, the relevance is questionable. It might be more meaningful to compare infants of professionals or children of alcoholic fathers or single-parent families across two or more cultures. Studies should be based on samples comparable in terms of roles rather than ethnicity.

Psychiatric tools include interviews, observations, and questionnaires. They should be sharpened by population-specific norms, judicious wording, inclusion of specific context, use of observer-based ratings, and inclusion of scales of global impairment. Test and retest reliability must be ensured (Fegert 1989; Uma et al. 1992).

The future focus must be on studying effective community strategies for providing care to the underprivileged sections of society. Training should be directed toward the utilization of fewer professionals and more trained health workers, thereby bringing down the cost of care and simultaneously increasing patient access (Krishnamurthy and Bhageerathi 1986; Srinivasa Murthy and Burns 1987).

In the last years of the twentieth century, cultures have been created, assimilated, alienated, and extinguished at an alarming rate. India's aim perhaps should be to achieve an optimum state of synergistic pluralism (Pareek 1989). The study of the human predicament is an exciting one for psychiatry, whose pivotal position between social and medical disciplines gives it unique opportunities in studying global phenomena. As Waldron and McDermott (1979) have said, every therapist should become more flexible and ultimately grow in understanding and skill from a multicultural to a cross-cultural and finally to a transcultural approach.

References

Agarwal DIL, Awasthy A, Upadhyay SK, et al: Growth, behavior, development, and intelligence in rural children between 1–3 years. Indian Pediatr 4:467–480, 1992

Agarwal G, Sarcar NIL, Saxena RP: Maternal child rearing attitudes and behavior problems among children. Child Psychiatry Quarterly 12:61–65, 1979

Anandalaxmi S: The female child in a family setting. Indian Journal of Social Work 52:29–36, 1991

Aphale C: Growing Up in an Urban Complex. National Publishing House, 1976

Baig T: Our Children. Publication Division, Ministry of Information and Broadcasting, Government of India, 1979

Bhatia AT: Language development in a child in a multilingual environment: a case study. ICSSR Research Abstract Quarterly 19:171–176, 1990

Birchwood M, Cochrane R, Macmillan F, et al: The influence of ethnicity and family structure on relapse in first-episode schizophrenia: a comparison of Asian, Afro-Carribean, and white patients. Br J Psychiatry 161:783–790, 1992

Blair EM: Communication of the rap music subculture youth. Subculture Journal of Popular Culture 27:21–34, 1993

Carney MWP: Vitamin deficiency and mental symptoms. Br J Psychiatry 156:878–882, 1990

Census of India 1991. Office of the Registrar General and Census Commissioner, Government of India, 1991

Devos GA: Ethnic adaptation and minority status. Journal of Cross-Cultural Psychiatry 2:101–124, 1980

Dube KC: A study of prevalence and biosocial variables in mental illness in a rural and urban community in UP, India. Acta Psychiatr Scand 46:327–359, 1970 du Toit BM: People on the move: rural urban migration with special reference to the third world. Human Organization 49:305–317, 1990

Fegert JH: Bias factors in the translation of questionnaires and classification systems in international comparative child and adolescent psychiatric research. Acta Paedopsychiatrica 52:279–286, 1989

Flaskerud JM, Liu PU: Effects of an Asian client therapist language, ethnicity on utilization and outcome of therapy. Community Ment Health J 27:31–42, 1991

Fry PS, Ghosh R: Attribution of success and failure: comparison of cultural differences between Asian and Caucasian children. Journal of Cross-Cultural Psychiatry 3:220–237, 1992

Garbarino J: The meaning of poverty in the world of children. American Behavioral Scientist 35:220–237, 1992

Gill S, Singh MB, Ghauhan N: Effect of an intervention programme on selected cognitive abilities of preschool children. Indian Journal of Social Science 1:97–106, 1990

Graves PK: Infant behavior and maternal attitudes: early sex differences in W. Bengal India. Journal of Cross-Cultural Psychiatry 9:45–60, 1978

Hackett L, Hackett R: Parental ideas of normal and deviant child behavior: a comparison of two ethnic groups. Br J Psychiatry 162:351–357, 1991

Hoskote R: Requiem for a culture. Times of India Sunday Review, February 27, 1994

Isley B, Langford CG: Gender in parent-child interaction: observation of proximity in two Thanjavur villages. Indian Journal of Social Work, 1991, pp 399–410

Jahoda G, Lewis IM: Acquiring culture, in Cross-Cultural Studies in Child Development. Edited by Jahoda G, Lewis IM. London, Croom Helm, 1988

Jiloha MC, Srinivasa Murthy R: An epidemiological study of psychiatric morbidity in primary school children. Child Psychiatry Quarterly 14:108–119, 1981

Kakar S: The Inner World: A Psychoanalytic Study of Childhood and Society in India. Families and Children. Delhi, Oxford University Press, 1990, pp 114–133

Kapur M, Cariapa I, Parthasarthy R: Evaluation of an orientation course for teachers on emotional problems amongst school children. Indian Journal of Clinical Psychiatry 7:103–107, 1980

Kartal M: Invisibility of the girl child in India. Indian Journal of Social Work 52:5–12, 1991

Krishnamurthy K, Bhageerathi K: Child mental health services through ICDS. Child Psychiatry Quarterly 19:26–35, 1986

Lamb K: Biased tidings: the media and the Cyril Burt controversy. Mankind Quarterly, Vol 33, 1992

Littlewood R: From categories to contexts: a decade of the new cross cultural psychiatry. Br J Psychiatry 156:308–327, 1990

Malhotra S: Stability of temperamental characteristics over time. Child Psychiatry Quarterly 21:43–50, 1988

Malhotra S, Randhava A: Temperament, emotional disorders of childhood: applicability in the Indian population. Child Psychiatry Quarterly 16:59–60, 1983

Mane P: Mental health of Indian women: realities and needed response, in Mental Health in India: Issues and Concerns. Edited by Mane P, Gandevia K. Bombay, TISS, 1993

Marriott K: Towards constructing an Indian ethnosociology. Contributions to Indian Sociology 23:1–39, 1989

Mayuri K, Monite P: Television: children's viewing patterns. Social Changes 22:55–64, 1992

Nadkarni VM: Ecosystems perspective, in Mental Health in India: Issues and Concerns. Edited by Mane P, Gandevia K. Bombay, TISS, 1993

Naik US, Plumber GR: Early Intervention With Infants at Risk for Developmental Disorders. APAWMR-UNICEF, 1992

Narang RL, Jain BK, Gupta MS, et al: Spectrum of psychiatric symptomatology in children in high and low socioeconomic groups in Ludhiana. Indian Pediatr 8:1489–1496, 1991

Neki JS: Guru chela relationship: the possibility of therapeutic paradigm. Am J Orthopsychiatry Vol 43, 1973

Nigam A, Singh SB, Srivastava JR: A comparative study of the personality traits of relapsed and non-relapsed cases. . . . Child Psychiatry Quarterly 11:98–105, 1978

Pareek U: Synergic pluralism: psychosocial dimensions of ethnicity in India. Indian Journal of Social Work 50:303–315, 1989

Sareender S, Reddy GC, Baburajan PK: Divorce in India: a macro-level analysis. Social Change 22:3–8, 1992

Saxena AK, Mehrotra SN, Singh SB: A psychosocial study of children of working mothers. Child Psychiatry Quarterly 19:128–137, 1986

Segal U: Child abuse in India: a theoretical overview. Indian Journal of Social Work 52:293–302, 1991

Seth M, Srivastava KK, Seth K: Personality patterns of Indian deprived and nondeprived boys and girls on Cattells' 16PF Test. Child Psychiatry Quarterly 15:124–130, 1992

Sharma A: Constructing an Indian ethnosociology: some comments. Contributions to Indian Sociology 226:132–141, 1992

Sharma U: Contextualizing alternative medicine. Anthropology Today 9:15–18, 1993

Shiva M: Women and health, in State of India's Health. Edited by Muhopadhyay A. Voluntary Health Association of India, 1992

Silver LB, Silver BJ: Clinical practice of child psychiatry: a survey. Journal of the American Academy of Child Psychiatry 276:573–579, 1983

Singh R: Steps away from an Indian ethnosociology. Contributions to Indian Sociology 26:141–148, 1992

Sinha JBP: Salient Indian values and their socioecological roots. Indian Journal of Social Sciences 3:477–487, 1990

Sinha SD: Cognitive and psychomotor skills in India: a review of research. Journal of Cross-Cultural Psychiatry 10:324–355, 1979

Somen KS: Behavioral problems of school children and viewed by teachers. Child Psychiatry Quarterly 17:113–122, 1989

Someswarananda S: Cultivating concentration power by using simple yoga and pranayama techniques. Indian Journal of Social Work 50:435–437, 1989

Srinivasa Murthy R, Burns BJ: Community Mental Health Proceedings of the Indo-U.S. Symposium. Bangalore, NIMHANS, 1987

Stern G, Cottrell D, Holmes J: Patterns of attendance of child psychiatry outpatients with special reference to Asian families. Br J Psychiatry 156:384–387, 1990

Subramaniam D, Subramaniam K, Devaki MN, et al: A clinical study of 276 patients diagnosed as suffering from hysteria. Indian Journal of Psychiatry 22:65–68, 1980

Thara R, Rajkumar S: Gender differences in schizophrenia: results of a follow-up study in India. Schizophr Res 7:65–90, 1992

Tonge BT: The impact of television on children and clinical practice. Aust N Z J Psychiatry 40:552–560, 1990

Uma H, Kapur M, Girimaji SR, et al: A screening tool for assessment of home environment and psychosocial development of preschool children. Indian J Pediatr 59:417–422, 1992

UNICEF: The Progress of Nations. New York, UNICEF, 1994a

UNICEF: The State of the World's Children. New York, Oxford University Press for UNICEF, 1994b

Upadhyay SK, Saran A, Agarwal DK: Growth and development in relation to malnutrition and environment. Indian Pediatr 29:595–605, 1992

Varghese A, Baig A: Psychiatric disturbances in children: an epidemiological study. Indian J Med Res 62:1538–1542, 1974

Varghese A, Baig A, Senseman LA, et al: A social and psychiatric study of a representative group of families in Vellore town. Indian J Med Res 61:608–620, 1973

Venkoba RA: Sociocultural factors of marriage and suicide behavior in India, in Proceedings of the 20th Annual Conference of APA and IASP. Edited by Yufit RI. San Francisco, 1987

Venkoba RA, Nammalvar N: Death orientation in depression. Indian Journal of Psychiatry 21:199–205, 1979

Wadley S: Women and the Hindu tradition, in Women in Indian Society. Edited by Gradially R. New Delhi, Sage, 1988

Waldron J, McDermott JF: Transcultural conditions, in Basic Handbook of Child Psychiatry, Vol 3. Edited by Noshpitz J. New York, Basic Books, 1979, pp 433–444

Westermeyer J: Working with an interpreter in psychiatric assessment and treatment. J Nerv Ment Dis 178:745–749, 1990

Wig NN, Varma VK, Khanna BC: Diagnostic characteristics of a general hospital psychiatric adult out-patient clinic. Indian Journal of Psychiatry 20:647, 1978

Wong CK: Child psychiatry in Hong Kong: an overview. Aust N Z J Psychiatry 24:331–338,1990

Epilogue

The preceding chapters have attempted to draw a kaleidoscopic tapestry that depicts the multifaceted nature and essence of transcultural psychiatry. I hope that the concept of transcultural psychiatry I have suggested in this volume will fully provide for its lasting and legitimate use and help instill some coherence to clinical practice and research in this area of human endeavor, steeped as it is in uncertainties, ambivalences, and ambiguities. This definitional approach, though not completely ignoring the history of the concept, prefers to emphasize the nature of the experience and encounter as a healer engages a patient against a complex background of dazzling similarities and differences. The definition is pragmatic and tactical and in its simplicity can lead to a wider degree of understanding than has heretofore been achieved.

My hope is that this attempt, therefore, will not be sterile but indeed can be fruitful, because it provides a framework and orientation that helps to reduce excess energy and time spent on linguistic and semantic debates that detract from the central issues of relief of pain and suffering.

I also must acknowledge that a cookbook approach in this area is likely to be unwieldy or of limited usefulness, because human problems are protean and unique in their genesis and relief. If we are sensitive about differences of age, gender, religious belief, and socioeconomic class, then understanding transcultural psychiatry becomes a daily task for mental health workers. It should no longer be seen as an esoteric discipline and exercise. This sentiment is expressed by Pedersen et al. in *Counseling Across Cultures* (1976): "Multicultural counseling is not an exotic topic that applies to remote regions but is the heart and core of good counseling with any client." This point deserves special emphasis when we discuss psychotherapy. Good psychotherapy that has as its central elements mutual respect between patient and therapist and opportunities for resonance, empathy, and participant observation by the therapist is likely to be sensitive to differences and similarities between the participants. The sociocultural factors and personal experiences of the patient constitute the subjective, transpersonal, and objective world of the patient that the therapist, with his or her corresponding world, must engage and encounter.

As various contributors to this volume have suggested, we do not treat a culture but rather help individuals with their unique life experiences and idiosyncrasies, with their here-and-now difficulties within a familial, cultural, and environmental matrix. From that point of view, this volume could not be complete without a statement on stereotyping. In this regard, I recall an argument I had with the late John Speigel, M.D., a prominent cultural and family psychiatrist and a past president of the American Psychiatric Association (APA). The occasion was a meeting of the American Society for the Study of Culture and Psychiatry. Dr. Speigel had suggested that stereotypes are true. While such may be the case with positive stereotypes, generally stereotypes tend to be negative or conceal negative aspects. His remarks at the time were probably of the same enormity as those of one of his predecessors, a past president of the APA, who opposed desegregation of state mental hospitals.

The issue of stereotypes leads to the question of the ethics of transcultural psychiatry. The relationship between a therapist and his or her patient is an ethical situation even when the individuals are matched in every other forgeable variable. The potential for abuse of the power relationship is probably greater when one is dealing with disenfranchised and minority individuals. Mental health workers, therefore, have to be mindful of the potential abuse of their positions. On a similar note, we should be aware that our patients may harbor stereotypes of their own about their therapists. Some elder scholars have alluded to this issue in the past, as have Lipsedge et al. in this volume.

A related fact is the issue of therapist acculturation in foreign lands, which has clinical implications. On the macrolevel, a good percentage of psychiatrists and other mental health workers in the United Kingdom, United States, and Canada are international medical graduates and allied professionals. In fact, 45% of first-year United States psychiatry residents are international medical graduates (Brown 1994). Their ability to optimize their contribution depends on their ability to come close to their hosts, which, in turn, depends on their lifestyles and personalities and the characteristics of the host environment, such as friendliness, openness, and acceptance of strangers. These characteristics may vary in different parts of the country, since friendliness within a homogeneous culture may not extend to strangers of that culture. Although the university environment is usually congenial and protective, these qualities are by no means guaranteed. The foreign worker's acculturation to the wider community is imperative. Fluency in language is another important requirement. Difficulty in communication may be burdensome for the psychically disturbed, and, in some instances, it may fuel the denial of patients, who are likely to ignore important interpretations by a refrain of "I cannot understand what the therapist is saying." Mental health workers working with immigrant and foreign individuals and families should do their best to enmesh themselves in and attempt to know such communities. Since normality is not defined by the sick state, opportunities to come close to these families by knowing about their histories, cultures, and daily family experiences can be gratifying.

Lastly, the majority of the preceding chapters have assumed the provision of services by an individual provider. Mental health services are usually offered by institutions such as mental health centers, child guidance clinics, and family centers. Such institutions must recognize the role of cultural factors in the reception and effectiveness of their services. For individuals who are interested in developing culturally competent systems of service delivery, a useful reference is the monograph *Towards a Culturally Competent System of Care: A Monograph on Effective Services for Minority Children Who Are Severely Emotionally Disturbed* (Cross et al. 1989). Although the work focuses on children, some of the basic principles outlined apply to other groups of patients as well. For example, essential elements that contribute to a system, institution, or agency's ability to become more culturally competent are identified. These approaches include to "1) value diversity; 2) have the capacity for cultural self-assessment; 3) be conscious of the dynamics inherent when cultures interact; 4) have institutionalized cultural knowledge; and 5) have developed adaptations to diversity" (Cross et al. 1989, p. v).

The authors of the monograph further assert that the preceding factors must exist at all levels of the system, along with congruence within these levels among attitudes, policies, and practices. Agencies should recognize a basic set of values and principles. For example, as indicated in the monograph, an agency providing authoritative, competent services to minority children should be guided by a set of principles and values such as the following:

- The family as defined by each culture is the primary system of support and preferred point of intervention.
- The system must recognize that minority populations have to be at least bicultural and that this status creates a unique set of mental health issues to which the system must be equipped to respond.
- Individuals and families make different choices based on cultural forces; these choices must be considered if services are to be helpful.
- Inherent in cross-cultural interactions are dynamics that must be acknowledged, adjusted to, and accepted.
- The system must sanction and in some cases mandate the incorporation of cultural knowledge into practice and policy making.
- Cultural competence involves working in conjunction with natural, informal support and helping networks within the minority community (e.g., neighborhoods, churches, spiritual leaders, and healers).
- Cultural competence extends the concept of self-determination to the community. Only when a community recognizes and owns a problem does it take responsibility for creating solutions that fit the context of the culture.
- Community control of service delivery through minority participation on boards of directors, administrative teams, and program planning and evaluation committees is essential to the development of effective services.
- An agency staffing pattern that reflects the makeup of the potential patient population, adjusted for the degree of community need, helps ensure the delivery of effective services.
- Culturally competent services incorporate the concept of equal and nondiscriminatory services but go beyond that approach to include responsive services matched to the patient population (Cross et al. 1989, pp. v–vi).

Cross et al. (1989, p. vii) also suggest that in designing services to meet the needs of minority patients in the context of their culture, several factors must be considered:

- The concept of least-restrictive alternatives.
- The community-based approaches with strong outreach components.
- Strong interagency collaboration, including natural helpers and community systems.
- Early intervention and prevention.
- Intake and patient identification to reduce differential treatment of minority youth.
- Assessment and treatment processes that define "normal" in the context of the patient's culture.
- Development of adequate cross-cultural communication skills.
- The case management approach as a primary service modality.
- The use of home-based services.

Clearly it is difficult to prescribe or design a guidebook for all patient groups and cultures. However, the model espoused in the previously cited monograph can at least encourage involvement in the right directions.

A significant barrier to a wider appreciation of transcultural psychiatry may be associated with presumptions about the training needed for this type of approach. A prerequisite is sensitivity to differences, which we have previously espoused. A healthy and open-minded attitude toward our patients regarding their backgrounds and beliefs is also singularly important. Continued self-reassessment and willingness to seek consultation from individuals familiar with the subcultural groups are a sine qua non. Finally, the humanistic origins of transcultural psychiatry should remain at the forefront of these transactions.

References

Brown SJ: IMGs keep residency program enrollment up. Clinical Psychiatry News 22:1–2, 1994

Cross TL, Bazron BJ, Dennis KW, et al: Towards a Culturally Competent System of Care: A Monograph on Effective Services for Minority Children Who Are Severely Emotionally Disturbed. Washington, DC, CASSP Technical Assistance Center, 1989

Pedersen P, Lonner WJ, Draguns JG (eds): Counseling Across Cultures. Honolulu, HI, University of Hawaii Press, 1976

Index

Boldface page references indicate information located in tables or figures.